FDA REGULATORY AFFAIRS

A Guide for Prescription Drugs,
Medical Devices, and Biologics

FDA REGULATORY AFFAIRS

A Guide for Prescription Drugs, Medical Devices, and Biologics

EDITED BY

Douglas J. Pisano
David Mantus

CRC PRESS

Boca Raton   London   New York   Washington, D.C.

Library of Congress Cataloging-in-Publication Data

FDA regulatory affairs : a guide for prescription drugs, medical devices, and biologics /
   edited by Douglas J. Pisano, David Mantus.
       p. cm.
   Includes bibliographical references and index.
   ISBN 1-58716-007-2
     1. Drug development—United States. 2. United States Food and Drug
   Administration—Rules and practice. 3. Pharmaceutical industry—United States. I. Pisano,
   Douglas J. II. Mantus, David.

   RM301.25.F37 2003
   615′.19′00973—dc22   2003055779

Preface

This book is a roadmap to the FDA, and drug, biologic, and medical device development. It is written in plain English with an emphasis on easy access to understanding how this agency operates with respect to practical aspects of U.S. product approval. It is meant to be a concise reference offering current, real-time information. It has been written as a handy reference to be used by students, staff, and professionals at corporations, organizations, and schools and colleges across the United States who are in need of a simple, concise text from which to learn and teach. The topics are covered in a simple and concise format. It is a compilation and commentary of selected laws and regulations pertaining to the development and approval of drugs, biologics, and medical devices in the United States. It is *not* intended to take the place of an actual reading of the laws of the United States of America or the regulations of the United States Food and Drug Administration, its agencies, or any body that regulates the development or approval of drugs, biologics, and medical devices in the United States.

Douglas J. Pisano, Ph.D., R.Ph.
Dean, School of Pharmacy – Worcester
Director, M.S. Degree Program in Regulatory Affairs and Health Policy
Massachusetts College of Pharmacy and Health Sciences
Worcester, MA

David Mantus, Ph.D.
Adjunct Assistant Professor
M.S. Degree Program in Regulatory Affairs and Health Policy
Massachusetts College of Pharmacy and Health Sciences
Vice President, Regulatory Affairs
Sention, Inc.
Providence, RI

Editors

Douglas J. Pisano is an Associate Professor of Pharmacy Administration and the dean of the newly established Massachusetts College of Pharmacy and Health Sciences, Worcester Campus. The mission of the Worcester Campus is to educate future pharmacists to be advanced level clinical practitioners with special emphasis on community practice.

In addition, he serves as the Director of the Master of Science Degree Program in Regulatory Affairs and Health Policy at the Boston campus of the college. Since the Fall of 1984, he has maintained a full-time faculty appointment and is a member of the graduate faculty.

Dr. Pisano earned a Bachelor of Science degree in Pharmacy from the Massachusetts College of Pharmacy and Health Sciences, and state licensure in 1981. He earned his Master of Science degree in Public Policy/Public Affairs from the John W. McCormack Institute, University of Massachusetts at Boston in 1989, and Doctor of Philosophy degree in Law, Policy, and Society from Northeastern University in 1997.

His graduate and undergraduate teaching responsibilities include required courses in pharmacy law, FDA regulation, pharmacy management, and health policy. In 1999, Dr. Pisano was the recipient of the Trustee's Award for Teaching Excellence. In 2000, he received the Special Recognition Award for Increasing Understanding of Regulatory Affairs from the Regulatory Affairs Professionals Society.

Professor Pisano has numerous professional and peer-reviewed publications to his credit, including The Practical Guide to Pharmacy Law Series, continuing education programs, two books, and numerous chapters in areas relating to pharmacy law, drug regulation, professional malpractice, risk management, drug utilization review, health policy, and other topics in healthcare. He also has one book in development.

Professor Pisano's research interests and grants cover studies in legal/regulatory issues, cost effectiveness, professional malpractice, pharmacist/patient communications, and healthcare practice dilemmas.

A national speaker and invited lecturer, Dr. Pisano has made several hundred presentations to varied audiences of pharmacy and nonpharmacy professionals, including the Judiciary Committee of the U.S. House of Representatives, on the areas of pharmacy education, state and federal pharmacy, drug and device law and regulation, professional liability, pharmacy practice, health policy, and other related topics.

David Mantus is an Adjunct Assistant Professor in the Master of Science degree program in Regulatory Affairs and Health Policy at the Massachusetts

College of Pharmacy and Health Sciences (MCPHS). In addition, he serves as Vice President, Regulatory Affairs at Sention Inc., a pharmaceutical development company focused on the discovery and development of drugs to treat memory impairment and other central nervous system disorders.

Dr. Mantus received his Bachelor of Science degree in Chemistry from the College of William and Mary, and his Master of Science and Doctorate in Chemistry from Cornell University. He was also a postdoctoral fellow in Biomedical Engineering at the University of Washington, conducting research on the surface properties of biomaterials intended for medical implants.

Dr. Mantus has previously held regulatory and project management positions at Procter and Gamble Pharmaceuticals, the Massachusetts Public Health Biological Laboratories, PAREXEL, and Shire Biologics. In these positions he has worked on a range of drug development issues, from initial concept and strategy review up to and including post-approval issues in advertising, promotion, and manufacturing and compliance. Dr. Mantus has shepherded multiple products through development, and while at Shire Biologics managed their first product approval in the United States.

Dr. Mantus has published and presented on a range of topics, including analytical chemistry, materials science, clinical trial design, clinical data quality assurance, project management and regulatory affairs. He was recognized by the World Health Organization (WHO) for his contributions teaching regulatory authorities from the developing world as part of the International Vaccine Program. He has both presented and chaired conferences in the U.S. and abroad. In his academic capacity, Dr. Mantus teaches a two-semester course at MCPHS on drug development and regulation, affectionately referred to as "FDA I and II." His students hold, and have gone on to hold, a variety of regulatory and quality assurance positions at pharmaceutical companies and the Food and Drug Administration (FDA).

Contributors

Josephine C. Babiarz Massachusetts College of Pharmacy and Health Sciences, Worcester, MA

Robert Buckley GelTex Pharmaceuticals, Waltham, MA

Thomas Class Millennium Pharmaceuticals, Inc., Cambridge, MA

Jacqueline A. Dombroski Telik, Inc., South San Francisco, CA

Vahe Ghahraman Datafarm, Inc., Marlboro, MA

Alberto Grignolo PAREXEL International, Waltham, MA

Marlene E. Haffner U.S. Food & Drug Administration, Rockville, MD

Catherine Hay Massachusetts Biologic Laboratory, Boston, MA

John J. Jessop The Biologics Consulting Group, Alexandria, VA

Florence Kaltovich SAIC, Frederick, MD

James G. Kenimer The Biologics Consulting Group, Alexandria, VA

Shylendra Kumar Medical Imaging Perceptive Informatics Inc., Waltham, MA

David S. Mantus Sention, Providence, RI

Robert G. Pietrusko Millennium Pharmaceuticals, Inc., Cambridge, MA

Douglas J. Pisano Massachusetts College of Pharmacy & Health Sciences, Worcester, MA

David J. Pizzi PAREXEL International Corp., Waltham, MA

Janet C. Rae PAREXEL International Corp., Waltham, MA

Barry Sall PAREXEL International Corp., Waltham, MA

Contents

1

Overview of Drug Development and the FDA

Douglas J. Pisano

CONTENTS

Regulations and laws are central social constructs that provide guidance for all societies around the globe. Governments create laws in a number of ways with various intents for a myriad of purposes. In the U.S., laws are created by the Congress, a body of officials elected by the citizenry, who are charged with the governance of the country by representing the common, public good. The Congress proposes and passes laws that are relatively general in nature and intended to address some particular issue in a fashion that can be consistently applied by all who are affected by them. Once passed, laws are remanded to the appropriate government or administrative agency

1-58716-007-2/04/$0.00+$1.50
© 2004 by CRC Press LLC

which then decides on how these laws are to be applied. These "applications of law" are called regulations. Regulations serve as the practical foundation from which citizens adhere to the law as it was originally intended.

In the U.S., all food, drugs, cosmetics, and medical devices for both humans and animals are regulated under the authority of the Food and Drug Administration (FDA). The FDA and all of its regulations were created by the government in response to the pressing need to address the safety of the public with respect to its foods and medicinals. The purpose of this chapter is to describe and explain the nature and extent of these regulations as they apply to drugs in the U.S. An historical perspective is offered as a foundation for regulatory context. In addition, the chapter will discuss the FDA's regulatory oversight and that of other agencies, the drug approval and development process, and the mechanisms used to regulate manufacturing and marketing as well as various violation and enforcement schema.

1.1   Brief History of Drug Laws and Regulations

Prior to 1902, the U.S. government took a hands-off approach to the regulation of drugs. Many of the drugs available were so-called "patent medicines" which were so named because each had a more or less descriptive or patent name. No laws, regulations or standards existed to any noticeable extent even though the United States Pharmacopeia (USP) became a reality in 1820 as the first official compendium of the U.S. The USP set standards for strength and purity that could be used by physicians and pharmacists who needed centralized guidelines to extract, compound, and otherwise utilize drug components that existed at the time.[1]

However, in 1848, the first American drug law, the Drug Importation Act, was enacted when American troops serving in Mexico became seriously affected when adulterated quinine, an antimalarial drug, was discovered. This law required laboratory inspection, detention, and even destruction of drugs that did not meet acceptable standards. Later, in 1902, the Virus, Serum and Toxins Act (Biologics Control Act) was passed in response to tetanus-infected diphtheria antitoxin which was manufactured by a small laboratory in St. Louis, MO. Thirteen school children died as a result of the tainted serum. No national standards were as yet in place for purity or potency. The Act authorized the Public Health Service to license and regulate the interstate sale of sera, vaccines, and related biologic products used to prevent or treat disease.

This Act also spurred Dr. Harvey W. Wiley, chief chemist for the Bureau of Chemistry, a branch of the U.S. Department of Agriculture (USDA) and

---

[1] Valentino, J., Practical Uses for the USP: A Legal Perspective, in Strauss' *Federal Drug Laws and Examination Review*, 5th ed., Technomic Publishing Co., Lancaster, PA, 1999, p. 38.

the forerunner for today's U.S. Food and Drug Administration (FDA), to investigate the country's foods and drugs. He established the Hygienic Table, a group of young men who volunteered to serve as human guinea pigs, and who would allow Dr. Wiley to feed them a controlled diet laced with a variety of preservatives and artificial colors. More popularly known as the "Poison Squad," they helped Dr. Wiley gather enough data to prove that many of America's foods and drugs were adulterated, the products' strength or purity was suspect or misbranded, or products had inadequate or inaccurate labeling. Dr. Wiley's efforts, along with publication of Upton Sinclair's *The Jungle* (a book revealing the putrid conditions in America's meat industry), were rewarded when Congress passed America's first food and drug law in 1906, the Pure Food and Drug Act (USPFDA, also known as the Wiley Act). The Wiley Act prohibited interstate commerce of misbranded foods or drugs based on their labeling. It did not affect unsafe drugs in that its legal authority would come to bear only when a product's ingredients were falsely labeled. Even intentionally false therapeutic claims were not prohibited.

This began to change in 1911 with the enactment of the Sherley Amendment which intended to prohibit the labeling of medications with false therapeutic claims that were intended to defraud the purchaser. These amendments, however, required the government to find proof of intentional labeling fraud. Later, in 1937, a sentinel event occurred that changed the entire regulatory picture. Sulfa became the miracle drug of the time and was used to treat many life-threatening infections. It tasted bad and was hard to swallow which led entrepreneurs to seek a palatable solution. S.E. Massingill Co. of Bristol, TN, developed what the company thought was a palatable, raspberry favored liquid product. However, they used diethylene glycol to solubilize the sulfa. A volume of 6 gal of this dangerous mixture, Elixir of Sulfanilamide, killed 107 people, mostly children.

The result was the passage of one of the most comprehensive statutes in the history of American health law. The Federal Food, Drug, and Cosmetic Act of 1938 (FDCA) repealed the Sherley Amendments and required that all new drugs be tested by their manufacturers for safety and that those tests be submitted to the government for marketing approval via the New Drug Application. The FDCA also mandated that drugs be labeled with adequate directions if they were shown to have had harmful effects. In addition, the FDCA authorized the FDA to conduct unannounced inspections of drug manufacturing facilities. Though amended many times since 1938, the FDCA is still the broad foundation for statutory authority for the FDA as it exists today.

However, a new crisis loomed. Throughout the late 1950s, European and Canadian physicians began to encounter a number of infants born with a curious birth defect called phocomelia, a defect that resulted in limbs resembling flippers similar to those found on seals. These birth defects were traced back to mothers who had been prescribed the drug thalidomide in an effort to relieve morning sickness while pregnant. The manufacturer of this drug applied for U.S. marketing approval of the drug as a sleep aid. However, due to the efforts of Dr. Frances O. Kelsey, FDA's chief medical officer at the time, the case was made that the drug was not safe, and therefore not effective for release to the U.S. marketplace.

Dr. Kelsey's efforts and decisive work by the U.S. Congress resulted in yet another necessary amendment to the FDCA in 1962, the Kefauver–Harris Act. This act essentially closed many of the loopholes regarding drug safety in American law. Its drug efficacy amendments now required drug manufacturers to prove safety and efficacy of their drug products, register with the FDA, and be inspected at least every 2 years, have their prescription drug advertising approved by the FDA (this authority being transferred from the Federal Trade Commission), and provide and obtain documented "informed consent" to research subjects prior to human trials. An increase in controls over manufacturing and testing was added to determine drug effectiveness.

In an effort to address these new provisions of the act, the FDA contracted the National Academy of Sciences, along with the National Research Council, to examine some 3,400 drug products approved between 1938 and 1962 based on safety alone. Called the Drug Efficacy Study Implementation Review of 1966 (DESI), it charged these organizations to make a determination as to whether post-1938 drug products were "effective" for the indications claimed in their labeling, "probably effective," "possibly effective," or "ineffective." Those products not deemed "effective" were either removed from the marketplace, reformulated, or sold with a clear warning to prescribers that the product was not deemed effective.

Later, in 1972, the FDA began to examine over-the-counter (OTC) drug products. Phase II of the Drug Efficacy Amendments required the FDA to determine the efficacy of OTC drug products. This project was much larger in scope than the analysis of prescription drugs. The 1970s American consumer could choose from more than 300,000 OTC drug products. The FDA soon realized that it did not have the resources to evaluate each and every one. Hence, it created advisory panels of scientists, medical professionals, and consumers who were charged with evaluating active ingredients used in OTC products within 80 defined therapeutic categories. After examining both the scientific and medical literature of the day, the advisory panels made decisions regarding active ingredients and their labeling. The result was a monograph that described in detail acceptable active ingredients and labeling for products within a therapeutic class. Products that complied with monograph guidelines were deemed "Category I: Safe and Effective, Not Misbranded." However, products not in compliance with monograph guidelines were deemed "Category II: Not Safe and Effective or Misbranded." Category II products were removed from the marketplace or reformulated. Products for which data was insufficient for classification were deemed Category III and were allowed to continue on the market until substantive data could be established or until they were reformulated and in compliance with the monograph. The OTC Drug Review took approximately 20 years to complete.

Though there were numerous other federal laws and regulations that were passed throughout the 1970s, many were based on regulating the practice of medical professionals or were for the direct protection of consumers. For example, The Federal Controlled Substances Act (CSA), part of the Comprehensive Drug Abuse and Prevention Act of 1970, placed drugs with a relatively high potential for abuse into five federal schedules along with a closed record-keeping system designed to track federally controlled substances via a definite paper trail as they were ordered, prescribed, dispensed and utilized throughout the healthcare system.

The 1980s also passed with significant regulatory change. Biotechnology had begun on a grand scale and the pharmaceutical industry was on its cutting edge. Many of the medicinal compounds being discovered were shown to be very expensive and have limited use in the general U.S. population. However, these compounds could prove life saving to demographically small patient populations who suffered from diseases and conditions that were considered rare. In an effort to encourage these biotech pharmaceutical companies to continue to develop these and other products, Congress passed the Orphan Drug Act in 1983. The Act continues to allow manufacturers to gain incentives for research, development and marketing of drug products used to treat rare diseases or conditions that would otherwise be unprofitable via a system of breaks and deductions in a manufacturer's corporate taxes. Though the success of the Orphan Drug Act provided great medical benefit for a few, a scandal was looming in other parts of the pharmaceutical industry.

The generic pharmaceutical industry experienced steady growth as many of the exclusive patents enjoyed by major pharmaceutical companies for brand-named products were beginning to expire. Generic versions of these now freely copied products were appearing much more frequently in the marketplace. However, these generic copies were required to undergo the same rigorous testing that brand-name, pioneer or innovator products did. This led to a very public scandal in which a few unscrupulous generic pharmaceutical companies took short cuts in reporting data, submitted fraudulent samples and offered bribes to FDA officials to gain easy and rapid market approval of their products. As a result, Congress passed the Price Competition and Patent Restoration Act of 1984. This Act, also called the Waxman–Hatch Act after its sponsors, was designed to level the playing field in the prescription drug industry with regard to pioneer/innovator/ brand name prescription drug products and their generic copies. The Act was composed of two distinct parts or "titles." Title I was for the benefit of the generic pharmaceutical industry. It extended the scope of the Abbreviated New Drug Application to cover generic versions of post-1962 approved drug products. It required that generic versions of pioneer or innovator drugs have the same relevant aspects as those with regard to bioequivalence (rate and extent of absorption of the active drug in the human body) and pharmaceutical equivalence (same dosage form as the pioneer drug to which it is compared). Though somewhat simplified, the Waxman–Hatch Act permitted easier market access to generic copies of pioneer drugs provided they were not significantly different from the pioneer drug in their absorption, action, and dosage form. In addition, Title II of the Act was designed to aid and encourage research based on innovator pharmaceutical companies in continuing their search for new and useful medicinal compounds by extending the patent life of pioneer drug products while in the FDA review period.

However, the patent extension benefit has become somewhat moot due to an overall reduction in FDA review time as a result of prescription drug user fees. In 1992, Congress passed the Prescription Drug User Fee Act (PDUFA). The Act was intended to help FDA generate additional funds to upgrade and modernize its operations and to accelerate drug approval. It authorized FDA to charge pharmaceutical manufacturers a "user fee" to accelerate drug review. As a result of the PDUFA legislation, FDA has been able to reduce approval time of new pharmaceutical products from greater than 30 months to approximately 13 to 15 months today. However, the Act had a "sunset" provision that limited FDA authority to charge user fees until the year 1997.

After reviewing the successes of the PDUFA legislation, Congress extended the user fee provisions during passage of the FDA Modernization Act (FDAMA) of 1997. FDMA reauthorized the fees till the year 2002 in an effort to further reduce prescription drug approval time. The Act however, not only extended user fee provisions, it gave FDA the authority to conduct "fast track" product reviews to further speed life-saving drug therapies to market, permitted an additional 6-month patent exclusivity for pediatric prescription drug products, and required the National Institutes of Health to build a publicly accessible database on clinical studies of investigational drugs or life-threatening diseases.

American drug law has come quite far since the early 1900s. Today, the FDA continues to work with Congress and the pharmaceutical industry to regulate and evaluate new and existing drug, biologic, and device products. The overriding regulatory challenge that the FDA will face will be to keep current, through regulation and policy, future technological advances by science and industry.

1.2   Regulatory Oversight of Pharmaceuticals

The primary responsibility for the regulation and oversight of pharmaceuticals and the pharmaceutical industry lies with the FDA. The FDA was created in 1931 and is one of several branches within the U.S. Department of Health and Human Services (HHS). FDA's counterparts within HHS include agencies such as the Centers for Disease Control and Prevention (CDC), the National Institutes of Health (NIH), and the Healthcare Financing Administration (HCFA).

FDA is organized into a number of offices and centers headed by a commissioner who is appointed by the President with the consent of the

Senate. It is a scientifically based law enforcement agency whose mission is to safeguard public health and to ensure honesty and fairness between the consumer and health-regulated industries, involved with pharmaceuticals, devices, and biologics.[2] It licenses and inspects manufacturing facilities, tests products, evaluates claims and prescription drug advertising, monitors research, and creates regulations, guidelines, standards, and policies. It does all of this through its office of operations which contains component offices and centers such as the Center for Drug Evaluation and Research (CDER), Center for Biologics Evaluation and Research (CBER), Center for Devices and Radiological Health (CDRH), Center for Food Safety and Applied Nutrition (CFSAN), the Center for Veterinary Medicine (CVM), Office of Orphan Products Development, Office of Biotechnology, Office of Regulatory Affairs, and the National Center for Toxicological Research. Each of these entities has a defined role, though sometimes their authorities overlap. For example, if a pharmaceutical company submits a drug that is contained and delivered to a patient during therapy by a device not comparable to any other, CDER and CDRH may need to coordinate that product's approval. Though most prescription drugs are evaluated by CDER, any other center or office may become involved with its review. One of the most significant resources to industry and consumers is the FDA's website www.fda.gov. Easily accessible and navigable, each center and office has its own HTML within the site.

The FDA is not the only agency within the U.S. government with a stake in pharmaceutical issues. The Federal Trade Commission (FTC) has authority over general business practices such as deceptive and anticompetitive practices, e.g., false advertising. In addition, the FTC regulates the advertising of OTC drugs, medical devices, and cosmetics. To a lesser degree, the Consumer Product Safety Commission (CPSC) regulates hazardous substances and the containers of poisons and other harmful agents; the Environmental Protection Agency (EPA) regulates pesticides used in agriculture and FDA-regulated food products; the Occupational Safety and Health Administration (OSHA) regulates the working environment of employees who may use FDA-regulated commodities, e.g., syringes, chemotherapy, and chemical reagents; and the Healthcare Financing Administration (HCFA) regulates the federal Medicaid and Medicare programs. The Drug Enforcement Administration (DEA), which enforces the Federal Controlled Substances Act, is charged with controlling and monitoring the flow of licit and illicit controlled substances, as well as various state and local drug control agencies that establish their own regulations and procedures for manufacturing, research, and development of pharmaceuticals.

---

[2] Strauss, S, Food and Drug Administration: An Overview, Strauss' *Federal Drug Laws and Examination Review*, 5th ed., Technomic Publishing Co., Lancaster, PA, 1999, p. 323.

1.3   New Drug Approval and Development

Prior to any discussion of how pharmaceuticals make their way through the FDA for market approval, one needs to have an understanding of what constitutes a drug. A drug is a substance that exerts an action on the structure or function of the body by chemical action or metabolism and is intended for use in the diagnosis, cure, mitigation, treatment, or prevention of disease.[3] The concept of "new drug" stems from the Kefauver–Harris Amendments to the FDCA. A new drug is defined as one that is not generally recognized as safe and effective for the indications proposed. However, this definition has much greater reach than simply a new chemical entity. The term new drug also refers to a drug product already in existence though never approved by the FDA for marketing in the U.S.; new therapeutic indications; a new dosage form; a new route of administration; a new dosing schedule, or any other significant clinical differences than those approved.[4] Therefore, any chemical substance intended for use in humans or animals for medicinal purposes, or any existing chemical substance that has some significant change associated with it is considered not safe or effective and a "new drug" until proper testing and FDA approval is met.

FDA approval can be a fairly lengthy and expensive process. In order for a pharmaceutical manufacturer to place a product on the market for human use, a multiphasic procedure must be followed. It must be remembered that the mission of the FDA is to protect the public and they take that charge very seriously. Hence, all drug products must at least follow the step-wise process.

1.4   Preclinical Investigation

Human testing of new drugs cannot begin until there is solid evidence that the drug product can be used with reasonable safety in humans. This phase is called the *preclinical investigation*. The basic goal of preclinical investigation is to assess potential therapeutic effects of the substance on living organisms and to gather sufficient data to determine reasonable safety of the substance in humans through laboratory experimentation and animal investigation.[5] FDA requires no prior approval for investigators or pharmaceutical industry sponsors to begin a preclinical investigation on a potential drug substance. Investigators and sponsors are, however, required to follow Good Labora-

---

[3] FDCA, Sec. 21(g)(1).
[4] Strauss, S., Food and Drug Administration: An Overview, Strauss' *Federal Drug Laws and Examination Review*, 5th ed., Technomic Publishing Co., Lancaster, PA, 1999, pp. 176, 186.
[5] Pinna, K. and Pines, W., The Drugs/Biologics Approval Process, *A Practical Guide To Food and Drug Law and Regulation*, FDLI, Washington, D.C., 1998, p. 96.

tory Practices (GLP) regulations.[6] GLPs govern laboratory facilities, personnel, equipment, and operations. Compliance with GLPs requires procedures and documentation of training, study schedules, processes, and status reports that are submitted to facility management and included in the final study report to FDA. Preclinical investigation usually takes 1 to 3 years to complete. If at that time enough data is gathered to reach the goal of potential therapeutic effect and reasonable safety, the product sponsor must formally notify FDA of their wishes to test the potential new drug on humans.

1.5   Investigational New Drug Application (INDA)

Unlike the preclinical investigation stage, the INDA phase has much more direct FDA activity throughout. Since a preclinical investigation is designed to gather significant evidence of reasonable safety and efficacy of the compound in live organisms, the IND phase is the clinical phase where all activity is used to gather significant evidence of reasonable safety and efficacy data about the potential drug compound in humans. Clinical trials in humans are carefully scrutinized and regulated by the FDA to protect the health and safety of human test subjects and to ensure the integrity and usefulness of the clinical study data.[7] Numerous meetings between both the agency and sponsor will occur during this time. As a result, the clinical investigation phase may take as many as 12 years to complete. Only 1 in 5 compounds tested may actually demonstrate clinical effectiveness and safety and reach the U.S. marketplace.

The sponsor will submit the INDA to the FDA. The INDA must contain information on the compound itself and information of the study. All INDAs must have the same basic components: a detailed cover sheet, a table of contents, an introductory statement and basic investigative plan, an investigators' brochure, comprehensive investigation protocols, the compound's actual or proposed chemistry, manufacturing and controls, any pharmacology and toxicology information, any previous human experience with the compound and any other pertinent information the FDA deems necessary. After submission, the sponsor company must wait 30 days to commence clinical trials. If FDA does not object within that period, the trials may begin.

Prior to the actual commencement of the clinical investigations however, a few ground rules must be established. For example, a clinical study protocol must be developed, proposed by the sponsor, and reviewed by an Institutional Review Board (IRB). An IRB is required by regulation[8] and is a committee of medical and ethical experts designated by an institution such

---

[6] 21CFR58.

[7] Pinna, K. and Pines, W., The Drugs/Biologics Approval Process, *A Practical Guide To Food and Drug Law and Regulation*, FDLI, Washington, D.C., 1998, p. 98.

[8] 21CFR56.

as a university medical center in which the clinical trial will take place. The charge of the IRB is to oversee the research to ensure that the rights of human test subjects are protected and that rigorous medical and scientific standards are maintained.[9] IRBs must approve the proposed clinical study and monitor the research as it progresses. It must develop written procedures of its own regarding its study review process and its reporting of any changes to the ongoing study as they occur. In addition, an IRB must also review and approve documents for informed consent prior to commencement of the proposed clinical study. Regulations require that potential participants are informed adequately about the risks, benefits, and treatment alternatives before participating in experimental research.[10] An IRB's membership must be sufficiently diverse in order to review the study in terms of the specific research issue, community and legal standards, professional conduct, and practice norms. All of its activities must be well documented and open to FDA inspection at any time.

Once the IRB is satisfied that the proposed trial is ethical and proper, it will begin. The clinical trial phase has three steps or phases. Each has a purpose, requires numerous patients, and can take longer than 1 year to complete.

1.6   Phase I

A Phase I study is relatively small (less than 100 subjects) and brief (1 year or less). Its purpose is to determine toxicology, metabolism, pharmacologic actions and, if possible, any early evidence in effectiveness. The results of the Phase I study are used to develop the next step.

1.7   Phase II

Phase II studies are the first controlled clinical studies using several hundred subjects who are afflicted with the disease or condition being studied. The purpose of Phase II is to determine the compound's possible effectiveness against the targeted disease or condition and its safety in humans. Phase II may be divided into two subparts: Phase IIa, a pilot study that is used to determine initial efficacy, and Phase IIb which uses controlled studies on several hundred patients. At the end of the Phase II studies, the sponsor and FDA will usually confer to discuss the data and plans for Phase III.

---

[9] Pinna, K. and Pines, W., The Drugs/Biologics Approval Process, *A Practical Guide To Food and Drug Law and Regulation*, FDLI, Washington, D.C., 1998, p. 98.
[10] 21CFR50.

1.8   Phase III

Phase III studies are considered "pivotal" trials that are designed to collect all of the necessary data to meet the safety and efficacy standards FDA requires to approve the compound for the U.S. marketplace. Phase III studies are usually very large, consisting of several thousand patients in numerous study centers with a large number of investigators who conduct long term trials over several months or years. Also, Phase III studies establish final formulation, marketing claims and product stability, packaging, and storage conditions. On completion of Phase III, all clinical studies are complete, all safety and efficacy data has been analyzed, and the sponsor is ready to submit the compound to the FDA for market approval. This process begins with submission of a New Drug Application (NDA).

1.9   New Drug Application (NDA)

An NDA is a regulatory mechanism that is designed to give the FDA suffi-cient information to make a meaningful evaluation of a new drug.[11] All NDAs must contain the following information: preclinical laboratory and animal data, human pharmacokinetic and bioavailability data, clinical data, methods of manufacturing, processing and packaging, a description of the drug product and substance, a list of relevant patents for the drug, its man-ufacture or claims, and any proposed labeling. In addition, an NDA must provide a summary of the application's contents and a presentation of the risks and benefits of the new drug.[12] Traditionally, NDAs consisted of hun-dreds of volumes of information, in triplicate, all cross referenced. Since 1999, the FDA has issued final guidance documents that allow sponsors to submit NDAs electronically in a standardized format. These electronic submissions facilitate ease of review and possible approval.[13]

The NDA must be submitted complete in the proper form and with all critical data. If the FDA considers it "accepted," it will then determine the application's completeness. If "complete," the agency considers the applica-tion "filed" and will begin the review process within 60 days.[14] The purpose of an NDA from the FDA's perspective is to ensure that the new drug meets the criteria to be "safe and effective." Safety and effectiveness are determined

---

[11] 21CFR314.

[12] Pinna, K. and Pines, W., The Drugs/Biologics Approval Process, *A Practical Guide To Food and Drug Law and Regulation*, FDLI, Washington, D.C., 1998, pp. 102–103.

[13] Fed Reg, V. 64(18), January 28, 1999.

[14] Pinna, K., and Pines, W., The Drugs/Biologics Approval Process, *A Practical Guide To Food and Drug Law and Regulation*, FDLI, Washington, D.C., 1998, p. 103.

through the Phase III pivotal studies based on "substantial evidence" gained from a well-controlled clinical study. Since the FDA realizes there are no absolutely safe drugs, FDA looks to the new drug's efficacy as a measure of its safety. It weighs the risks vs. benefits of approving the drug for use in the U.S. market.

Also, the NDA must be very clear about the manufacture and marketing of the proposed drug product. The application must define and describe manufacturing processes, validate Current Good Manufacturing Practices (CGMPs), provide evidence of quality, purity, strength, identity, and bio-availability (a preinspection of the manufacturing facility will be conducted by the FDA). Finally, the FDA will review all product packaging and labeling for content and clarity. Statements on a product's package label, package insert, media advertising, or professional literature must be reviewed. Of note, "labeling" refers to all of the above and not just the label on the product container.

The FDA is required to review an application within 180 d of filing. At the end of that time, the agency is required to respond with an "action letter." There are three kinds of action letters. An Approval Letter signifies that all substantive requirements for approval are met with and that the sponsor company can begin marketing the drug as of the date on the letter.

An Approvable Letter signifies that the application substantially complies with the requirements but has some minor deficiencies that must be addressed before an approval letter is sent. Generally, these deficiencies are minor in nature and the product sponsor must respond within 10 days of receipt. At this point, the sponsor may amend the application and address the agency's concerns, request a hearing with the agency, or withdraw the application entirely.

A Non-Approvable Letter signifies that FDA has a major concern with the application and will not approve the proposed drug product for marketing as submitted. The remedies a sponsor can take for this type of action letter are similar to those as in the Approvable Letter.

1.10　PDUFA/FDAMA Effects

The New Drug Application review has been significantly affected by both the PDUFA and FDAMA legislation. The Prescription Drug User Fee Act (PDUFA) allows the FDA to collect fees from sponsor companies who submit applications for review. The fees are used to update facilities and hire and train reviewers. The fees apply only to NDA drug submissions, biologic drug submissions, and any supplement thereto. The fees do not apply to generic drugs or medical devices. The results of the PDUFA legislation were significant; approval rates have increased from approximately 50% to nearly

80% and the review times have decreased to under 15 months for most applications.[15]

Later, in 1997, the FDA Modernization Act (FDAMA) reauthorized PDUFA until the year 2002. It waives the user fee to small companies that have less than 500 employees and are submitting their first application. It allows payment of the fee in stages and permits a small percentage of refund if the application is refused. Also, it exempts applications for drugs used in rare conditions (Orphan Drugs), supplemental applications for pediatric indications, and applications for biologicals used as precursors for other biologics manufacture. In addition, FDMA permits a "fast track" approval of compounds that demonstrate significant benefit to critically ill patients such as those which suffer from AIDS.[16]

1.11 Biologics

Biologics are defined as substances derived from or made with the aid of living organisms that include vaccines, antitoxins, sera, blood, blood products, therapeutic protein drugs derived from natural sources (i.e., anti-thrombin III) or biotechnology (e.g., recombinantly derived proteins), and gene or somatic cell therapies.[17] As with the more traditionally derived drug products, biologics follow virtually the same regulatory and clinical testing schema with regard to safety and efficacy. A Biologics License Application (BLA) is used rather than a New Drug Application (NDA) though the official FDA form is designated 356h and is identical. The sponsor merely indicates in a check box if the application is for a drug or a biologic. Compounds characterized as biologics are reviewed by CBER.[18]

1.12 Orphan Drugs

Orphan drugs are approved using many of the same processes as any other application. However, there are several significant differences. An orphan drug as defined under the Orphan Drug Act of 1993 is a drug used to treat a rare disease that would not normally be of interest to commercial manufacturers in the ordinary course of business. A rare disease is defined in the

[15] Strauss, S., Food and Drug Administration: An Overview, Strauss' *Federal Drug Laws and Examination Review*, 5th ed., Technomic Publishing Co., Lancaster, PA, 1999, p. 280.
[16] Food and Drug Administration Modernization Act of 1997, PL. 105, 1997.
[17] 42USC, Sec. 262
[18] Form FDA 356h.

law as any disease that affects fewer than 200,000 persons in the U.S. or one in which a manufacturer has no reasonable expectation of recovering the cost of its development and availability in the U.S. The act creates a series of financial incentives that manufacturers can take advantage of. For example, the act permits grant assistance for clinical research, tax credits for research and development, and a 7-year market exclusivity to the first applicant to obtain market approval for a drug designated as an orphan. This means that if a sponsor gains approval for an orphan drug, the FDA will not approve any application by any other sponsor for the same drug for the same disease or condition for 7 years from the date of the first applicant's approval, provided certain conditions are met such as an assurance of sufficient availability of the drug to those in need, or a revocation is made of the drug's orphan status.[19,20]

1.13   Abbreviated New Drug Applications (ANDA)

Abbreviated New Drug Applications (ANDAs) are used when a patent has expired for a product that has been on the U.S. market, and a company wishes to market a copy. In the U.S. a drug patent lasts 20 years. After that time, a manufacturer is able to submit an abbreviated application for that product provided they certify that the product patent in question has already expired, is invalid, or will not be infringed.

The generic copy must meet certain other criteria as well. The drug's active ingredient must have already been approved for the conditions of use proposed in the ANDA, and nothing has changed to call into question the basis for approval of the original drug's NDA.[21] Sponsors of ANDAs are required to prove that their version meets with the standards of bio and pharmaceutical equivalence. The FDA publishes a list of all approved drugs called *Approved Drug Products with Therapeutic Equivalence Evaluations*, also called the "Orange Book" because of its orange-colored cover. It lists marketed drug products that are considered by the FDA to be safe and effective, and provides monthly information on therapeutic equivalence evaluations for approved multisource prescription drug products.[22] The Orange Book rates drugs based on their therapeutic equivalence. For a product to be considered therapeutically equivalent, it must be both *pharmaceutically equivalent* (i.e., the same dose, dosage form, strength, etc.), and *bioequivalent* (i.e., rate and extent of its absorption are not significantly

[19] The Orphan Drug Act of 1982, PL 97-414.
[20] The Orphan Drug Amendments of 1985, PL 99-91.
[21] Pinna, K. and Pines, W., The Drugs/Biologics Approval Process, *A Practical Guide To Food and Drug Law and Regulation*, FDLI, Washington, D.C., 1998, p. 119.
[22] USP/DI, Volume III, 13th ed., Preface, v.

different from the rate and extent of absorption of the drug with which it is to be interchanged).

Realizing that there may be some degree of variability in patients, FDA allows pharmaceuticals to be considered bioequivalent in either of two methods. The first method studies the rate and extent of absorption of a test drug which may or may not be a generic variation, and a reference or brand name drug under similar experimental conditions and in similar dosing schedules where the test results do not show significant differences. The second approach uses the same method but the results determine that there is a difference in the test drugs' rate and extent of absorption, considered to be medically insignificant for the proper clinical outcome of that drug. The regulation reads:

> Bioequivalence of different formulations of the same drug substance involves equivalence with respect to the rate and extent of drug absorption. Two formulations whose rate and extent of absorption differ by 20% or less are generally considered bioequivalent. The use of the 20% rule is based on a medical decision that, for most drugs, a 20% difference in the concentration of the active ingredient in blood will not be clinically significant.[23]

The FDA's Orange Book uses a two-letter coding system that is helpful in determining which drug products are considered therapeutically equivalent. The first letter, either an "A" or a "B," indicates a drug product's therapeutic equivalence rating. The second letter describes dose forms and can be any one of a number of different letters.

The "A" codes are described in the Orange Book as follows:

Drug products that FDA considers to be therapeutically equivalent to other pharmaceutically equivalent products, i.e., drug products for which:

1. There are no known or suspected bioequivalence problems. These are designated AA, AN, AO, AP, or AT, depending on the dose form.
2. Actual or potential bioequivalence problems have been resolved with adequate *in vivo* and/or *in vitro* evidence supporting bioequivalence. These are designated AB.[24]

The "B" codes are much less desirable ratings when compared with a rating of "A." Products that are rated "B" may still be commercially marketed, however, they may not be considered therapeutically equivalent. The Orange Book describes "B" codes as follows:

---

[23] USP/DI, p.I/7.
[24] USP/DI, p.I/9.

Drug products that FDA at this time does not consider to be therapeutically equivalent to other pharmaceutically equivalent products, i.e.,
drug products for which actual or potential bioequivalence problems
have not been resolved by adequate evidence of bioequivalence.
Often the problem is with specific dosage forms rather than with
the active ingredients. These are designated BC, BD, BE, BN, BP,
BR, BS, BT, or BX.[25]

FDA has adopted an additional subcategory of "B" codes. The designation
"B*" is assigned to former "A" rated drugs "if FDA receives new information
that raises a significant question regarding therapeutic equivalence."[26] Not
all drugs are listed in the Orange Book. Drugs obtainable only from a single
manufacturing source, DESI-drugs or drugs manufactured prior to 1938 are
not included. Those that do appear are listed by generic name.

1.14 Phase IV and Postmarketing Surveillance

Pharmaceutical companies that successfully gain marketing approval for
their products are NOT exempt from further regulatory requirements. Many
products are approved for market on the basis of a continued submission of
clinical research data to the FDA. This data may be required to further
validate efficacy or safety, detect new uses or abuses for the product, or to
determine its effectiveness per labeled indications under conditions of wide-
spread usage.[27] The FDA may also require a Phase IV study for drugs
approved under FDAMA's "fast track" provisions.

Any changes to the approved product's indications, active ingredients,
manufacture, and labeling require the manufacturer to submit a supplemental NDA (SNDA) for agency approval. Also, "adverse drug reports" are
required to be reported to the agency. All reports must be reviewed by the
manufacturer promptly, and if found to be serious, life-threatening or unexpected (not listed in the product's labeling), the manufacturer is required to
submit an "alert report" within 15 working days of receipt of the information.
All adverse reactions thought not to be serious or unexpected must be
reported quarterly for 3 years after the application is approved, and annually
thereafter.[28]

---

[25] USP/DI, p.I/10.

[26] USP/DI, p.I/12.

[27] Pinna, K and Pines, W., The Drugs/Biologics Approval Process, *A Practical Guide To Food and Drug Law and Regulation*, FDLI, Washington, D.C., 1998, p. 111.

[28] Pinna, K., and Pines, W., The Drugs/Biologics Approval Process, *A Practical Guide To Food and Drug Law and Regulation*, FDLI, Washington, D.C., 1998, p. 111.

1.15 Over-The-Counter (OTC) Regulations

The 1951 Durham–Humphrey Amendments of the FDCA specified three criteria to justify prescription-only status. If the compound is shown to be habit-forming, to require a prescriber's supervision, or has a NDA prescription-only limitation, it will require a prescription. The principles used to establish *OTC status* (nonprescription required) are a wide margin of safety, method of use, benefit-to-risk ratio, and adequacy of labeling for self-medication. For example, injectable drugs may not be used OTC with certain exceptions such as insulin. OTC market entry is less restrictive than that for Rx drugs and do not require premarket clearance. This poses many fewer safety hazards than Rx drugs because they are designed to alleviate symptoms rather than disease. Easier access far outweighs the risks of side effects that can be adequately addressed through proper labeling.

As previously discussed, OTC products underwent a review in 1972. Though reviewing the 300,000+ OTC drug products in existence at the time would have been virtually impossible, FDA created OTC advisory panels to review data based on some 26 therapeutic categories. OTC drugs would be examined only by active ingredient within a therapeutic category. Inactive ingredients would be examined only provided they were shown to be safe and suitable for the product and not interfering with effectiveness and quality.

This review of active ingredients would result in the promulgation of a regulation or a "monograph" which is a "recipe" or set of guidelines applicable to all OTC products within a therapeutic category. OTC monographs are general and require that OTC products show "general recognition of the safety and effectiveness of the active ingredient." OTC products do not fall under prescription status if their active ingredients (or combinations) are deemed by FDA to be "Generally Recognized as Safe and Effective" (GRASE). The monograph system is a public system with a public comment component included after each phase of the process. Any products for which a final monograph has not been established may remain on the market until one is determined.

There are four phases in the OTC monograph system. In Phase I, an expert panel is selected to review data for each active ingredient in each therapeutic category for safety, efficacy, and labeling. Their recommendations are noted in the *Federal Register.* A public comment period of 30 to 60 d was permitted and supporting or contesting data was accepted for review. Then the panel reevaluated the data and published a "proposed monograph" in the *Federal Register* which publicly announced the conditions for which the panel believed that OTC products in a particular therapeutic class were GRASE and not misbranded. A "tentative final monograph" was then developed and published, stating the FDA's position on safety and efficacy of a particular ingredient within a therapeutic category and acceptable labeling with indications, warnings, and directions for use. Active ingredients were deemed Category I — GRASE for claimed therapeutic indications and not misbranded; Category II — not GRASE and/or misbranded; or Category III — insufficient data for determination.

After public comment, the final monograph was established and published with the FDA's final criteria for which all drug products in a therapeutic class become GRASE and not misbranded. Following the effective date of the final monograph, all covered drug products that failed to conform to requirements were considered misbranded and/or unapproved new drugs.[29]

However, since the monograph panels are no longer convened, many current products are switched from prescription status. A company who wishes to make this switch and offer a product to the U.S. marketplace can submit an amendment to a monograph to the FDA which will act as the sole reviewer. They may also file an SNDA provided that they have 3 years of marketing experience with the drug as a prescription product, can demonstrate a relative high use during that period, and can validate that the product has a mild profile of adverse reactions. The last method involves a "citizen's petition" which is rarely used.[30]

1.16   Regulating Marketing

FDA has jurisdiction over prescription drug advertising and promotion. The basis for these regulations lies within the 1962 Kefauver–Harris Amendments. Essentially, any promotional information, in any form, must be truthful, fairly balanced, and fully disclosed. The FDA views this information as either "advertising" or "labeling." Advertising includes all traditional outlets in which a company places an ad. Labeling encompasses everything else, including brochures, booklets, lectures, slide kits, letters to physicians, company-sponsored magazine articles, etc. All information must be truthful and not misleading. All material facts must be disclosed in manner that is fairly balanced and accurate. If any of these requirements are violated, the product is considered misbranded for the indications for which it was approved under its NDA. FDA is also sensitive to the promotion of a product for "off-label" use. Off-label use occurs when a product is in some way presented in a manner that does not agree with or is not addressed in its approved labeling. Also, provisions of the Prescription Drug Marketing Act (PDMA) of 1987 apply. The Act prohibits company representatives from directly distributing or reselling prescription drug samples. Companies are required to establish a closed system of record keeping that will be able to

---

[29] Strauss, S., Food and Drug Administration: An Overview, Strauss' *Federal Drug Laws and Examination Review*, 5th ed., Technomic Publishing Co., Lancaster, PA, 1999, p. 285.
[30] Strauss, S., Food and Drug Administration: An Overview, Strauss' *Federal Drug Laws and Examination Review*, 5th ed., Technomic Publishing Co., Lancaster, PA, 1999, p. 285.

track a sample from their control to that of a prescriber in order to prevent diversion. Prescribers are required to receive these samples and record and store them appropriately.[31]

1.17 Violations and Enforcement

FDA has the power to enforce the regulations for any product as defined under the FDCA. It has the jurisdiction to inspect a manufacturer's premises and records. After a facilities inspection, an agency inspector will issue an FDA Form 483s which describes observable violations. Response to the finding as described on this form must be made promptly. A warning letter may be used when the agency determines that one or more of a company's practices, products, and procedures are in violation of the FDCA. The FDA district has 15 days to issue a warning letter after an inspection. The company has 15 days in which to respond. If the company response is satisfactory to the agency, no other action is warranted. If the response is not, the agency may request a recall of the violated products. However FDA has no authority to force a company to recall a product. But, it may force removal of a product through the initiation of a seizure.

Recalls can fall into one of three classes. A Class I recall exists when there is a reasonable possibility that the use of a product will cause either serious adverse effects on health or death. Class II recall exists when the use of a product may cause temporary or medically reversible adverse effects on health, or where the probability of serious adverse effects on health is remote, and a Class III recall exists when the use of a product is not likely to cause adverse health consequences. Recalls are also categorized as Consumer Level, where the product is requested to be recalled from the consumers' homes or control; Retail Level, where the product is to be removed from retail shelves or control, and Wholesale Level, where the product is to be removed from wholesale distribution. Companies that conduct recall of their products are required to conduct "effectiveness checks" to determine the effectiveness of recalling the product from the marketplace.

If a company refuses to recall the product, the FDA will seek an injunction against the company.[32] An injunction is recommended to the Department of Justice (DOJ) by the FDA. The DOJ takes the request to federal court which issues an order that forbids a company from carrying out a particular illegal act, such as marketing a product that the FDA considers a violation of the FDCA. Companies can either comply with the order or sign a consent agreement that will specify changes required by the FDA in order for the company to continue operations or to litigate.

---

[31] 21USC301, et seq.
[32] 21USC301, et seq.

The FDA may also initiate a seizure of violative products.[33] A seizure is ordered by the federal court in the district where the products are located. The seizure order specifies products, their batch numbers, and any records as determined by the FDA as violative. The U.S. Marshals carry out this action. The FDA institutes a seizure to prevent a company from selling, distributing, moving, or otherwise tampering with the product.

The FDA may also debar individuals or firms from assisting or submitting an ANDA, or directly providing services to any firm with an existing or pending drug product application. Debarment may last for up to 10 years.[34]

However, one of the more powerful deterrents that the FDA uses is adverse publicity. The agency has no authority to require a company to advertise adverse publicity. It does publish administrative actions against a company in any number of federal publications such as the *Federal Register*, the *FDA Enforcement Report*, the *FDA Medical Bulletin*, and the *FDA Consumer*.[35]

1.18 Summary

The laws and regulations that govern the U.S. pharmaceutical industry are both vast and complicated. Interpretation of the FDCA is in a constant state of flux. FDA is charged with this interpretation based on the rapid technological changes that are everyday occurrences within the industry. Many may suggest that more rapid drug approval places the citizenry in greater danger of adverse events. Others may reply that technology offers newer and more effective therapies for deadly disease.

Historically, the U.S. Congress has passed laws governing our medication based on a reaction to a crisis. The Pure Food and Drug Act, the Food, Drug and Cosmetic Act, and the Price Competition and Patent Restoration Act are only a few. One hopes that this method of regulation will not continue as the norm. We can be proud of proactive legislation such as the Kefauver–Harris Amendments, the Orphan Drug Act, PDUFA, and FDAMA. These acts have paved the way for meaningful change within the drug investigation process as we continue in our battle against disease. The U.S. system of investigating new drugs is one that continues to have merit by allowing enough time to investigate benefit vs. risk. The American public can look forward to great advances from the industry and should be comfortable that FDA is watching.

2

Regulatory Strategy

Jacqueline A. Dombroski

CONTENTS

> *strat-e-gy* 1. a plan, method, or series of maneuvers or stratagems for obtaining a specific goal or result. 2. Also, *strategics*, the science or art of planning or directing large military movements and operations. 3. The use or an instance of using this science or art. 4. Skillful use of a stratagem.

> *strat-a-gem* 1. A plan, scheme, or trick for surprising or deceiving an enemy. 2. Any artifice, ruse, or trick to attain a goal or to gain an advantage over an adversary.

1-58716-007-2/04/$0.00+$1.50
© 2004 by CRC Press LLC

2.1 Introduction

Regulatory affairs professionals have an important influence in the premarketing development, regulatory submissions, and post-approval product lifecycles of pharmaceutical products. Their knowledge and experience can have a positive effect on the efficiency of a development program, the timing and success of marketing approval applications, and the safe and effective marketing for pharmaceutical products. To be most effective, regulatory affairs knowledge and experience must be applied before and during the various phases of pharmaceutical product development and marketing.

Given the complex and costly nature of pharmaceutical product development, it is a common, industry-wide practice to design product development plans that identify the critical steps and the resources required to meet the goals of marketing a product, thereby obtaining a return on the original investment. The product development plan (or its appropriate abstracts) is an important tool for communication, not only for planning and implementing research and development studies and regulatory submission activities, but also for business purposes because a clear and realistic product development plan may enhance fund-raising activities. The overall product development plan for a specific product may incorporate multiple strategies and stratagems, all with the aim of meeting the ultimate goal of a marketed product. The regulatory strategy is a fundamental part of a pharmaceutical product development plan and it is also the cornerstone upon which all of the other contributing parts of the plan must be based because of the requirement for regulatory approval for clinical testing and marketing for the majority of pharmaceutical products. However, a regulatory strategy must be used as a dynamic, reactive plan. It will need to be modified, perhaps frequently, during product development to take account of the growing body of knowledge about the product and to accommodate any changes in legislation and regulatory authority requirements for clinical trials and marketing.

An effective regulatory strategy cannot be developed in isolation from other aspects of a product development plan. A thorough understanding of the pharmaceutical product, its intended clinical indication and the potential market is required. Therefore, the preparation of a regulatory strategy is an interesting and challenging task that requires a variety of skills including the ability to research, analyze, and interpret pertinent literature and data, and effectively communicate with people from all of the disciplines that contribute to product development inside and outside of the company. Thus, a regulatory affairs professional developing a regulatory strategy will communicate not only with the scientific, regulatory affairs and clinical staff within product research and development groups but also with personnel from corporate functions such as advertising, marketing, legal, and finance. All levels of regulatory affairs personnel can contribute to the development and implementation of a regulatory strategy although the overall responsibility for this task is usually assigned to a person with moderate to long-term experience in regulatory affairs. Training and experience in contributing to or developing a regulatory strategy is frequently used as a career development and evaluation goal for regulatory affairs staff, and its importance is reflected in the increasing level of regulatory strategy experience required to attain senior regulatory affairs positions.

The remainder of this chapter will focus on aspects of developing a regulatory strategy for the marketing of human drug products, although the general concepts are equally applicable for other regulated products such as medicinal devices, foods, and cosmetics. The phases of product development and the details of the design of regulatory strategies for medicinal devices, foods, and cosmetics differ from those for drugs because the requirements for marketing approval are different. Although the establishment and protection of intellectual property rights are important in pharmaceutical product development, these activities also require a strategy, which is beyond the scope of this chapter.

2.2   Overview of a Regulatory Strategy

A regulatory strategy can be defined as a plan that identifies the series of tasks that must be completed and data that must be generated to achieve the goal of obtaining and maintaining regulatory authority approval for marketing a pharmaceutical product. A regulatory strategy may also include information on when the tasks should be performed in relation to other tasks, and estimates of the resources that may be needed to achieve the goal. Information in a regulatory strategy should be presented in a way that it may be incorporated into a pharmaceutical product development plan. To aid the understanding of a regulatory strategy and the rationale for the recommendations made in the strategy it is usually necessary to prepare a report that summarizes the background information reviewed while preparing the strategy and the analysis and interpretation of that information.

The broad definition of a regulatory strategy given above applies to the whole life cycle of a pharmaceutical product; however, it is not usually either practical or possible to design a detailed regulatory strategy for the whole life cycle of a product at the outset of a pharmaceutical development program because of the long time periods involved. It may take 8 to 10 years of development and regulatory agency review time before a product is approved for marketing, and the total life cycle of a product, including additional indications for use and postapproval improvements in the dosage form may readily span more than 20 years. Therefore, a series of regulatory strategies may be required during the life cycle of a product so that the complexity of the choices that could be made during each phase of product development can be thoroughly addressed. Also, because alternative pathways may exist to meet the goal of a marketed product and the data generated during development may produce unexpected results, it is advisable to incorporate alternate or contingency plans in the regulatory strategy at each stage. A regulatory strategy that covers the anticipated future life cycle of a product would be useful, however, at the critical transition point when the product is first approved for marketing. Thus, a regulatory strategy for a specific pharmaceutical product should be customized for the phases of its product development program as outlined later in this chapter. Some general principles that apply to any regulatory strategy are discussed first.

2.2.1   The Goal of a Regulatory Strategy

The main goal of any regulatory strategy for a pharmaceutical product is to achieve a regulatory affairs milestone. Thus, a regulatory strategy must identify which regulatory milestone the plan is intended to cover. Some common regulatory milestones during pharmaceutical product development include:

- The assignment of an established name by a regulatory authority [e.g., the United States Approved Name (USAN) or British Approved Name (BAN)] and the subsequent assignment of the International Nonproprietary Name (INN) by the World Health Organization.

- The agreement of a regulatory authority that a clinical study research program may begin in humans following the submission of a clinical trial application or notification such as an Investigational New Drug Exemption Application (IND) in the U.S. or a Clinical Trial Exemption Application (CTX) in the United Kingdom (U.K.).

- The approval of inclusion of the drug product in a special category by a regulatory authority to attain either faster regulatory review (e.g., designation as an Orphan Drug in the U.S. or European Union (E.U.), or designation as a Fast Track Development Program or assignment for Accelerated Approval in the U.S) or other benefits such as a regulatory authority agreement to provide "Special Protocol Assessment," or access to scientific advice during product development market exclusivity, access to government funding for research and development, or application review fee waivers that are available for some classes of drugs in the U.S. and E.U. as well as other countries.

- Certification of regulatory or quality compliance following inspections or audits conducted by regulatory authorities either prior to marketing approval or under a periodic, routine compliance monitoring program.

- The approval of a marketing authorization application by a regulatory authority after reviewing an application such as a New Drug Application (NDA) in the U.S. or a Marketing Authorization Application (MAA) in the E.U.

- The approval of a regulatory submission that changes or expands the product labeling in a beneficial way, for example, to include additional therapeutic indications, additional patients eligible for treatment, new information on the use of the drug or its safety profile, a new dose regimen, or a new dosage form. Typical regulatory submissions include NDA Supplements and NDA Amendments in the U.S. and Product License Variations in the E.U.

- The approval of a regulatory submission that changes or expands the nonclinical information available for a marketed drug product such as changes in the chemistry, manufacturing, quality control testing, or stability data for the drug substance or drug product, or additional information about the safety of the drug substance or drug product in animals.

2.2.2 Background Information for a Regulatory Strategy

In preparing a regulatory strategy it is necessary to take into account the current and proposed legislation for pharmaceutical products of the applicable class, regulatory guidelines, regulatory and quality compliance practice requirements, pharmacopeial requirements, and other types of recommendations available from the regulatory authorities and trade organizations in the countries where regulatory submissions are to be made. This information may be obtained either directly from the regulatory agencies or other organizations either as paper copies or, in some countries, as electronic files. In addition, a literature research should be performed to find any available information on the plans or prior actions of regulatory authorities, companies, or academic research centers that may be relevant to the drug product that is in development. Great care should be taken in designing the literature search strategy and selecting keywords because it is relatively easy to become overwhelmed with information that is of limited value if the search is too broad or the key words too general.

Using the information described above, it is possible to prepare a background report that summarizes the key features of the "regulatory environment" in which the pharmaceutical product is being developed as well as "competitive intelligence" information about drugs that are being developed by other organizations and that are categorized in the same pharmacological class or are being developed for the same or a related therapeutic indication. The regulatory strategy should make recommendations that are specifically applicable to the pharmaceutical development plan of the drug product being developed, based on the analysis and interpretation of the regulatory environment and competitive intelligence information gathered.

Generally, more information that will be relevant to a regulatory strategy is available publicly in the U.S. than in other countries because of the provisions of the Freedom of Information (FOI) Act and the availability of a wide variety of reporting mechanisms. For example, in the U.S., the Food and Drug Administration (FDA) maintains and routinely updates a Website from which it is possible to obtain electronic copies of the reports written by the FDA's scientific and technical reviewers about recent original NDAs, as well as the NDA Supplements and Amendments that affect product labeling. Paper copies of these NDA review reports can be purchased either by sending a written request and the applicable fee to the FDA under the FOI Act or, usually more rapidly, through a commercial organization. It is possible to attend the meetings of the FDA's advisory committees where some (but not all) NDAs or other relevant regulatory affairs topics are discussed in a public forum. For some Advisory Committee meetings it is possible to purchase audio or video tapes of the public discussions (but not the closed sessions) relatively quickly after the meeting, and paper copies of the transcripts of the meetings may be purchased several months after the meeting has occurred. Representatives of the FDA's review divisions also participate in public meetings and Webcasts held by a variety of organizations. As well, copies of their presentation materials are generally posted to the relevant sections of the FDA's Website. There is also a wide variety of newspapers, direct mail, and other publications that report rapidly on regulatory affairs news from the FDA and pharmaceutical and other industries regulated by the FDA. Fewer such sources are generally available outside of the U.S.

2.2.3 Regulatory Strategy and Timelines

Time and other resources are important features of any pharmaceutical development plan and are also important considerations for a regulatory strategy. A regulatory strategy should identify the key summary information, data, and completed study reports that must be available and the regulatory and document management tasks that must be performed to prepare an adequate regulatory submission that will be accepted by the regulatory agency for review. The regulatory strategy should also identify milestone meetings such as those with key investigators or regulatory agencies that may be needed before a regulatory submission can be made. Realistic timelines should be suggested by all contributing authors for the preparation of briefing documents for meetings, and for the preparation of summaries and study reports for regulatory submissions. The timelines should be analyzed and incorporated into the regulatory strategy because these have a direct influence on the timelines for the preparation of regulatory submissions. Resources may then be identified and assigned via the product development plan to achieve the desired timeline for the regulatory submission.

The time that will be taken to prepare a regulatory strategy must also be carefully considered because if the preparation of a regulatory strategy is delayed while every possible source is reviewed for regulatory and competitive intelligence, pharmaceutical development will most likely proceed without the regulatory strategy. As mentioned above, a regulatory strategy is a dynamic plan that should be frequently reviewed and revised, therefore, it is generally better to prepare an outline for the regulatory strategy and summarize the key regulatory requirements to provide initial guidance than to wait for background research on the regulatory environment and competitive intelligence to be completed. The regulatory background report and regulatory strategy should be revised, as necessary, to take account of new data and information from all sources including those within the company as well as outside the company, but the timing of such revisions should be based on the importance of the new information available. For example, the therapeutic indication(s) for clinical research studies in humans may not have been decided at the outset of pharmaceutical development, or the intended indication may change due to the results of pharmacological or toxicological studies. Market analysis data may also change the direction or emphasis of clinical research studies. As a result of this kind of information, the regulatory strategy should be rapidly reviewed and revised, especially if different regulatory agency requirements or guidelines must be followed. In a rapidly progressing and competitive area of research, rapid refinement of clinical research study designs and the regulatory strategy may be needed to keep ahead or abreast of other products being developed for the same or similar indications if it is important for the company to be the first or among the earliest to receive regulatory approval. Information that does not directly affect the timing or types of research studies required may not need to be incorporated into a regulatory strategy.

2.2.4 Multiple Regulatory Strategies

A regulatory strategy could recommend more than one plan that will meet the business goals of the corporation or may comprise parallel strategies with different outcomes. Due to the range of pharmacological activities of many drugs, organizations may have to decide to perform research in some but not all of the therapeutic areas in which a drug may be effective. In this case, the comparison of multiple regulatory strategies for the different research and business opportunities may be a key factor in the decision-making process. For example, presentation of the differing regulatory strategies that are possible for a drug with the potential for therapeutic use in a variety of oncology indications and in rheumatoid arthritis will give an organization valuable information to choose the indication for which it will seek marketing approval first, and it may influence other business decisions such as licensing agreements that could provide funding for research or other business needs. In this case, in the U.S. it is likely that an effective drug with a good safety profile would be approved more quickly for marketing for some oncology indications rather than, for example, for rheumatoid arthritis. This is due to less cumulative patient data required and well-established regulatory initiatives in place to speed the development and review of oncology drugs. If an organization has a limited budget for development, it is more likely to initially develop the drug for an oncology indication than for rheumatoid arthritis, which would probably require longer clinical research studies in a wider selection and greater numbers of potentially eligible patients. The special regulatory initiatives (such as Orphan Drug designation, Fast Track Development Programs, Accelerated Approval, and Special Protocol Assessment) are discussed in more detail in other chapters.

2.3   Regulatory Strategies for Different Phases of Product Development

The major phases of pharmaceutical product development may be summarized in three general categories as follows:

- Preclinical Development Phase
- Clinical Development Phase
- Postapproval Development and Marketing Phase

A summary of the major pharmaceutical product development activities and a discussion of the key points for a regulatory strategy for each phase follow.

2.3.1   Regulatory Strategy during the Preclinical Development Phase

During the preclinical development phase, preliminary data on the chemistry, manufacturing, quality control, and stability of the drug substance and drug product are generated. The drug substance and drug product are characterized and analytical methods are developed to control them. Reference standards may be set up. *In vitro* and *in vivo* pharmacology studies are performed to characterize the effects of the drug and attempt to elucidate the mechanism of action. The toxicology study program is initiated to study the pharmacological and toxicological effects of the drug substance and/or drug product in animal species. The results from the preclinical development phase are evaluated and verified. Clinical researchers select the pharmacological activity (or activities) that may warrant further research in humans and design a clinical research study to investigate the tolerability, overall safety, and dose-response of the drug product. A summary of the preclinical data and the proposed clinical research study design is prepared according to regulatory authority requirements. The summary data and other appropriate documents such as a cover letter and application form are submitted to one or more regulatory authorities to notify the authority of the company's intention to initiate clinical research studies in humans. The regulatory authorities acknowledge the receipt of the notification and indicate whether or not the clinical study or studies may proceed.

The major goals at this stage of drug product development will be to provide an adequate body of evidence to initiate or continue the submission of patent applications to establish and protect intellectual property rights, and to support the first human clinical trials. The regulatory strategy for the preclinical development phase focuses on assembling the appropriate data and making the necessary regulatory submissions to obtain regulatory agency clearance to perform the first clinical research studies in humans.

Although a regulatory strategy could be developed at any time during the preclinical phase of product development, there are advantages in preparing a regulatory strategy as early as possible. However, a regulatory strategy is probably most useful after the compound has passed from discovery research to pharmacological testing. The advantages of developing a regulatory strategy early in preclinical development include opening channels of communication with all disciplines involved in product development about the type, scope, and quality of data that will be required for the regulatory submissions for clinical trials and facilitating the early identification of gaps in the body of evidence that may impact the timing of regulatory authority applications for the initiation of clinical trials or approval for marketing. There should be frequent discussions within product development teams about which studies may be performed during the clinical trial phase of product development, guided by the regulatory strategy. Nonclinical researchers who have not been involved with research on a drug that is the subject of a clinical trial application may be unaware of the regulatory requirement to report to the FDA and other regulatory agencies, important safety findings from animal studies performed during the course of parallel clinical development. For example, in the U.S., a clinical research program may be put on "clinical hold" pending the investigation of unexpected deaths in large numbers of animals at doses that may be pertinent to the clinical dose even though the pharmacology or toxicology study was not intended to support the IND.

During this phase of development the regulatory strategy should focus on the near-term regulatory goals and milestones. For example, the most common regulatory goals are:

- Obtaining an established name (e.g., the USAN) and the INN
- Submission of a clinical trial notification application (e.g., an IND or CTX)

In the U.S., examples of important regulatory milestones in this phase include:

- Determination or confirmation of whether the product is regulated by the FDA
- Confirmation of which FDA division will review the IND application
- A pre-IND Meeting with the FDA
- A meeting with the FDA about designation under the Orphan Drug program
- Submission of a Drug Master File (DMF) describing the manufacture of a drug substance

Generally, an analysis of the regulatory environment is necessary for developing a regulatory strategy for this phase of development, however, an in-depth analysis of competitive intelligence may be less important. It will also be important to consider the advantages and disadvantages of specific regulatory submissions when preparing the regulatory strategy. The questions that could be asked that would have an impact on the regulatory strategy include the following examples:

- Is an IND needed for this product?
- Should more than one IND be submitted (for indications that are reviewed by different FDA division)?
- Does the company need a pre-IND meeting with the FDA?
- Is this the best time to apply for Orphan Drug designation?
- Is a DMF needed at this stage of development?
- In the absence of a USAN/INN, what will the company call the drug substance?
- Should the trade name (if available) be used for the drug product in the IND?
- Is there enough drug substance to prepare adequate quantities of clinical trial supplies that will meet the applicable Good Manufacturing Practice requirements for this stage of development?
- Are there sufficient data on the chemistry, characterization, quality control testing, and stability of the drug substance and drug product to meet the regulatory requirements and also to convince the reviewers that the clinical trial materials will be of good quality and raise no concerns about obvious physical or chemical safety hazards for the human subjects?
- Are the data from the pharmacology studies sufficient to provide a scientific rationale for the product to progress to clinical studies in humans?
- Are the pharmacological data relevant to a human disease or deficiency so that there is an established target population for the intended therapeutic use of the drug product?

- Is there enough information available from the animal studies to predict a dose and dose regimen that may be relatively safe (free of catastrophic, life-threatening, or disabling adverse effects) for first use in human subjects?
- Is there an investigator willing to perform a clinical study with this product?
- Does the company have access to properly qualified staff to monitor and perform the study?

An estimate of the time it may take to complete the major tasks that are required to meet the regulatory and/or product development goals may also be included in the regulatory strategy at this phase. Frequently, the timeline is of great interest to the senior management of organizations who are most likely to be interested in resource and cost management.

2.3.2   Regulatory Strategy during the Clinical Development Phase

During the clinical development phase, the nonclinical research study programs initiated in the preclinical development phase continue. Further characterizations of the drug substance and drug product occur during a study program generally referred to as pharmaceutical development. The manufacturing processes may be improved, scaled up, and the robustness of the manufacturing steps tested for consistency and reproducibility. Analytical test methods that are used for quality control and stability testing studies are tested for robustness, sensitivity, reproducibility, and transferability between laboratories, and if necessary, changed or improved. Additional analytical methods may be developed to monitor the key characteristics of the drug substance and drug product. Specifications and acceptance criteria are developed for the routine testing and quality control of the drug substance and drug product. In-process analytical data and end-of-process batch analysis data are collected for each batch of drug product and drug substance to enable a review of the consistency and reproducibility of the data. Stability studies are initiated and data collected to characterize the stability of the drug substance and drug product under a variety of storage conditions. The manufacturing processes and analytical quality control test methods that have been shown to consistently produce a high quality drug substance and drug product with a suitable shelf-life are selected for the manufacture and testing of the materials for the pivotal clinical research studies that will form the basis of the therapeutic claim for the marketing approval application.

Clinical research studies are performed to characterize the dose regimen, safety, and efficacy of the drug product in humans for one or more therapeutic indications. The design of the clinical studies has the goal of providing specific information in the following general areas (as described in the Note for Guidance on General Considerations for Clinical Trials, International Conference on Harmonization Topic E8; effective date in the U.S.: December, 1997):

2.3.2.1   Phase I

Phase I studies are typically human pharmacology studies conducted with either healthy volunteer subjects or patients involving one or a combination of the following objectives: estimation of initial safety and tolerability; determination of pharmacokinetics; assessment of pharmacodynamics; or early measurement of activity or potential therapeutic benefit. Open label, uncontrolled study designs are common. Statistical and other detailed analyses may be comprehensive, limited, or absent, depending upon the objectives and design of the study.

2.3.2.2   Phase II

Phase II studies usually have a primary objective of exploring therapeutic effectiveness in patients; exploratory analysis techniques may also be evaluated. A variety of uncontrolled or controlled study designs may be used. Subjects may be randomized to predetermined treatment groups and either blinded or open label designs may be used. Another important objective is to determine the dose and dose regimen for Phase III clinical studies. Additional objectives may include evaluation of potential study endpoints, characterization or comparison of therapeutic regimens, and collection of safety and efficacy data in different subject populations.

2.3.2.3   Phase III

The primary objectives of Phase III studies are selected to confirm the therapeutic effectiveness of the drug and to collect safety data in the intended indication and the intended patient population for the drug product for which marketing authorization will be sought. Phase III studies extend the knowledge gained from the Phase I and Phase II studies and provide for the treatment of subjects in much larger numbers than in the Phase I and Phase II studies. Studies are controlled to either provide a comparison with a subject's individual baseline data or a comparator product that may contain an active drug product or placebo may be used. Studies are designed to eliminate or minimize bias in the selection of patients for treatment, their evaluations, and the subsequent analysis of data. The treatment response variables and a comprehensive statistical analysis plan are determined prospectively before the study begins. Extensive data are collected according to predetermined schedules.

    The level of documentation and verification of the accuracy of data collected and analyzed increases progressively through each phase of clinical development. Representatives of the sponsor of the clinical investigations and/or staff from the compliance monitoring groups of regulatory agencies may audit the documents related to any clinical trial, although audits of Phase III and some Phase II trials are most frequent. Deficiencies in study designs, collection, and documentation of data, therapeutic or other patient care issues at the investigational sites, or significant deviations from regulatory reporting or compliance requirements may lead to substantial penalties during this phase of clinical research, sometimes causing substantial delays in approval or outright rejection of a marketing authorization application.

During this phase of development the regulatory strategy should focus on both the near-term and long-term regulatory goals and milestones. For example, some common regulatory goals are:

- To meet regulatory requirements for maintaining an effective and active clinical trial application by revision of information already submitted and the addition of new information pertinent to ongoing clinical investigations (IND amendments in the U.S. or variations in the E.U.)
- To maintain compliance with regulatory and quality requirements for studies, techniques, data management, and documentation (for example, expedited reporting of serious, unexpected adverse events, annual progress reports, compliance with Good Clinical Practice, Good Laboratory Practice, and Good Manufacturing Practice)
- To maintain the availability of clinical study materials (import or export applications may be needed in some countries)
- To identify and verify the regulatory authorities' requirements for approval of a marketing authorization application and launch of the product
- To identify and apply for consideration under special regulatory initiatives
- To seek regulatory practices and techniques that will shorten or enhance the preparation of the marketing authorization application and the regulatory authorities' review cycles

In the U.S., examples of important regulatory milestones during the clinical development phase include:

- Meetings with the FDA; for example:
  - End of Phase II Meeting(s)
  - Orphan Drug Designation meeting
  - Fast Track Development Program or Accelerated Approval meeting (if applicable)
  - Pre-NDA Meeting
  - Pre-Electronic Submission Guidance Meeting

- Submission of a Drug Master File (DMF) describing the manufacture of a drug substance or drug product
- Submission of completed sections of a "Rolling NDA"
- Preapproval inspections of manufacturing sites
- Submission of the paper or electronic NDA
- Payment of review fees
- Audits of clinical investigators' sites
- Drug Establishment Listing
- Application for an NDC code
- Provision of mock-ups of final labeling, advertising, and samples of the drug product

Ongoing and frequent analysis of the regulatory environment is necessary for developing a regulatory strategy for the clinical development phase because the impact of changes in regulatory requirements, new guidelines, or new interpretations by the regulatory agencies during clinical development can lead to costly changes in study designs, additional studies, or delays in completing clinical studies. An in-depth analysis of competitive intelligence is also important because the successes or failures of organizations with similar or competing products can also have wide ranging effects on clinical studies. It will also be important to consider or reconsider the advantages and disadvantages of specific regulatory submissions when preparing the regulatory strategy. The questions that are typically asked that may have an impact on the regulatory strategy and/or clinical development include the following examples:

- Does the organization need to have a legal corporate entity within each country where the marketing applications will be submitted or can a local representative be employed?
- Will one well-controlled clinical study be adequate for regulatory approval?
- Are the comparator products that were used in the pivotal Phase III registration studies available in each country where a marketing authorization application will be submitted?
- Does the therapeutic indication exist in each country where a marketing authorization application will be submitted?
- Will approval be sought for more than one therapeutic indication?
- Will approval be sought for more than one dose or dosage form?
- Where will applications be made for marketing approval?
- Will multinational applications be made nearly simultaneously or in staggered sequence?

- What is the projected review time for each stage of the process for each regulatory agency?
- What are the local regulatory requirements for each regulatory agency?

An estimate of the time it may take to complete the major tasks that are required to meet the regulatory goals will need to be included in the regulatory strategy at this phase. Data, information, or documents on the critical path to meet the regulatory goals should be identified and contingency plans put in place. The regulatory strategy should not focus on detailed tracking of completion of study reports, availability of specific data, document management issues, or any other topics that can be more effectively handled by project or functional management teams.

2.3.3 Regulatory Strategy for the Postapproval Phase

During the phase that follows the first approval for marketing, pharmaceutical product and clinical development may continue in a very active mode to provide data for revised labeling or line extensions to increase market share. Generally, new nonclinical information and data (primarily changes in the chemistry, manufacturing, quality control testing, and stability data but occasionally additional animal data) are submitted to the regulatory authorities to revise the original marketing application. Clinical studies that explore new indications, new doses, some new dosage forms, or involve new patient populations have the same characteristics as the Phase I, Phase II, and Phase III studies described previously in this chapter, and for regulatory strategy purposes are generally submitted to the regulatory authorities under the existing or new clinical trial applications. However, a Phase IV clinical study that is carried out under the conditions of the existing marketing approval (e.g., same dose, same dose regimen, same therapeutic indication, and same target population) may or may not need to be submitted to the regulatory authorities where the study will be performed, depending on the local regulatory requirements and the design and objectives of the study.

As the life cycle of the drug product reaches maturity, it is common for pharmaceutical product development and clinical research to be substantially scaled back or minimized. Typically, the routine activities for a product that has been marketed for some time include minor revisions of analytical methods, the submission of data on stability monitoring of representative batches, expedited reporting of unexpected, serious adverse events; periodic safety update reports to revise the data and analysis in the original marketing authorization application; and revision of product labeling. Annual progress reports and periodic renewals of product licenses may also be required in some countries.

The changing business environment may also require that other administrative types of regulatory submissions are made — for example, transfer of company ownership or responsibility for a product (as occurs with out-licensing agreements, company closures, or mergers), changes in the trade name of a product, and co-marketing agreements. Regulatory submissions are also required for changes in the legal status of a product (such a change from a prescription medicine to an over-the-counter medicine), product recalls, and product withdrawals from the market.

During this phase of development the scope of potential regulatory affairs activities and goals are so broad that a discussion of all of the possibilities is outside the scope of this chapter. However, a regulatory strategy for a marketed product should focus on the both near-term and longer-term regulatory submissions. The major goals and milestones of the regulatory strategy for a marketed product will be:

- To prepare and submit adequate data and information to permit line extensions

- To maintain compliant and active regulatory approvals for marketing

- To meet regulatory requirements for safety reporting, advertising and labeling, annual progress reports, periodic safety updates and renewals and

- To meet regulatory requirements for submissions for a change in the legal status of a product

The general concepts and steps involved in preparing a regulatory strategy for a new drug product are equally applicable to a marketed product although the details of the regulatory submissions and the analyses of the regulatory environment and competitive intelligence may be considerably different.

2.4   Conclusions

In summary, the regulatory strategy is a fundamental part of a pharmaceutical product development plan and the cornerstone upon which the other contributing parts of the plan must be based because of the requirement for regulatory approval for clinical testing and marketing for the majority of pharmaceutical products. A regulatory strategy must be a dynamic, reactive plan that is modified, perhaps frequently, during product development and throughout the life cycle of a drug product to take account of the growing body of knowledge about the product and to accommodate any changes in legislation and regulatory authority requirements for clinical trials and marketing. The tasks and data required to meet and maintain the goal of regulatory authority approval for marketing are defined within a regulatory strategy or its supporting documents. Analysis of the regulatory environment for a specific drug product and competitive intelligence information provides valuable background information for focusing the regulatory strategy on the most effective steps to achieve a competitive advantage in the marketing of a pharmaceutical product without undermining compliance with regulatory or quality requirements. A successful regulatory strategy is a skillfully designed plan that achieves the best possible outcomes for the marketing of a pharmaceutical product. Typically, a successful outcome involves a compromise with the regulatory authority that includes a rapid approval of the most beneficial or desirable product labeling with minimal restrictions, achieved with minimal delays during regulatory authority review.

3

What Is an IND?

Robert G. Pietrusko and Thomas Class

CONTENTS

1-58716-007-2/04/$0.00+$1.50
© 2004 by CRC Press LLC

3.1   What is an IND?

An Investigational New Drug Application (IND) is a submission to the U.S. Food and Drug Administration requesting permission to initiate a clinical study of a new drug product in the U.S. The Federal Food, Drug, and Cosmetic Act (the Act) requires that all drugs have an approved marketing application (NDA, BLA, ANDA) before they can be shipped in interstate commerce. From a legal perspective, the IND is a request for exemption from the Act's prohibition from introducing any new drug into interstate commerce without an approved application. The IND allows you to legally ship an unapproved drug or import the new drug from a foreign country.

In reality the IND is much more than a legal tool allowing a company to ship a drug. The IND application allows a company to initiate and conduct clinical studies of their new drug product. The IND application provides the FDA with the data necessary to decide whether the new drug and the proposed clinical trial pose a reasonable risk to the human subjects participating in the study. The Act directs the FDA to place investigations on *clinical hold* if the drug involved presents unreasonable risk to the safety of the subjects. The safety of the clinical trial subjects is always the primary concern of the FDA when reviewing an IND, regardless of the phase of the clinical investigation. In later phases (Phase II and III), the FDA will also evaluate the study design in terms of demonstrating efficacy, but safety of the subjects is critical throughout the drug development process. When preparing an IND, and throughout the drug development process, the primary goal of the sponsor should be to demonstrate to the FDA that the new drug, the proposed trial, and the entire clinical development plan described in the IND is designed to minimize risk to the trial subjects.

IND Term

Clinical Hold — an order issued by the FDA to the sponsor to delay a proposed clinical investigation or to suspend an ongoing investigation. Subjects may not be given the investigational drug or the hold may require that no new subjects be enrolled into an ongoing study. The clinical hold can be issued before the end of the 30-day IND review period to prevent a sponsor from initiating a proposed protocol or at any time during the life of an IND.

3.1.1   When Do I Need an IND?

Simply put, an IND is required any time you want to conduct a clinical trial of an unapproved drug in the U.S. However, what is actually considered a new or unapproved drug and how the act defines a drug often makes the decision about filing an IND more complicated. The Act defines a drug in part, as "articles intended for use in the diagnosis, cure, mitigation, treatment, or prevention of disease in man or other animals; and articles (other than food) intended to affect the structure or any function of the body of man or other animals."[1] The Act further defines a new drug, in part, as "any drug the composition of which is such that such drug is not generally recognized as safe and effective for use under the conditions prescribed, recommended, or suggested in the labeling."[2] Because of these legal definitions, an approved drug can be considered a new drug and require an IND to conduct a study. An IND would be required to conduct a clinical trial if the drug is:

- A new chemical entity
- Not approved for the indication under investigation
- In a new dosage form
- Being administered at a new dosage level
- In combination with another drug and the combination is not approved

A less obvious situation in which a clinical study must be conducted under the authority of an IND is when the chemical compound being used will not be developed for therapeutic use but is being used as a "clinical research tool." Sometimes these "tools" are administered to human subjects to elicit specific physiologic responses that are being studied. In this context, these compounds are considered drugs because the Act states that compounds intended to affect the structure or any function of the body of man or other animals are drugs. There is no exemption from the IND requirements in the Act or Regulations for studies conducted with compounds considered drugs that are not being developed for a therapeutic use. All clinical studies where a new drug is administered to human subjects, regardless of whether the drug will be commercially developed, require an IND.

---

[1] The Federal Food, Drug and Cosmetic Act Chapter II Section 201 (g)(1).
[2] The Federal Food, Drug and Cosmetic Act Chapter II Section 201 (p)(1).

3.1.2   When Don't I Need an IND?

An IND is not required to conduct a study if the drug:

- Is not intended for human subjects, but is intended for *in vitro* testing or laboratory research animals (nonclinical studies)
- Is an approved drug and the study is within its approved indication for use

The regulations also exempt studies of *approved* drugs if *all* of the following criteria are satisfied:[3]

- The study will not be reported to the FDA in support of a new indication or other change in labeling or advertising for the product.
- The study will not utilize a route of administration, dose level, or patient population that increases the risks associated with the use of the drug.
- The studies are to be conducted in compliance with IRB and informed consent regulations.
- The studies will not be used to promote unapproved indications.

The FDA will not accept an IND application for investigations that meet these exemption criteria.

The IND regulations also provide an exemption for studies that utilize placebos,[4] as long as the study would not otherwise require submission of an IND. The use of a placebo in a clinical study does not automatically necessitate an IND.

In April of 2002, the FDA published a draft guidance document clarifying under what circumstances an IND would not be required for the study of marketed cancer drugs.[5] The guidance specifically discusses how investigators assess increased risk to cancer patients when there is scientific literature or other clinical experience available to support the proposed uses. The guidance states that studies may be considered exempt from the IND requirements if the studies involve a new use, dosage, schedule, route of administration, or new combination of marketed cancer drugs in a patient population with cancer if the four exemption criteria for approved products listed above are met. They also clarified that as a basis for assessing whether there is an increased risk associated with the proposed use, the investigators and their IRBs must determine that, based on the scientific literature and generally known clinical experience, there is no significant increase in the risk associated with the use of the drug product.

---

[3] Code of Federal Regulations Title 21 Section 312.2.
[4] Code of Federal Regulations Title 21 Section 312.2 (b)(5).
[5] FDA Draft Guidance for Industry: IND Exemptions for Studies of Lawfully Marketed Cancer Drug or Biologic Products. FDA, Rockville, MD, April 2002.

The guidance also provides a clarification for drug manufacturers who provide approved cancer drugs to sponsor investigators for clinical study, providing an approved cancer drug for an investigator sponsored trial would not, in and of itself, be considered promotional activity on the part of the manufacturer if it is for a bona fide clinical investigation.

Whenever a sponsor or investigator considers conducting a clinical study, careful consideration should be given to the need for an IND. Companies should consult with their regulatory affairs staff to determine if an IND is required and investigators can consult with the *institutional review board* at their institution. If, after consultation, it is still unclear whether an IND is required, potential sponsors should contact the FDA for advice. Conducting a study without an IND when one is required can lead to regulatory action by the FDA.

IND Term

Institutional Review Board (IRB) — a board or committee formally designated by an institution to review and approve the initiation of biomedical research involving human subjects. The primary purpose of the IRB is to protect the rights and welfare of human subjects.

IND Facts

In 2002, the FDA received 2,374 Original INDs. Of these, 428 were commercial INDs and 1,946 were noncommercial INDs.[6] At the close of the 2002 calendar year there were 11,544 active INDs (4,158 commercial and 7,386 noncommercial).[7]

3.2   Pre-IND Meeting

A meeting between the sponsor and the FDA frequently is useful in resolving questions and issues raised during the preparation for an IND. The FDA encourages such meetings to the extent that they aid in the solution of scientific problems and to the extent that the FDA has available resources. To promote efficiency, all issues related to the submission of the IND should be included if practical since the FDA generally expects to grant only one pre-IND meeting. On occasion, when there are complex manufacturing

---

[6] Original INDs received calendar years 1986–2002. FDA website http://www.fda.gov/cder/rdmt/cyindrec.htm.

[7] Number of active INDs at the close of the calendar year (calendar years 1986–2002). FDA website http://www.fda.gov/cder/rdmt/cyactind.htm.

issues, a separate CMC meeting can be granted. Meetings at this stage regarding CMC information are often unnecessary when the project is straightforward. A pre-IND meeting is considered a Type B meeting. It is a "formal" meeting requiring a written request that includes, among other things, a list of specific objectives and outcomes, and a list of specific questions, grouped by discipline. Most issues and questions are usually related to the design of animal studies needed to initiate clinical trials as well as the scope and design of the initial study in humans. Type B meetings should be scheduled to occur within 60 days of the FDA's receipt of the written request for the meeting. A briefing document is required at least 4 weeks prior to the meeting. The briefing document should provide summary information relevant to the product and supplementary information that the FDA can use to provide responses to the questions that have been identified by the sponsor for the IND submission. There should be free, full, and open communication about the scientific or medical issue to be discussed during the meeting. The meeting may be a face-to-face meeting or the FDA may prefer to have a telephone conference call to serve as the meeting. Frequently, the FDA will have a pre-meeting to address the issues that have been raised and may provide initial feedback prior to the meeting. Usually the attendance at the pre-IND meeting is multidisciplinary, involving the FDA personnel in clinical, pharmacology/toxicology, biopharmaceutics, chemistry, statistics, microbiology, and other disciplines. At the conclusion of the meeting, there should be a review of all the issues, responses, and agreements. An assigned individual from the FDA, usually a project manager, will prepare the minutes of the meeting. In general, they should be available to the sponsor within 30 days after the meeting. It is most important that all issues and agreements be addressed in the IND submission. There are other meetings that can be held during the IND phases of development, including an End of Phase I meeting (generally for fast track products), an End of Phase II meeting, and a pre-NDA or pre-BLA meeting.

3.3   The Content and Format of an IND Application

The content and format of an initial IND is laid out in 21 CFR Part 312 and in two key guidance documents published by the FDA. This section outlines the required content and format of an initial IND based on the CFR requirements and the published guidance. The initial IND application to the FDA can be for a Phase I first-in-human study or it can be for a later-phase study where clinical studies of the compound have already been conducted in volunteers or patients. Although the basic content is the same, the expected level of detail is different. The information expected in later-phase studies is based on the phase of investigation, the amount of human experience with the drug, the drug substance, and the dosage form of the drug. In the outline, requirements for Phase I study INDs will be addressed as well as initial INDs for later stage studies. This section is not intended to be a recitation of CFR 312.23 or the guidance documents, but an overview of the key elements of the initial IND, regardless of the phase of the proposed study. We include the specific references to 312.23 for each of the sections of an IND.

3.3.1 Cover Sheet — *312.23(a)(1)* FDA Form 1571 — Investigational New Drug Application (IND)

The form 1571 (Figure 3.1) is a required part of the initial IND and every subsequent submission related to the IND application. Each *IND amendment, IND safety report, IND annual report,* or general correspondence with the FDA regarding the IND must include a 1571. The 1571 serves as a cover sheet for IND submissions and provides the FDA with basic information about the submission: name of the sponsor, IND number, name of the drug, type of submission, serial number, and the contents of the application. Each submission to the IND must be consecutively numbered, starting with the initial IND application which is numbered 0000. The next submission (response to clinical hold, correspondence, amendment, etc.) should be numbered 0001 with subsequent submissions numbered consecutively in the order they are submitted. It is important to note that the FDA expects every submission, even the most routine correspondence, to be submitted with a completed form 1571 and have a serial number. The FDA tracks all IND submissions based on serial numbers and will file them according to the serial number when received. This can lead to a situation where the FDA serial number for a submission does not match the sponsor's serial number, which can lead to confusion when referencing previous submissions to the IND file. If more than one group within a company submits IND amendments, for example a pharmacovigilance group may submit safety reports directly to the FDA, coordination of the serial numbers is essential.

The 1571 form provides a section for the sponsor to state whether a contract research organization (CRO) will conduct any parts of the study and if any sponsor obligations will be transferred to the CRO. If sponsor responsibilities will be transferred, a list of the obligations transferred and the name and address of the CRO must be attached to the 1571 form. Although the sponsor may transfer some of its obligations to a CRO, the sponsor of the IND is ultimately responsible for the conduct of the clinical investigation and the regulatory and legal requirements pertaining to a clinical trial.

When signing the 1571, the sponsor is also making three important commitments to the FDA, which are outlined on page two of the form.

1. The sponsor is committing not to initiate the clinical study until 30 days after the FDA receives the IND, unless otherwise notified by the FDA, and not to begin or continue clinical studies covered by the IND if they are placed on clinical hold.

DEPARTMENT OF HEALTH AND HUMAN SERVICES PUBLIC HEALTH SERVICE FOOD AND DRUG ADMINISTRATION **INVESTIGATIONAL NEW DRUG APPLICATION (IND)** *(TITLE 21, CODE OF FEDERAL REGULATIONS (CFR) PART 312)*	*Form Approved:* OMB No. 0910-0014. *Expiration Date: January 31, 2006* *See OMB Statement on Reverse.* **NOTE:** No drug may be shipped or clinical investigation begun until an IND for that investigation is in effect (21 CFR 312.40).

1. NAME OF SPONSOR	2. DATE OF SUBMISSION

3. ADDRESS *(Number, Street, City, State and Zip Code)*	4. TELEPHONE NUMBER *(Include Area Code)*

5. NAME(S) OF DRUG *(Include all available names: Trade, Generic, Chemical, Code)*	6. IND NUMBER *(If previously assigned)*

7. INDICATION(S) *(Covered by this submission)*

8. PHASE(S) OF CLINICAL INVESTIGATION TO BE CONDUCTED:
☐ PHASE 1   ☐ PHASE 2   ☐ PHASE 3   ☐ OTHER_____
(Specify)

9. LIST NUMBERS OF ALL INVESTIGATIONAL NEW DRUG APPLICATIONS (21 CFR Part 312), NEW DRUG OR ANTIBIOTIC APPLICATIONS *(21 CFR Part 314)*, DRUG MASTER FILES *(21 CFR Part 314.420)*, AND PRODUCT LICENSE APPLICATIONS (21 CFR Part 601) REFERRED TO IN THIS APPLICATION.

10. ***IND submission should be consecutively numbered. The initial IND should be numbered "Serial number: 0000." The next submission (e.g., amendment, report, or correspondence) should be numbered "Serial Number: 0001." Subsequent submissions should be numbered consecutively in the order in which they are submitted.***	SERIAL NUMBER _ _ _ _

11. THIS SUBMISSION CONTAINS THE FOLLOWING: *(Check all that apply)*
☐ INITIAL INVESTIGATIONAL NEW DRUG APPLICATION (IND)   ☐ RESPONSE TO CLINICAL HOLD

PROTOCOL AMENDMENT(S):	INFORMATION AMENDMENT(S):	IND SAFETY REPORT(S):
☐ NEW PROTOCOL	☐ CHEMISTRY/MICROBIOLOGY	☐ INITIAL WRITTEN REPORT
☐ CHANGE IN PROTOCOL	☐ PHARMACOLOGY/TOXICOLOGY	☐ FOLLOW-UP TO A WRITTEN REPORT
☐ NEW INVESTIGATOR	☐ CLINICAL	

☐ RESPONSE TO FDA REQUEST FOR INFORMATION   ☐ ANNUAL REPORT   ☐ GENERAL CORRESPONDENCE

☐ REQUEST FOR REINSTATEMENT OF IND THAT IS WITHDRAWN, INACTIVATED, TERMINATED OR DISCONTINUED   ☐ OTHER _____
(Specify)

CHECK ONLY IF APPLICABLE

JUSTIFICATION STATEMENT MUST BE SUBMITTED WITH APPLICATION FOR ANY CHECKED BELOW. REFER TO THE CITED CFR SECTION FOR FURTHER INFORMATION.

☐ TREATMENT IND 21 CFR 312.35(b)   ☐ TREATMENT PROTOCOL 21 CFR 312.35(a)   ☐ CHARGE REQUEST/NOTIFICATION 21 CFR 312.7(d)

FOR FDA USE ONLY

CDR/DBIND/DGD RECEIPT STAMP	DDR RECEIPT STAMP	DIVISION ASSIGNMENT:
		IND NUMBER ASSIGNED:

FORM FDA 1571 (1/03)   PREVIOUS EDITION IS OBSOLETE.   **PAGE 1 OF 2**

PSC Media Arts (301) 443-1090   EF

FIGURE 3.1
Form 1571.

---

12.   **CONTENTS OF APPLICATION**
                          This application contains the following items: *(Check all that apply)*

☐ 1. Form FDA 1571 *[21 CFR 312.23(a)(1)]*
☐ 2. Table of Contents *[21 CFR 312.23(a)(2)]*
☐ 3. Introductory statement *[21 CFR 312.23(a)(3)]*
☐ 4. General Investigational plan *[21 CFR 312.23(a)(3)]*
☐ 5. Investigator's brochure *[21 CFR 312.23(a)(5)]*
☐ 6. Protocol(s) *[21 CFR 312.23(a)(6)]*
    ☐ a. Study protocol(s) *[21 CFR 312.23(a)(6)]*
    ☐ b. Investigator data *[21 CFR 312.23(a)(6)(iii)(b)]* or completed Form(s) FDA 1572
    ☐ c. Facilities data *[21 CFR 312.23(a)(6)(iii)(b)]* or completed Form(s) FDA 1572
    ☐ d. Institutional Review Board data *[21 CFR 312.23(a)(6)(iii)(b)]* or completed Form(s) FDA 1572
☐ 7. Chemistry, manufacturing, and control data *[21 CFR 312.23(a)(7)]*
    ☐ Environmental assessment or claim for exclusion *[21 CFR 312.23(a)(7)(iv)(e)]*
☐ 8. Pharmacology and toxicology data *[21 CFR 312.23(a)(8)]*
☐ 9. Previous human experience *[21 CFR 312.23(a)(9)]*
☐ 10. Additional information *[21 CFR 312.23(a)(10)]*

---

13. IS ANY PART OF THE CLINICAL STUDY TO BE CONDUCTED BY A CONTRACT RESEARCH ORGANIZATION? ☐ YES ☐ NO

    IF YES, WILL ANY SPONSOR OBLIGATIONS BE TRANSFERRED TO THE CONTRACT RESEARCH ORGANIZATION? ☐ YES ☐ NO

    IF YES, ATTACH A STATEMENT CONTAINING THE NAME AND ADDRESS OF THE CONTRACT RESEARCH ORGANIZATION,
    IDENTIFICATION OF THE CLINICAL STUDY, AND A LISTING OF THE OBLIGATIONS TRANSFERRED.

---

14. NAME AND TITLE OF THE PERSON RESPONSIBLE FOR MONITORING THE CONDUCT AND PROGRESS OF THE CLINICAL
    INVESTIGATIONS

---

15. NAME(S) AND TITLE(S) OF THE PERSON(S) RESPONSIBLE FOR REVIEW AND EVALUATION OF INFORMATION RELEVANT TO THE
    SAFETY OF THE DRUG

I agree not to begin clinical investigations until 30 days after FDA's receipt of the IND unless I receive earlier notification by FDA that the studies may begin. I also agree not to begin or continue clinical investigations covered by the IND if those studies are placed on clinical hold. I agree that an Institutional Review Board (IRB) that complies with the requirements set fourth in 21 CFR Part 56 will be responsible for initial and continuing review and approval of each of the studies in the proposed clinical investigation. I agree to conduct the investigation in accordance with all other applicable regulatory requirements.

---

16. NAME OF SPONSOR OR SPONSOR'S AUTHORIZED REPRESENTATIVE	17. SIGNATURE OF SPONSOR OR SPONSOR'S AUTHORIZED REPRESENTATIVE	
18. ADDRESS *(Number, Street, City, State and Zip Code)*	19. TELEPHONE NUMBER *(Include Area Code)*	20. DATE

(**WARNING**: A willfully false statement is a criminal offense. U.S.C. Title 18, Sec. 1001.)

Public reporting burden for this collection of information is estimated to average 100 hours per response, including the time for reviewing instructions, searching existing data sources, gathering and maintaining the data needed, and completing reviewing the collection of information. Send comments regarding this burden estimate or any other aspect of this collection of information, including suggestions for reducing this burden to:

Food and Drug Administration	Food and Drug Administration	"An agency may not conduct or sponsor, and a
CBER (HFM-99)	CDER (HFD-94)	person is not required to respond to, a
1401 Rockville Pike	12229 Wilkins Avenue	collection of information unless it displays a
Rockville, MD 20852-1448	Rockville, MD 20852	currently valid OMB control number."

Please **DO NOT RETURN** this application to this address.

FORM FDA 1571 (1/03)   PAGE 2 OF 2

FIGURE 3.1
Form 1571 Continued.

2. The sponsor is committing to ensure that an IRB will be responsible for initial and continuing review and approval of each study in the proposed clinical investigation.

3. The sponsor is committing to conduct the investigation in accordance with all other applicable regulatory requirements.

These are significant commitments and the sponsor should be aware that signing the 1571 is more than a formality and that making a willfully false statement on the 1571 is a criminal offense. Detailed information on completing the 1571 form can be found on the FDA website,[8] in Section 312.23 (a)(1) and from the FDA review division responsible for reviewing the IND.

IND Term

IND Amendment — A submission to the IND file that adds new or revised information to the file. Every submission adds to, revises, or affects the body of information within the IND and is therefore considered an IND amendment. Protocol amendments and information amendments are two examples of information that is filed to an IND in the course of clinical development. A protocol amendment is submitted when a sponsor intends to conduct a new study, wishes to modify the design or conduct of a previously submitted study protocol, or adds a new investigator to a protocol. An information amendment is used to submit new CMC, toxicology, pharmacology, clinical or other information that does not fall within the scope of a protocol amendment, annual report or IND safety report.

IND Term

IND Safety Report — An expedited report to the FDA and all participating investigators of a serious and unexpected adverse experience associated with use of the drug or findings from nonclinical studies that suggest a risk to human subjects.

IND Term

IND Annual Report — A brief report to the FDA of the progress of the clinical investigations. It is submitted each year within 60 days of the anniversary date that the IND went into effect.

---

[8] FDA Center for Drug Evaluation and Research Information for Sponsor-Investigators Submitting Investigational New Drug Applications. FDA, Rockville, MD, March 8, 2001.

3.3.2 Table of Contents — *313.23(a)(2)*

This should be a comprehensive listing of the contents of the IND broken down by volume and page number. The TOC should include all required sections, appendices, attachments, reports, and other reference material. The TOC must be accurate and building the table should not be a last-minute task. An accurate, well laid out TOC will allow the FDA reviewers to quickly find the information they need and ultimately speed review of the IND application. Many sponsors begin planning the IND submission by laying out the table of contents first. This allows the team to clearly see what information is required for the submission and how the document will be structured and it allows the TOC to be updated as the application is being built.

3.3.3 Introductory Statement and General Investigational Plan — *312.23(a)(3)*

This section should provide a brief, three- to four-page overview of the investigational drug and the sponsor's investigational plan for the following year. The goal of this section is simply to provide a brief description of the drug and lay out the development plan for the drug.

For a Phase I first-in-person (FIP) IND, two to three pages may be sufficient if the sponsor is attempting to determine early pharmacokinetic and pharmacodynamic properties of the drug. The sponsor should not attempt to develop and present a detailed development plan that will, in all likelihood, change considerably should the product proceed to further development.[9]

The introductory statement should begin with a description of the drug and the indication(s) to be studied and include the pharmacologic class of the compound, the name of the drug and all active ingredients, the structural formula of the drug and the dosage form and route of administration. This section must also describe the sponsor's plan for investigating the drug during the following year and should include a rationale for the drug and the research study proposed, the general approach to be followed in studying the drug, the indication(s) to be studied, the type of clinical studies to be conducted, the estimated number of patients receiving the drug and any risks anticipated based on nonclinical studies or prior studies in humans.

If the drug has been previously administered to humans, the introductory statement should include a brief summary of human clinical experience to date, focusing mainly on safety of the drug in previous studies and how that supports studies proposed in the IND. If the drug was withdrawn from investigation or marketing in any country for safety reasons, the name of the country and the reasons for withdrawal should also be briefly discussed in the introductory statement.

---

[9] FDA Guidance for Industry: Content and Format of Investigational New Drug Applications (INDs) for Phase I Studies of Drugs, Including Well-Characterized, Therapeutic, Biotechnology Drugs. FDA, Rockville, MD, November 1995.

3.3.4   Investigator's Brochure — *312.23(a)(5)*

The content and format of the Investigator's Brochure (IB) is described in 21 CFR 312.23 (a)(5) and in greater detail in the ICH E6 Good Clinical Practice guidance document.[10] We do not present an exhaustive discussion of the IB here, preferring to focus more broadly on the purpose of the document and the general content required by the regulations.

The investigator's brochure is a key document provided to each clinical investigator and the institutional review board at each of the clinical sites. The IB presents, in summary form, the key nonclinical, clinical and *CMC* data that support the proposed clinical trial. The IB provides the clinical investigators with the information necessary to understand the rationale for the proposed trial and to make an unbiased risk–benefit assessment of the appropriateness of the proposed trial.[11]

IND Term

CMC — Stands for chemistry, manufacturing, and controls, describing the chemical structure and chemical properties of the compound, the composition, manufacturing process and control of the raw materials, drug substance, and drug product that ensure the identity, quality, purity, and potency of the drug product.

The type and extent of information provided in the IB will be dependent on the stage of development of the drug product but the IB must contain the following information:

1. A brief summary of CMC information including the physical, chemical, and pharmaceutical properties of the drug and the chemical name and chemical structure, if known. It should also include a description of the formulation and how the drug is supplied and the storage and handling requirements.

2. A summary of all relevant nonclinical pharmacology, toxicology, pharmacokinetic, and drug metabolism information generated to support human clinical studies. It should include a tabular summary of each nonclinical study conducted, outlining the methodology used and the results of each study.

3. If human clinical studies have been conducted with the drug, a summary of information relating to safety and effectiveness should be presented, including any information from those studies on the

---

[10] FDA Guidance for Industry: E6 Good Clinical Practice: Consolidated Guidance. FDA, Rockville, MD, April 1996.
[11] FDA Guidance for Industry: E6 Good Clinical Practice: Consolidated Guidance. FDA, Rockville, MD, April 1996.

metabolism, pharmacokinetics, pharmacodynamics, dose response, or other pharmacological activities.

4. A summary of data and guidance for the investigator in the management of subjects participating in the trial. An overall discussion of the nonclinical and clinical data presented in the IB and a discussion of the possible risks and adverse reactions associated with the investigational drug product, and the specific tests, observations, and precautions that may be needed for the clinical trial.

It is important to remember that the IB is a living document and must be updated by the sponsor as new information becomes available from ongoing clinical and nonclinical studies. At a minimum, the IB should be reviewed and updated annually. However, important safety information should be communicated to the investigator, the IRB, and the FDA, if required, before it is included in the IB.

3.3.5   Clinical Protocol — *312.23(a)(6)*

As with the IB, the content and format of the protocol is described in 21 CFR 312.23 and in greater detail in the ICH E6 Good Clinical Practice guidance document,[12] so we will not present an exhaustive discussion of the protocol here. We will focus more broadly on the general content required, based on the phase of the proposed trial.

A clinical protocol describes how a particular clinical trial is to be conducted. It describes the objectives of the study, the trial design, how subjects are selected and how the trial is to be carried out. The initial IND is required to have a clinical protocol for each planned study. However, the IND regulations specifically allow Phase I protocols to be less detailed and more flexible than protocols for Phase II or III studies.[13] The regulations state that Phase I protocols should be directed primarily at providing an outline of the investigation: an estimate of the number of subjects to be included; a description of safety exclusions; and a description of the dosing plan, including duration, dose, or method to be used in determining dose. Phase I protocols should specify in detail only those elements for the study that are critical to subject safety, such as necessary monitoring of vital signs and blood chemistries, and toxicity-based stopping or dose adjustment rules.[14]

Although the regulations allow Phase I protocols to be less detailed, the sponsor can not submit a protocol summary in lieu of a complete protocol

---

[12] FDA Guidance for Industry: E6 Good Clinical Practice: Consolidated Guidance. FDA, Rockville, MD, April 1996.

[13] FDA Guidance for Industry: Content and Format of Investigational New Drug Applications (INDs) for Phase I Studies of Drugs, Including Well-Characterized, Therapeutic, Biotechnology Drugs. FDA, Rockville, MD, November 1995.

[14] FDA Guidance for Industry: Content and Format of Investigational New Drug Applications (INDs) for Phase I Studies of Drugs, Including Well-Characterized, Therapeutic, Biotechnology Drugs. FDA, Rockville, MD, November 1995.

as part of the initial IND. Although a protocol summary may be acceptable in some instances, submission of a summary should be discussed and agreed to by the reviewing division at the FDA during the pre-IND meeting. Later-phase protocols should be more detailed than a Phase I protocol and contain efficacy parameters, the methods and timing for assessing and analyzing the efficacy parameters, and detailed statistical sections describing the statistical methods to be employed and the timing of any planned interim analysis.

The regulations require any protocol submitted as part of an IND to contain the following elements.

1. A statement of the objectives and the purpose of the study.

2. Name, address, and qualifications (*curriculum vitae*) of each investigator and each subinvestigator participating in the study; the name and address of each clinical site; and the name and address of each institutional review board responsible for reviewing the proposed study. The required information regarding all investigators is collected on the FDA form 1572 Statement of Investigator (Figure 3.2). The 1572 form collects basic information about the investigator such as the name and address of the investigator, a description of the education and training of the investigator (a copy of the investigator's CV is usually attached), the name and address of the IRB at the site and the names of any sub-investigators at the site. For Phase II or Phase III studies, copies of the case report forms should be included with the 1572. The 1572 includes a series of commitments (see Box 9 in Figure 3.2) that the investigator agrees to by signing the form. These commitments include, among others, agreeing to conduct the study according to the protocol, agreeing to personally conduct or supervise the investigation, agreeing to report adverse events to the sponsor, and agreeing to maintain accurate records and agreeing to comply with all other obligations and requirements outlined in the regulations. Investigators and sponsors should be aware that making willfully false statements on the 1572 is a criminal offense.

3. Study subject inclusion and exclusion criteria and an estimate of the number of subjects to be enrolled in the study.

4. A description of the study design, control groups to be used, and a description of methods employed to minimize bias on the part of the subjects, investigators, and analysts.

5. The planned maximum dose, the duration of patient exposure to the drug, and the methods used to determine the doses to be administered.

6. A description of the measurements and observations to be made to achieve the study objectives.

7. A description of the clinical procedures and laboratory tests planned to monitor the effects of the drug in the subjects.

DEPARTMENT OF HEALTH AND HUMAN SERVICES PUBLIC HEALTH SERVICE FOOD AND DRUG ADMINISTRATION **STATEMENT OF INVESTIGATOR** ***(TITLE 21, CODE OF FEDERAL REGULATIONS (CFR) PART 312)*** (See instructions on reverse side.)	Form Approved: OMB No. 0910-0014. Expiration Date: January 31, 2006. *See OMB Statement on Reverse.*
	NOTE: No investigator may participate in an investigation until he/she provides the sponsor with a completed, signed Statement of Investigator, Form FDA 1572 (21 CFR 312.53(c)).

1. NAME AND ADDRESS OF INVESTIGATOR

2. EDUCATION, TRAINING, AND EXPERIENCE THAT QUALIFIES THE INVESTIGATOR AS AN EXPERT IN THE CLINICAL INVESTIGATION OF THE DRUG FOR THE USE UNDER INVESTIGATION. ONE OF THE FOLLOWING IS ATTACHED.

☐ CURRICULUM VITAE   ☐ OTHER STATEMENT OF QUALIFICATIONS

3. NAME AND ADDRESS OF ANY MEDICAL SCHOOL, HOSPITAL OR OTHER RESEARCH FACILITY WHERE THE CLINICAL INVESTIGATION(S) WILL BE CONDUCTED.

4. NAME AND ADDRESS OF ANY CLINICAL LABORATORY FACILITIES TO BE USED IN THE STUDY.

5. NAME AND ADDRESS OF THE INSTITUTIONAL REVIEW BOARD (IRB) THAT IS RESPONSIBLE FOR REVIEW AND APPROVAL OF THE STUDY(IES).

6. NAMES OF THE SUBINVESTIGATORS *(e.g., research fellows, residents, associates)* WHO WILL BE ASSISTING THE INVESTIGATOR IN THE CONDUCT OF THE INVESTIGATION(S).

7. NAME AND CODE NUMBER, IF ANY, OF THE PROTOCOL(S) IN THE IND FOR THE STUDY(IES) TO BE CONDUCTED BY THE INVESTIGATOR.

FORM FDA 1572 (1/03)   PREVIOUS EDITION IS OBSOLETE.   PAGE 1 OF 2

PSC Media Arts (301) 443-1090   EF

FIGURE 3.2
Form 1572.

8. ATTACH THE FOLLOWING CLINICAL PROTOCOL INFORMATION:

☐ FOR PHASE 1 INVESTIGATIONS, A GENERAL OUTLINE OF THE PLANNED INVESTIGATION INCLUDING THE ESTIMATED DURATION OF THE STUDY AND THE MAXIMUM NUMBER OF SUBJECTS THAT WILL BE INVOLVED.

☐ FOR PHASE 2 OR 3 INVESTIGATIONS, AN OUTLINE OF THE STUDY PROTOCOL INCLUDING AN APPROXIMATION OF THE NUMBER OF SUBJECTS TO BE TREATED WITH THE DRUG AND THE NUMBER TO BE EMPLOYED AS CONTROLS, IF ANY; THE CLINICAL USES TO BE INVESTIGATED; CHARACTERISTICS OF SUBJECTS BY AGE, SEX, AND CONDITION; THE KIND OF CLINICAL OBSERVATIONS AND LABORATORY TESTS TO BE CONDUCTED; THE ESTIMATED DURATION OF THE STUDY; AND COPIES OR A DESCRIPTION OF CASE REPORT FORMS TO BE USED.

9. COMMITMENTS:

I agree to conduct the study(ies) in accordance with the relevant, current protocol(s) and will only make changes in a protocol after notifying the sponsor, except when necessary to protect the safety, rights, or welfare of subjects.

I agree to personally conduct or supervise the described investigation(s).

I agree to inform any patients, or any persons used as controls, that the drugs are being used for investigational purposes and I will ensure that the requirements relating to obtaining informed consent in 21 CFR Part 50 and institutional review board (IRB) review and approval in 21 CFR Part 56 are met.

I agree to report to the sponsor adverse experiences that occur in the course of the investigation(s) in accordance with 21 CFR 312.64.

I have read and understand the information in the investigator's brochure, including the potential risks and side effects of the drug.

I agree to ensure that all associates, colleagues, and employees assisting in the conduct of the study(ies) are informed about their obligations in meeting the above commitments.

I agree to maintain adequate and accurate records in accordance with 21 CFR 312.62 and to make those records available for inspection in accordance with 21 CFR 312.68.

I will ensure that an IRB that complies with the requirements of 21 CFR Part 56 will be responsible for the initial and continuing review and approval of the clinical investigation. I also agree to promptly report to the IRB all changes in the research activity and all unanticipated problems involving risks to human subjects or others. Additionally, I will not make any changes in the research without IRB approval, except where necessary to eliminate apparent immediate hazards to human subjects.

I agree to comply with all other requirements regarding the obligations of clinical investigators and all other pertinent requirements in 21 CFR Part 312.

INSTRUCTIONS FOR COMPLETING FORM FDA 1572
STATEMENT OF INVESTIGATOR:

1. Complete all sections. Attach a separate page if additional space is needed.

2. Attach curriculum vitae or other statement of qualifications as described in Section 2.

3. Attach protocol outline as described in Section 8.

4. Sign and date below.

5. FORWARD THE COMPLETED FORM AND ATTACHMENTS TO THE SPONSOR. The sponsor will incorporate this information along with other technical data into an Investigational New Drug Application (IND).

10. SIGNATURE OF INVESTIGATOR	11. DATE

(**WARNING:** A willfully false statement is a criminal offense. U.S.C. Title 18, Sec. 1001.)

Public reporting burden for this collection of information is estimated to average 100 hours per response, including the time for reviewing instructions, searching existing data sources, gathering and maintaining the data needed, and completing reviewing the collection of information. Send comments regarding this burden estimate or any other aspect of this collection of information, including suggestions for reducing this burden to:

Food and Drug Administration	Food and Drug Administration	"An agency may not conduct or sponsor, and a
CBER (HFM-99)	CDER (HFD-94)	person is not required to respond to, a
1401 Rockville Pike	12229 Wilkins Avenue	collection of information unless it displays a
Rockville, MD 20852-1448	Rockville, MD 20852	currently valid OMB control number."

Please **DO NOT RETURN** this application to this address.

FORM FDA 1572 (1/03)   PAGE 2 OF 2

FIGURE 3.2
Form 1572 Continued.

3.3.6 Chemistry Manufacturing and Controls Information — *312.23(a)(7)*

This key section of an IND describes the composition, manufacturing process, and control of the drug substance and drug product. The CMC section must provide sufficient detail and information to demonstrate the identity, quality, purity, and potency of the drug product. The amount of information needed to accomplish this is based on the phase of the proposed study, the duration of the study, the dosage form of the investigational drug, and the amount of additional information available.[15] For a Phase I IND the CMC information provided for the raw materials, drug substance, and drug product should be sufficiently detailed to allow the FDA to evaluate the safety of the subjects participating in the trial. A safety concern or a lack of data making it impossible for the FDA to conduct a safety evaluation are the only reasons for a clinical hold based on the CMC section. Safety concerns may include:

1. Product made with unknown or impure components.
2. Product has a chemical structure(s) of known or highly likely toxicity.
3. Product does not remain chemically stable throughout the testing program.
4. Product has an impurity profile indicative of a potential health hazard or an impurity profile insufficiently defined to assess potential health hazard.
5. A poorly characterized master or working cell bank.[16]

A key aspect to assuring the safety of the subjects participating in clinical trials is adherence to current good manufacturing practices (cGMP). The FDA requires that any drug product intended for administration to humans be manufactured in conformance with cGMP. Adherence to GMP provides a minimum level of control over the manufacturing process and final drug product and helps to ensure the identity, quality, purity, and potency of the clinical trial material. The GMP controls used to manufacture drug products for clinical trials should be consistent with the stage of development and they should be manufactured in suitable facilities using appropriate production and control procedures to ensure the quality of the drug product.[17]

---

[15] FDA Guidance for Industry: Content and Format of Investigational New Drug Applications (INDs) for Phase I Studies of Drugs, Including Well-Characterized, Therapeutic, Biotechnology Drugs. FDA, Rockville, MD, November 1995.

[16] FDA Guidance for Industry: Content and Format of Investigational New Drug Applications (INDs) for Phase I Studies of Drugs, Including Well-Characterized, Therapeutic, Biotechnology drugs. FDA, Rockville, MD November 1995.

[17] FDA Guidance for Industry: Q7A Good Manufacturing Practice Guidance for Active Pharmaceutical Ingredients. FDA, Rockville, MD, August 2001.

INDs for later phase studies must contain the CMC information outlined in 312.23 but the focus should be on safety issues relating to the proposed phase and expanded scope of the investigation. The FDA will expect that the CMC section for a later phase IND will be more detailed than a Phase I IND and demonstrate a higher level of characterization of the drug substance and drug product and greater control over the raw materials and manufacturing process. For Phase II studies, the sponsor should be able to document that the manufacturing process is controlled at predetermined points and yields a product meeting tentative acceptance criteria.[18]

The regulations require the CMC section of an IND to contain the following sections.

1. CMC Introduction

   This section should provide a brief overview of the investigational drug product. In this section the sponsor should state whether there are any signals of potential risk to human subjects because of the chemistry of the drug substance or drug product or the manufacturing process for the drug substance or drug product. If potential risks are identified, the risks should be discussed, steps to monitor the risks should be described, or the reasons the potential risks are acceptable should be presented. In the introduction the sponsor should also describe any differences between the drug product to be used in the proposed study and the drug product used in the nonclinical toxicology studies that support the clinical investigations. How these differences affect the safety profile should be discussed and if there are no differences, that should be stated.

2. Information on the drug substance in the form of a summary report containing the following information:

   • A brief description of the drug substance and evidence to support its chemical structure. INDs for later phase trials should include a more complete description of the physical, chemical, and biological characteristics of the drug substance and provide additional supporting evidence characterizing the chemical structure.

   • The name and address of the manufacturer.

   • A brief description of the manufacturing process. The description should include a detailed flow diagram of the process and a list of all the reagents, solvents, and catalysts used in the process. INDs for later phase trials will include a more detailed description of the manufacturing process and the controls. A process flow diagram that includes chemical structures and configurations, and significant side products should be included, and acceptance criteria for the product should be described.

---

[18] FDA Guidance for Industry: INDs for Phase 2 and Phase 3 Studies. Chemistry, Manufacturing and Controls Information. FDA, Rockville, MD, May 2003.

- A brief description of the acceptable limits (specifications) and ana-lytical methods used to assure the identity, strength, quality, potency, and purity of the drug substance. This section should include a description of the test methods used and outline the proposed accep-tance criteria. The proposed acceptance criteria should be based on analytical data (e.g., IR spectrum to prove identity and HPLC chro-matograms to support purity level and impurities profile).[19] Valida-tion data and established specifications are not required for Phase I studies; however, a certificate of analysis for the lot(s) of clinical trial material should be included with the initial IND. Initial INDs for later phase studies should provide the same type of information as for earlier phase studies but analytical procedures and acceptance criteria should be better defined and validation data should be avail-able if requested by theFDA.

- Data to support the stability of the drug substance. For a Phase I IND, a brief description of the stability studies conducted and the methods used to monitor stability should be provided, including a table outlining stability data from representative lots of material. For later phase studies, a stability protocol should be submitted includ-ing a list of all tests, analytical procedures, sampling time points for each test, and the duration of the stability studies. Preliminary sta-bility data should be submitted along with stability data from clinical material used in earlier phase studies.

3. Information on the drug product in the form of a summary report containing the following information.

- A list of usually no more than two or three pages of all components used in the manufacture of the drug product, including components intended to be in the drug product and those that may not appear, but are used in the manufacturing process. The components should be identified by their established name (chemical name) and their compendial status (NF, USP) should be listed, if it exists. Analytical procedures and acceptance criteria should be presented for noncom-pendial components. If applicable, the quantitative composition of the drug product should be summarized and any expected varia-tions should be discussed. The same type of information should be presented in an IND for a phase later phase study.

- The name and address of the manufacturer of the drug product.

- A brief, step-by-step description of the manufacturing and packag-ing procedures including a process flow diagram. For sterile prod-ucts, a description of the sterilization process should be included.

---

[19] FDA Guidance for Industry: Content and Format of Investigational New Drug Applications (INDs) for Phase I Studies of Drugs, Including Well-Characterized, Therapeutic, Biotechnology Drugs. FDA, Rockville, MD, November 1995.

The same type of information should be included in an IND for a later phase study.

- A description of the proposed acceptable limits (specifications) for the drug product and the test methods used. Validation data and established specifications are not required in the Phase I IND; however, a complete description of the analytical procedures and validation data should be available on request for later phase studies. For sterile products, sterility and endotoxin tests should be submitted in the initial IND. A certificate of analysis for the drug product lot(s) to be used in the proposed investigation should also be provided.

- A description of the proposed container closure system and a brief description of the stability study and test methods. Stability data on representative material should be presented in a tabular format. A copy of the stability protocol is not required for a Phase I study. An initial IND for a later phase study should include a copy of the stability protocol that includes a list of tests, analytical procedures, sampling time points and the expected duration of the stability program. When applicable, stability data on the reconstituted drug product should be included in the initial IND.

4. Information on any placebo that will be utilized in the proposed clinical study. This should include a brief written description of the composition, manufacture, and control of the placebo. Process flow diagrams and tabular summaries can be utilized in the description.

5. Copies of all proposed product labels and any other proposed labeling that will be provided to the investigators. Mock-ups of the proposed labeling are acceptable or actual printed labeling can be submitted. The investigational drug must be labeled with the caution statement: "Caution: New Drug — Limited by Federal (or U.S.) law to investigational use."[20]

6. A claim for categorical exclusion from an environmental assessment. The National Environmental Policy Act of 1969 (NEPA) requires all federal agencies to assess the environmental impacts of their actions and to ensure that the interested and affected public is informed of environmental analyses.[21] The FDA is required to consider the environmental impacts of approving drug and biologic applications and requires all such applications to include an environmental assessment or a claim for categorical exclusion. IND applications are categorically excluded from the requirement to prepare and submit an environmental assessment.[22] In this section of the IND the sponsor

---

[20] Code of Federal Regulations Title 21 Section 312.6(a).

[21] FDA Guidance for Industry: Environmental Assessment of Human Drug and Biologics Applications. FDA, Rockville, MD, July 1998.

[22] Code of Federal Regulations Title 21 Section 25.31(e).

should state that the action requested (approval of an IND application) qualifies for categorical exclusion in accordance with 21 CFR 25.31(e) and that to the sponsor's knowledge, no extraordinary circumstances exist (21 CFR 25.15(d)).

3.3.7 Pharmacology and Toxicology Information — *312.23(a)(8)*

The decision to proceed to the initial administration of the investigational drug to humans must include the careful conduct and review of the data from nonclinical *in vivo* and *in vitro* studies. These data must provide a good level of confidence that the new drug product is reasonably safe for administration to human subjects at the planned dosage levels. The goals of the nonclinical safety testing include: characterization of toxic effects with respect to target organs, dose dependence, relationship to exposure and potential reversibility.[23] Nonclinical safety information is important for the estimation of an initial safe starting dose for human trials and the identification of parameters for clinical monitoring for potential adverse events.[24]

The pharmacology and toxicology section of the IND includes the nonclinical safety data that the sponsor generated to conclude that the new drug is reasonably safe for clinical study. The amount and type of nonclinical data needed to support a new drug product depends on the class of the new drug, the duration of the proposed clinical trials and the patient population that will be exposed to the drug. Generally, the following nonclinical safety studies are required before initiating Phase I studies and the results of these studies must be included in the IND:

- Safety pharmacology studies (often conducted as part of the toxicity studies).
- Single dose and repeat dose toxicity studies (duration of the repeat dose studies should equal or exceed the duration human clinical trials).
- Genotoxicity studies (*in vitro* studies evaluating mutations and chromosomal damage).
- Reproduction toxicity studies (nonclinical animal studies conducted to reveal any effects the investigational drug may have on mammalian reproduction).
- Other supplementary studies may be needed if safety concerns are identified.

---

[23] FDA Guidance for Industry: M3 Nonclinical Safety Studies for the Conduct of Human Clinical Trials for Pharmaceuticals. FDA, Rockville, MD, July 1997.
[24] FDA Guidance for Industry: M3 Nonclinical Safety Studies for the Conduct of Human Clinical Trials for Pharmaceuticals. FDA, Rockville, MD, July 1997.

The CDER Guidance Documents Webpage[25] provides access to all of the key guidance documents discussing required nonclinical testing for new drugs.

The Pharmacology and Toxicology Information section of the initial IND should contain the following sections.

1. A summary report of five pages or less, describing the pharmacologic effects and mechanism of action of the drug and information on the absorption, distribution, metabolism, and excretion (ADME) of the drug. If this information is not known at the time the initial IND is submitted, it should be stated. Lack of this information should not generally be a reason for a Phase I IND to be placed on clinical hold.[26] However, most sponsors will have at least early pharmacologic data including exposure, half life of the drug, and an understanding of the major factors that influence the pharmacokinetics of the drug, e.g., the enzymes responsible for metabolism of the drug. Initial INDs for later-phase studies should be able to provide this pharmacology information, and it may be derived from earlier phase clinical investigations.

2. An integrated summary of the toxicologic effects of the drug in animals and *in vitro*. The summary presents the toxicologic findings from completed animal studies that support the safety of the proposed human investigation. The integrated summary is usually 10 to 20 pages in length, includes text and tables, and should contain the following information:

   - A brief description of the design of the trials and any deviations from the design in the conduct of the studies including the dates the studies were conducted.

   - A systematic presentation of the findings from the animal toxicology and toxicokinetic studies. This data should be presented by organ system (e.g., cardiovascular, renal, hepatic, etc.) and if a particular body system was not assessed, it should be noted.

   - The names and qualifications of the individuals who evaluated the animal safety data and concluded that it is reasonably safe to begin the proposed human studies.

   - A statement of where the studies were conducted and where the study records are stored and available for inspection.

   - A declaration that each nonclinical safety study reported in the IND was performed in full compliance with *good laboratory prac-*

---

[25] FDA Center for Drug Evaluation and Research Guidance Documents Web Page: http://www.fda.gov/cder/guidance/index.htm

[26] FDA Guidance for Industry: Content and Format of Investigational New Drug Applications (INDs) for Phase I Studies of Drugs, Including Well-Characterized, Therapeutic, Biotechnology Drugs. FDA, Rockville, MD, November 1995.

tices (GLP) or if a study was not conducted in compliance with GLP, a brief statement of why it was not and a discussion on how this might affect the interpretations of the findings.

The integrated summary can be developed based on unaudited draft toxicology reports of the completed animal studies. Final, fully quality-assured individual study reports are not required for submission of an initial IND. If the integrated summary is based on unaudited draft reports, the toxicology reports should be finalized and an update to the summary submitted to the FDA by 120 days after submission of the original integrated summary.[27] The updated summary, as well as the final study reports, should identify any differences found in the preparation of the final, fully quality-assured study reports and the information submitted in the initial integrated summary. If there were no differences found, that should be stated in the update. Although not required, many sponsors submit copies of the final toxicology reports at the time of the 120-day update. If the sponsor does not submit the reports at this time, they must be available to the FDA, upon request, by the 120-day time-frame and in any case, submitted with the NDA.

3. Full data tabulations for each animal toxicology study supporting the safety of the proposed trial. This should be a full tabulation of the data suitable for detailed review and consists of line listings of individual data points, including laboratory data for each animal in the trials and summary tabulations of the data points. This section will also include either a brief technical report or abstract for each study or a copy of the study protocol and amendments. These are provided to help the FDA reviewer interpret the data included in the line listings. Many sponsors will include copies of the final toxicology study reports in this section in lieu of the technical report or protocol. However, this is not required and submission of the initial IND does not need to be delayed until final, full quality-assured study reports are available.

IND Term

Good Laboratory Practice (GLP) — A quality system, that applies to the conduct of nonclinical safety studies used to support an IND, NDA, ANDA, or other regulatory submission. GLP regulations set standards for the organization of the laboratory, facilities, personnel,

---

[27] FDA Guidance for Industry Q&A: Content and Format of INDs from Phase 1 Studies of Drugs, Including Well-Characterized, Therapeutic, Biotechnology-Derived Products. FDA, Rockville, MD, October 2000.

and operating procedures. Clinical studies with human subjects, basic exploratory studies to determine potential utility of a compound, or tests to determine the chemical or physical characteristics of a compound are not subject to GLP regulations.

3.3.8   Previous Human Experience — *312.23 (a)(9)*

This section should contain an integrated summary report of all previous human studies and experiences with the drug. When the planned study will be the first administration to humans, this section should be indicated as not applicable. However, if initial clinical investigations have been conducted in other countries before the U.S. IND is filed, this section could be extensive. The summary should focus on presenting data from previous trials that are relevant to the safety of the proposed investigation (e.g., PK and PD data, the observed adverse event profile in previous studies, or other experiences, ADME data, etc.) and any information from previous trials on the drugs effectiveness for the proposed investigational use. Any published material relevant to the safety of the proposed investigation or assessment of the drug's effectiveness in the proposed indication should be provided in the IND. Other published material may be listed in a bibliography.

If the drug is marketed outside of the U.S., or was previously, a list of those countries should be provided as well as a list of any countries where the drug was withdrawn from marketing because of safety or effectiveness issues.

3.3.9   Additional Information — *312.23(a)(10)*

This section is used to present information on special topics. The following topics should be discussed, if relevant, in this section:

1. Drug dependence and abuse potential. If the drug is psychotropic or otherwise shows potential for abuse, data from clinical studies or animal studies that may be relevant to assessment of the investigational drug.
2. Radioactive drugs. Data from animal or human studies that allow calculation of radiation-absorbed dose to the whole body and critical organs upon administration to human subjects.
3. Pediatric studies. Any plans the sponsor has for assessing the safety and effectiveness of the drug in the pediatric population.
4. Other information. Any other relevant information that might aid in the evaluation of the proposed clinical investigations.

3.3.10   Relevant Information — *312.23(a)(11)*

- Any information specifically requested by the FDA that is needed to review the IND application.

3.3.11   Other Important Information about the Format, Content and Submission of an IND

- For clinical studies that will be submitted as part of an NDA or BLA, IND sponsors must collect *financial disclosure* information from each investigator or subinvestigator who is directly involved in the treatment or evaluation of clinical trial subjects. Each investigator or subinvestigator must supply sufficient and accurate financial information that will allow the sponsor to eventually submit certification or disclosure statements in an NDA or BLA. Each investigator or subinvestigator must commit to update this information if any changes occur during the course of the investigation and for one year following completion of the study. Most phase 1 studies, large, open safety studies conducted at multiple sites; treatment protocols; and parallel track protocols are exempted from financial disclosure requirements.[28,29,30]

- Although not a required component of an IND, some FDA review divisions may ask the sponsor to submit a copy of the informed consent form for the study.

- Within the IND application a sponsor may include references to other information pertinent to the IND that may have been previously submitted to the FDA, for instance in another IND or in a marketing application. Another IND might be referenced if the sponsor is submitting a treatment use protocol that references the technical sections of an open IND for the same drug, or a sponsor might be conducting a clinical study of an approved drug but for a new indication. In this instance the sponsor may reference the nonclinical and CMC sections of the NDA instead of submitting the same information in a new IND.

- The sponsor may also reference a *drug master file* (DMF) in the IND application that contains important information necessary to complete review of the IND. A DMF might contain proprietary information about a unique excipient or specialized drug delivery device that the manufacturer does not want to share with the sponsor of the IND. In this case the manufacturer will submit a DMF to the

---

[28] Code of Federal Regulations Title 21 Section 312.53(c)(4).
[29] Code of Federal Regulations Title 21 Part 54–Financial Disclosure By Clinical Investigators.
[30] FDA Guidance for Industry: Financial Disclosure By Clinical Investigators. FDA, Rockville, MD, March 20, 2001.

FDA and allow the sponsor to reference it in the IND. Reference to any DMF or other information submitted by an entity other than the sponsor must include a letter authorizing the sponsor to make the reference and giving the FDA permission to review the DMF in support of the IND.

IND Term

Financial Disclosure — When submitting a marketing application for a drug, device, or biologic product, the applicant is required to include a list of all clinical investigators who conducted clinical studies and certify and/or disclose certain financial arrangements that include: certification that no financial arrangements with an investigator have been made where study outcome could affect compensation; that the investigator has no proprietary interest in the product; that the investigator does not have significant equity interest in the sponsor; and that the investigator has not received significant payments of other sorts; and/or disclose specified financial arrangements and any steps taken to minimize the potential for bias. By collecting the financial disclosure information at the start of a study, the sponsor will be aware of potential conflicts and will be able to consult with the FDA early on, and take steps to minimize the potential for bias.

Drug Master File

A Drug Master File (DMF) is a submission to the FDA that is used to provide confidential detailed information about processes or articles used in the manufacturing, processing, packaging, and storing of one or more human drugs. The information contained in the DMF may be used to support an Investigational New Drug Application (IND), a New Drug Application (NDA), an Abbreviated New Drug Application (ANDA), another DMF, an Export Application, or amendments and supplements to any of these.

- Reports or journal articles in a foreign language must be accompanied by a complete and accurate English translation.
- Each IND submission must include a four-digit serial number. The initial IND must be numbered 0000 and each subsequent submission (correspondence, amendment, and safety report) must be numbered chronologically in sequence. This serial number is included on the

1571 form, any cover letter included with the submission, and on any labels affixed to the binders containing submission.

- The FDA requires sponsors to submit the original and two copies of all IND submissions, including the initial IND application and any amendments, correspondence, or reports. The FDA can request that a sponsor submit additional copies of a particular submission at any time.

- The initial IND and all subsequent submissions more than one page in length should be fully paginated, including all appendices and attachments.

- All IND submissions should be printed on good quality $8^1/_2 \times 11$ inch paper with a $1^1/_4$ inch left margin to allow for binding. Individual volumes should be no more than approximately 2 inches thick and bound in pressboard type binders. Three-ring binders are generally not used. The FDA requires the following types of binders for specific sections of IND submissions:
  - One copy of the submission will serve as an archive copy and should be bound in a red polyethylene binder.
  - The CMC section should be bound in a green pressboard binder.
  - Microbiology information should be bound in an orange press board binder.

- Each volume should be labeled with permanent adhesive labels printed in permanent black ink. The labels should contain the volume number of the submission (vol. X of XX vols.), name of drug, the IND number, and the sponsor's name.[31] Binders for a variety of the FDA submissions, including INDs, can be purchased from the Government Printing Office (U.S. Government Printing Office (GPO) Washington, D.C. 20404-0001).

- For complete traceability, and adequate documentation, the initial IND application and subsequent submissions to the IND should be sent to the FDA using an overnight delivery service such as FedEx, United Parcel Service, or DHL. Many of these services offer email notification to the sender upon delivery and other customer service tools that make routine shipments easier. Sponsors should keep records of receipt for all IND submissions as documented proof of submission should questions arise.

3.3.12 The FDA Review of the IND

When the initial IND submission is made to the FDA, it is logged in the Records Room and given an IND number. A sponsor can call in advance of

[31] FDA Center for Drug Evaluation and Research IND, NDA, ANDA or Drug Master File Binders Web Page http://www.fda.gov/cder/ddms/binders.htm.

the submission and receive the number, and this number can be used within the submission document. Many companies commonly call ahead to receive this information. Once the IND is stamped as received, it is sent to the review division within CDER or CBER. If there is any question about which division the IND will reside in, the Ombudsman Office is contacted. Once the IND arrives at the Review Division, it is critically evaluated by several reviewers of chemistry, biopharmaceutics, medical, statistics, and microbiology and pharmacology/toxicology sections as appropriate. All these areas review the data submitted with the primary purpose to ensure appropriate safety of the individuals who will be enrolled in the study. This differs from a review of the NDA or BLA (or CTD), in which both safety and efficacy are evaluated, and the manufacturing portion is reviewed for large-scale manufacturing.

Once an IND is submitted, the study cannot be initiated until a period of 30 days has passed or if the FDA has given agreement to start the study before the 30-day period expires. The usual practice is to contact the FDA shortly before the 30-day period has expired to see if there are any issues, rather than going ahead at day 30 if the FDA has not responded. If there are any major issues relating to the safety of the volunteers or patients in the proposed study, the FDA can institute a "clinical hold."[32] (MaPP 6030.1) A "clinical hold" is an order issued by the FDA to the sponsor of an IND to delay or to suspend a clinical investigation, i.e., to start a clinical trial. A clinical hold may be either a "complete clinical hold" — a delay or suspension of *all* clinical work requested under an IND, or a "partial clinical hold" — a delay or suspension of only part of the clinical work (e.g., a specific protocol or part of a protocol. If a clinical hold is imposed, the specific reasons for the clinical hold will be specified in the clinical hold letter to the sponsor of the IND. Also, if the FDA concludes that there may be grounds for imposing a clinical hold, the Agency will attempt to discuss and satisfactorily resolve the matter before issuing a clinical hold letter. A sponsor must respond to all clinical hold issues before the FDA will begin to review these responses. When all responses from the sponsor are received by the FDA, the FDA has 30 calendar days to review and respond in writing. Under no circumstances can the study be initiated unless the FDA lifts the clinical hold. Review Divisions differ in the frequency of clinical holds that are imposed. This depends to a certain extent on the nature of the disease being treated and the potential benefit of the drug to the patient or subject to be enrolled in the trial.

3.4 Maintaining an IND: IND Amendments and Other Required Reports

Clinical development of a new drug will take several years, and can take as many as 10 or 12 years, all the time requiring an active IND to conduct the

---
[32] Code of Federal Regulations Title 21 Section 312.42(a).

necessary clinical studies. Because of the long development times, the IND is continuously updated with new information and new protocols as the drug moves from one phase of investigation to the next. The IND regulations discuss two types of amendments — protocol amendments and information amendments — and two types of required reports: safety reports and annual reports. Most other routine communication with the FDA regarding an IND is referred to as general correspondence. It is important to remember, however, that the FDA considers any submission to the IND an amendment, and every submission must be labeled with the next sequential four-digit serial number. Even if the sponsor does not assign a submission the next serial number, the FDA will, and this very often leads to confusion in future submissions when, for example, the sponsor references amendment 0053 and the FDA spends time looking for information in 0053 that is actually in amendment 0056. The form 1571 cover sheet has an area for the sponsor to include the serial number and an area to designate specifically what type of submission it is they are submitting. Sponsors who maintain multiple INDs and other regulatory filings utilize electronic archiving systems that have powerful searching and cross referencing capabilities. This allows for searching a database based on key words or serial numbers.

In this section we will discuss the most common types of amendments and reports to the IND, and review the required content and timing for the submissions.

3.4.1 The IND Safety Report

The sponsor of an IND is responsible for continuously reviewing the safety of the investigational drug(s) under investigation. IND regulations require each sponsor to review and investigate all safety information obtained about the drug regardless of the source of the information. Safety information can come from a wide variety of sources including the clinical studies being conducted under the IND, animal studies, other clinical studies, marketing experience, and reports in scientific journals and unpublished reports. These can be foreign or domestic sources and may be information that is not generated by the sponsor. The ongoing safety review is also a critical component of the sponsor's responsibility to keep all participating investigators updated on new observations regarding the investigational drug, especially any information regarding potential adverse events.

The ICH E6 guidance[33] defines an adverse event (AE) as any unfavorable and unintended sign (including an abnormal laboratory finding) and symptom or disease temporally associated with the use of the investigational product, whether or not related to the investigational product. The ICH E6 guidance further defines a serious adverse drug reaction as any adverse event at any dose that:

---

[33] FDA Guidance for Industry: E6 Good Clinical Practice: Consolidated Guidance. FDA, Rockville, MD, April 1996.

- Results in death
- Is life threatening
- Requires inpatient hospitalization or prolongation of an existing hospitalization
- Results in persistent or significant disability/incapacity
- Is a congenital anomaly/birth defect

An adverse event that does not result in death, is not life threatening, or does not require hospitalization may still be considered serious if, in the opinion of the investigator, the event may have jeopardized the subject and medical intervention may be necessary to prevent one of the outcomes that defines a serious adverse event. The final key definition related to IND safety reports is what constitutes an unexpected adverse event. The IND regulations define an unexpected adverse event as any adverse drug experience, the specificity or severity of which is not consistent with the current investigator's brochure.[34] Essentially what this means is an adverse experience is unexpected if that event was not listed in the investigator's brochure as a possible side effect of the drug (not observed previously), or the event that occurred was listed in the brochure but it occurred in a more severe way than was expected.

Much of the safety information obtained by the sponsor will relate to safety data that the sponsor was already aware of and included in the investigator brochure or is nonserious in nature and does not require immediate notification of the investigators or the FDA; however, all new safety information should be included in the sponsor's safety database regardless of the reporting requirements.

The IND regulations require sponsors to notify all investigators and the FDA of certain types of safety events in an IND safety report. The IND regulations discuss two types of safety reports: a 15-day report and a more urgent 7-day report. When a reported adverse experience is considered related to the use of investigational drug and is a serious and unexpected event, the sponsor is required to notify all of the investigators in the study and the FDA within 15 calendar days of learning of the event. A 15-day safety report is submitted to the FDA on the FDA form 3500A or in a narrative format, and foreign events may be submitted on a *CIOMS I form.* IND safety reports are sent to the reviewing division at the FDA with jurisdiction over the IND. The reports should be submitted in triplicate (one original and two copies) with a 1571 form cover sheet and serial number. The more urgent safety report — the 7-day report or telephone report — is required when any unexpected fatal or life-threatening event associated with the use of the drug occurs. The FDA must be notified by telephone or facsimile within 7 calendar days of learning of a fatal or life-threatening event, and this contact must be followed up with a written report on form 3500A (or CIOMS I) within 15 days of learning of

---

[34] Code of Federal Regulations Title 21 Section 312.32(a).

the event. The telephone report or facsimile should be made to the FDA review division with jurisdiction over the IND. Other safety information that does not meet the requirements for expedited reporting should be submitted to the IND in an information amendment or in the annual report.

IND Term

CIOMS I Form — A standardized international reporting form used to report individual cases of serious, unexpected adverse drug reactions.

CIOMS (Council for International Organizations of Medical Sciences) — An international, nongovernmental, nonprofit organization established jointly by WHO and UNESCO in 1949. CIOMS has established a series of working groups that develop safety requirements for drugs and standardized guidelines for assessment and monitoring of adverse drug reactions.

The FDA interprets when the sponsor learns of the event to mean the sponsor's initial receipt of the information. If the sponsor's clinical associate learns of a serious adverse event while visiting a site, the 15-day clock begins as soon as the associate learns of the event and not when the associate reports the event to the clinical affairs or pharmacovigilance groups. The sponsor must have strict procedures and timelines in place for employees to report potential adverse events.

It is important to remember that these events may not come strictly from the sponsor's ongoing clinical trials. The IND regulations require 15-day IND safety reports for adverse findings from nonclinical studies that may indicate a risk to human subjects in the ongoing clinical trials. These could be adverse findings from carcinogenicity studies, reproductive toxicology studies, or any other nonclinical studies being conducted to support clinical trials.

The sponsor must continue to investigate the adverse experience after the IND safety report is submitted. Any additional or follow-up information obtained as part of the investigation must be submitted to the FDA as soon as the new information becomes available. In practice, most sponsors will submit follow up information to the FDA within a 15-calendar-day timeframe, as with the original safety report.

Submission of an IND safety report does not mean that the sponsor or the FDA has concluded that the information being reported constitutes an admission that the drug caused or contributed to the event. In fact, the IND regulations state that a sponsor need not admit, and may deny, that the report or information submitted constitutes an admission that the drug caused or contributed to an adverse event.[35]

---

[35] Code of Federal Regulations Title 21 Section 312.32(e).

IND Note

A sponsor who is conducting a clinical trial of a marketed drug product under an IND is not required to submit IND safety reports for adverse events that occur outside of the clinical study itself.

In the Federal Register of March 14, 2003, the FDA published a proposed rule[36] to amend the pre- and post-marketing safety reporting regulations for human drug and biological products. The proposed rule would harmonize the U.S. safety reporting requirements with international standards developed by CIOMS and ICH (International Conference on Harmonization) and provides new standards, definitions, and reporting formats. The proposed rule would amend the IND safety reporting requirements in a number of ways:

- Adverse drug experiences would be called suspected adverse drug reactions (SADR) and be defined as any noxious and unintended response to any dose of a drug product for which there is a reasonable possibility that the product caused the response.

- The definitions of serious, life-threatening, and unexpected adverse drug experiences would all be changed to include the term SADR.

- The proposed rule defines a minimum data set that is required for an IND safety report — identifiable patient, identifiable reporter, a suspect drug, and an SADR. The rule states that an IND safety report must not be submitted if the report does not contain the minimum data set.

- The decision of whether a SADR is considered serious and unexpected will be based on the opinion of the investigator or the sponsor. The current regulations are silent on who determines whether an event is serious and unexpected (most sponsors already make the determination in this fashion anyway).

- An IND safety report would be required if there is information sufficient to consider product administration changes. This would expand on the requirement to submit a safety report based on any findings from tests in laboratory animals that suggest a significant risk for human subjects. The proposed rule would require a safety report when a sponsor has information that, based on appropriate medical judgment, might influence the benefit–risk assessment of an investigational drug or that would be sufficient to consider changes in either product administration or the overall clinical investigation. This information could include unanticipated safety find-

---

[36] Safety Reporting Requirements for Human Drug and Biological Products; Proposed Rule. Federal Register Vol. 68, No. 50, March 14, 2003.

ings or data from *in vitro*, animal, epidemiological, or clinical studies
that suggest a significant human risk.

A final rule on safety reporting requirements is likely to be published
in 2004.

3.4.2 The Protocol Amendment

A protocol amendment is submitted to the FDA when a sponsor wants to
initiate a new clinical study that is not described in the existing IND or when
the sponsor makes changes to an existing protocol including adding a new
investigator to a trial. New protocols are submitted when clinical development of the drug advances to the next phase, e.g., from Phase I to Phase II,
or when an additional study is needed during the same phase of development, e.g., an additional Phase II study (Phase IIb) to evaluate dosing or a
clinical study to evaluate potential differences in pharmacokinetics or pharmacodynamics in response to changes in the formulation or route of administration of the investigational drug.

A protocol amendment for a new protocol must include a copy of the new
protocol and a brief description of the most clinically significant differences
between the new protocol and previous protocols. Although not specified
in the regulations, the FDA also expects Phase II and Phase III protocol
submissions to include information on how the data will be collected (case
report forms) to ensure that the study will achieve its intended scientific
purposes. When submitting a new protocol to an active IND, the sponsor
may initiate the study once the IRB has approved the protocol and it has
been submitted to the FDA. There is no 30-day review period for the FDA
and a sponsor can initiate a study once the protocol is submitted, if IRB
approval is in place. However, the FDA can still place the study on clinical
hold if it believes there is a safety issue or the protocol design is insufficient
to meet the stated objective. Sponsors may want to request feedback from
the FDA or specifically request in the amendment that the FDA notify the
sponsor if there are no objections to the proposed trial.

A protocol amendment is also required if a sponsor makes significant
changes to an existing protocol. For Phase I protocols an amendment is
required if the changes may affect the safety of the subjects participating in
the study. Other modifications that do not affect the safety of the subjects
should be submitted in the IND annual report and not in a protocol amendment. In the case of a Phase II or Phase III protocol, a protocol amendment
should be submitted for any change that may affect the safety of the subjects,
changes the scope of the trial, or affects the scientific validity of the study.
The IND regulations provide the following examples of changes that would
require a protocol amendment:

- An increase in drug dosage or duration of exposure of the subjects
  to the drug beyond that listed in the current protocol

- A significant increase in the number of subjects participating in the trial
- A change in the design of the protocol, such as adding or dropping a control group
- Adding a new test procedure to monitor for, or reduce the risk of, an adverse event
- Eliminating a test intended to monitor safety

When submitting a protocol amendment for a change to a protocol, the submission should include a description of the change, a brief discussion of the reason and justification for the change, and reference (date and serial number) to the submission that contained the protocol and other references to specific technical information in the IND or other amendments that supports the proposed change.

The IND regulations allow a sponsor to immediately implement a change to a protocol if the change is intended to eliminate an immediate hazard to the clinical trial subjects. In this case, the FDA must be notified of the change by a protocol amendment as soon as possible and the IRB at each site must also be notified of the change.

A protocol amendment is required when a new investigator or subinvestigator is added to conduct the clinical trial at a new or an existing site. The investigator is the person with overall responsibility for the conduct of the clinical trial at a trial site and a subinvestigator is any individual member of the clinical trial team designated and supervised by the investigator to perform trial related procedures or make trial related decisions (e.g., associates, residents, research fellows).[37] The required information regarding the new investigators is collected on the FDA form 1572 Statement of Investigator (Figure 3.2) and the sponsor must notify the FDA of new investigators and subinvestigators by submitting the 1572 as a protocol amendment within 30 days of the investigator being added to the study. An investigator may not participate in a study until he/she provides the sponsor with a completed and signed Statement of Investigator, form 1572.[38] Protocol amendments to add new investigators or to add additional information about an investigator or subinvestigator can be grouped and submitted at 30-day intervals.

All protocol amendments must be clearly labeled and identify specifically which type of protocol amendment is included, e.g., "Protocol Amendment: New Protocol" or "Protocol Amendment: New Investigator" and, as with all IND submissions, a 1571 cover sheet should be included with the submission. Box 11 on the 1571 should be marked, indicating that the submission is a protocol amendment.

---

[37] FDA Guidance for Industry: E6 Good Clinical Practice: Consolidated Guidance. FDA, Rockville, MD, April 1996.
[38] Code of Federal Regulations Title 21 Section 312.53.

3.4.3 Information Amendments

Information amendments are used to submit important information to the IND that is not within the scope of a protocol amendment, annual report, or IND safety report. An information amendment may include new toxicology or pharmacology information, final study reports for completed nonclinical or other technical studies, new chemistry manufacturing and controls information, notice of discontinuation of a clinical study, or any other information important to the IND. An information amendment can also include information that is specifically requested by the FDA. As with the protocol amendment, the FDA requests that information amendments be identified on the cover as an information amendment with the type of information being provided, e.g., "Information Amendment: Toxicology" and, as with all IND submissions, a 1571 cover sheet should be included. Information amendments should be submitted as needed but not more than once every 30 days, if possible.

Information typically submitted in an information amendment may also be required to support another type of amendment; for instance, a new protocol may require additional CMC information because of a change in formulation or change in manufacturing of the investigational drug. In these cases it is not necessary to submit a separate protocol amendment and a separate information amendment with two different serial numbers. All of the protocol and CMC information can be submitted in the same amendment but it should be clearly separated within the submission (by tabs or title pages), the submission should be labeled as containing a protocol amendment and an information amendment (Protocol Amendment: New Protocol and Information Amendment: CMC), and Box 12 on the 1571 form (Contents of Application) should indicate what is included with the submission.

3.4.4 IND Annual Reports

The IND regulations[39] require IND sponsors to submit an annual report that provides the FDA with a brief update on the progress of all investigations included in the IND. The regulations provide clear instruction as to the specific content and format of the annual report so we will only briefly summarize the content here. The annual report must contain the following information:

- Individual study information — a brief summary of the status of each study in progress, including the title of the study, total number of subjects enrolled to date, total number of subjects who completed the study, the number of subjects who dropped out for any reason, and a brief description of any study results if known.

---

[39] Code of Federal Regulations Title 21 Section 312.33.

- Summary Information — Nonclinical and clinical information obtained during the previous year. This section will include a table summarizing the most frequent and most serious adverse events, a listing of all IND safety reports submitted during the past year, a list of subjects who died during the investigation including cause of death, a list of patients who dropped out of the study because of adverse events, any new information about the mechanism of action, dose response, or bioavailability of the drug, a list of ongoing and completed nonclinical studies and a list of any manufacturing changes made during the previous year.
- The general investigational plan for the coming year.
- If the investigator brochure was modified during the year, a list of the changes along with a copy of the new brochure.
- If there is a Phase I protocol, any changes made to the protocol not reported in a protocol amendment.
- A listing of any significant foreign marketing developments with the drug, e.g., approval in another country or withdrawal or suspension of marketing approval.
- A log of any outstanding business for which the sponsor requests or expects a reply, comment, or meeting with the FDA.

As mentioned, the content of an annual report is well defined in the regulations and sponsors should not use the annual report as a substitute for an information amendment. Final nonclinical or clinical study reports, major CMC changes, or other important PK or PD data should be submitted in an information amendment and not held until the annual report. Information of this nature must be submitted to the IND when it becomes available, which allows the FDA to review it in a timely fashion, not several months after the information first became available. The annual report should not be used to report new information, e.g., new, serious, and unexpected adverse events that could change the risk/benefit profile of the investigation, perhaps necessitating a clinical hold. The annual report is a summary of the progress of the study over the past year and provides the general investigational plan for the coming year. The annual report must be submitted to the FDA review division with jurisdiction over the IND within 60 days of the anniversary date that the IND went into effect.

3.5 Other Types of INDs

In addition to the IND submitted by the commercial sponsor, there are investigator-sponsored INDs. They usually involve a single investigator who is performing a clinical trial. The investigator usually seeks permission from a commercial sponsor to "cross-reference" manufacturing data and nonclinical pharmacology and toxicology data. Letters from the commercial supplier of the product are required to allow the FDA to review the data contained in the supplier's IND or Drug Master File.

Additionally, there are "treatment INDs." These are reserved for investigational products for serious or immediately life-threatening diseases for whom no comparable or satisfactory alternative therapy is available. This IND would allow use in patients not in the clinical trials in accordance with a treatment protocol or treatment IND.[40] Special procedures apply for these INDs. Another type of IND is the "screening IND" (MaPP 6030.4). Generally, the FDA encourages separate INDs for different molecules and dosage forms. However, in the early phases of development, exploratory studies may be conducted on a number of closely related drugs to choose the preferred compound or formulation. These studies may be most efficiently conducted under a single IND. Its main benefit is the use of a single IND to avoid duplicative paperwork and to alert the FDA that the IND will be used to screen multiple compounds. The CMC and nonclinical pharmacology and toxicology data for each active moiety in the screening IND should be in accord with appropriate FDA guidances.

3.6 Promotion and Charging for Investigational Drugs

3.6.1 Promotion of Investigational Drug Products

The determination of safety and efficacy is made by the FDA based on all of the information submitted in a marketing application, and a drug cannot be represented as safe or effective until the FDA has approved the product for sale. Therefore, IND regulations specifically prohibit a sponsor or investigator from promoting or commercializing an investigational drug or stating that an investigational drug is safe or effective for the indication(s) under investigation. This includes commercial distribution of the investigational drug or test marketing the drug.[41] Sponsors must be particularly aware of this prohibition when issuing press releases about ongoing or completed clinical trials. The sponsor is often eager to publicly release positive information from trials, particularly pivotal trials, but a press release cannot state that the drug is safe or effective for its intended use no matter how positive the results of the trial may be. The FDA will consider statements like this in a press release or other public statements promotion of an unapproved drug. Sponsors can also run into trouble at professional meetings and trade shows.

---

[40] Code of Federal Regulations Title 21 Section 312.34.
[41] Code of Federal Regulations Title 21 Section 312.7 (a).

Company representatives cannot make claims about the safety or efficacy of an investigational drug, either verbally or in writing, or appear to be promoting an investigational drug in any way.

These prohibitions are not intended to restrict the dissemination of scientific information about the drug in scientific journals or other lay media. The results of clinical studies can be published in peer reviewed scientific journals, presented at medical or scientific meetings, and announced publicly in press releases. The information presented in these forums should be limited to scientific information and the actual results of a clinical study. Presenting the number of patients that met the primary efficacy measurements or other study outcomes is permissible as long as there is no conclusion of safety and efficacy based on the reported results.

3.6.2   Charging for Investigational Drugs

Charging for an investigational drug product in a clinical trial conducted under an IND is prohibited unless the sponsor has submitted a written request to the FDA seeking permission to charge for the drug and the FDA has issued a written approval.[42] In the request the sponsor must justify why charging for the drug is necessary to initiate or continue the trial and why the cost of providing the investigational product to trial subjects should not be considered a normal part of the cost of developing the drug. Although the regulations provide this mechanism, it is rare that a sponsor will charge for an investigational drug.

The regulations do permit a sponsor to charge for an investigational drug being administered under a treatment protocol or treatment IND if the following conditions are met:[43]

- There is adequate enrollment in the ongoing clinical trials under the IND.
- Charging does not constitute commercialization of the drug.
- The drug is not being commercially promoted or advertised.
- The sponsor is actively pursuing marketing authorization.
- The sponsor notifies the FDA in advance of its intent to charge for the drug in an information amendment.

The authorization to charge for the drug goes into effect automatically 30 days after the FDA receives the amendment, unless the sponsor is notified otherwise.

If the FDA allows the sponsor to charge for the drug, the price must not be greater than the costs of handling, distribution, manufacture, and research and development of the drug. The FDA can withdraw authorization to

---

[42] Code of Federal Regulations Title 21 Section 312.7 (d)(1).
[43] Code of Federal Regulations Title 21 Section 312.7 (d)(2).

charge for an investigational drug if it finds that any of the conditions of the authorization are no longer valid, e.g., the price being charged is greater than costs associated with the drug.

3.7 More Information About INDs

There is a great deal of additional information available about the IND application and much of it is now easily available via the internet. The most complete source of information about the IND application is the FDA Website itself (www.fda.gov). The CDER and CBER Websites contain a wealth of important information about preparing, submitting, and maintaining INDs. The most important documents to be familiar with are the guidance documents (Guidance for Industry) but there is significantly more IND information available on the FDA site than just the guidance documents. The FDA Website section below outlines a number of Web pages that provide significant information about INDs, how the FDA processes them, meeting with the FDA, and the drug development process in general.

The following list provides a selection of other IND resources found on the web, in journal articles, and in text books.

3.7.1 The Federal Food, Drug and Cosmetic Act

1. New Drugs Section 505 (i)
   www.fda.gov/opacom/laws/lawtoc.htm

3.7.2 The Regulations

1. Title 21 of the Code of Federal Regulations Part 312 — Investigational New Drug Application
   www.accessdata.fda.gov/scripts/cdrh/cfdocs/cfcfr/cfrsearch.cfm

3.7.3 The FDA Guidance for Industry

1. Content and Format of INDs for Phase 1 Studies of Drugs, Including Well-Characterized, Therapeutic, Biotechnology-Derived Products.
2. INDs for Phase 2 and 3 Studies of Drugs, Including Specified Therapeutic Biotechnology-Derived Products Chemistry Manufacturing and Controls Information.
3. IND Meetings for Human Drugs and Biologics Chemistry Manufacturing and Controls Information.

4. Guidance for Industry: Providing Regulatory Submissions to CBER in Electronic Format — Investigational New Drug Applications (INDs).

5. Guidance for Industry: Special Protocol Assessment.

6. Guidance for Industry: IND Exemptions for Studies of Lawfully Marketed Cancer Drug or Biologic Products (Draft).

3.7.4   The FDA Website

1. Compilation of Laws Enforced by the U.S. FDA
   www.fda.gov/opacom/laws/lawtoc.htm

2. Title 21 Code of Federal Regulations
   www.accessdata.fda.gov/scripts/cdrh/cfdocs/cfcfr/cfrsearch.cfm

3. CDER Guidance Documents
   www.fda.gov/cder/guidance/index.htm

4. CBER Guidance Documents
   www.fda.gov/cber/guidelines.htm

5. The CDER Handbook
   www.fda.gov/cder/handbook/

6. CDER Learn
   www.fda.gov/cder/learn/CDERLearn/default.htm. CDER's new site for online educational seminars.

7. IND Form Help: Information for Sponsor-Investigators Submitting Investigational New Drug Applications (INDs)
   www.fda.gov/cder/forms/1571-1572-help.html

8. Office of Drug Evaluation IV: Pre-IND Consultation Program
   www.fda.gov/cder/Regulatory/default.htm#Regulatory. A program offered by the **Office of Drug Evaluation IV (ODE IV)** designed to facilitate early informal communications between ODE IV and sponsors of new therapeutics for the treatment of bacterial infections, HIV, opportunistic infections, transplant rejection, and other diseases.

9. CDER Manual of Policies and Procedures (MaPPs)
   www.fda.gov/cder/mapp.htm

- MaPP 6030.1 IND Process and Review Procedures
- MaPP 6030.2 INDs: Review of Informed Consent Documents
- MaPP 6030.4 INDs: Screening INDs
- MaPP 6030.8 INDs: Exception from Informed Consent Requirements for Emergency Research

10. CBER Manual of Regulatory Standard Operating Procedures and Policies (SOPPs)
    www.fda.gov/cber/regsopp/regsopp.htm

    • SOPP 8201 Issuance of and Response to Clinical Hold Letters for Investigational New Drug Applications

11. Good Clinical Practice in FDA-Regulated Clinical Trials
    www.fda.gov/oc/gcp/default.htm

3.7.5 Other Websites

1. RegSource.com
   www.regsource.com/default.html
   A comprehensive site that contains a wealth of information on many topics within regulatory affairs including INDs.

3.7.6 Books

1. Mathieu, M., *New Drug Development: A Regulatory Overview*, 6th ed., Parexel International, Waltham, 2002, Chap. 4.

4

Formatting, Assembling, and Submitting the New Drug Application (NDA)

David J. Pizzi and Janet C. Rae

CONTENTS

The new drug application (NDA) is a critical component in the drug approval process. The U.S. Food and Drug Administration (FDA) requires drug sponsors to submit an NDA for review before a new pharmaceutical can be approved for marketing and sale in the U.S. The NDA contains clinical and nonclinical test data and analyses, drug chemistry information, and descriptions of manufacturing procedures.

An NDA consists of thousands of pages of information to be reviewed by FDA teams composed of highly qualified individuals with expertise in their respective technical fields. Usually, six different teams are responsible for reviewing an NDA. The teams are organized by technical reviewing responsibilities: clinical, pharmacology/toxicology, chemistry, statistics, biopharmaceutical, and microbiology.

To help speed the process of reviewing such a complex document with multiple sections, it is important that the information be presented clearly and consistently. The FDA has established guidelines for formatting, assembling, and submitting the NDA. Failure to follow these guidelines can result in deficiencies that could delay review, require an amended application, or result in a Refusal to File.

This chapter will provide an overview of preparing the NDA submission, insights into the FDA guidelines, and an understanding of potential problem areas.

4.1 FDA Guidelines

Most of the FDA guidelines regarding NDAs were written and implemented in early 1987. The guidelines address format, assembly, submission, and content of the overall NDA. Additional guidelines address format and content of specific sections within the NDA.

Note that the NDA shares many common elements with the Common Technical Document (CTD) developed by the International Conference on Harmonization (ICH) in order to streamline submissions for registration in all three ICH regions: the U.S., the European Union, and Japan. These documents can be developed in parallel. Although the FDA has adopted the CTD, the agency still requires specific regional administrative information in the NDA. (Refer to the end of this chapter for more information on the CTD.)

A list of the current FDA guidelines with their most recent revision dates follows:

- Guideline on Formatting, Assembling, and Submitting New Drug and Antibiotic Applications, February 1987
- Guideline for the Format and Content of the Summary for New Drug and Antibiotic Applications, February 1987
- Guideline for the Format and Content of the Nonclinical/Pharmacology/Toxicology Section of an Application, February 1987
- Guideline for the Format and Content of the Human Pharmacokinetics and Bioavailability Section of an Application, February 1987
- Guideline for the Format and Content of the Microbiology Section of an Application, February 1987

- Guideline for the Format and Content of the Clinical and Statistical Sections of New Drug Applications, July 1987
- Guideline for the Format and Content of the Chemistry, Manufacturing, and Controls Section of an Application, February 1987
- Guideline for Submitting Supporting Documentation in Drug Applications for the Manufacture of Drug Substances, February 1987
- Guideline for Submitting Documentation for the Manufacture of and Controls for Drug Products, February 1987
- Guideline for Submitting Samples and Analytical Data for Methods Validation, February 1987
- Guideline for Submitting Documentation for Packaging for Human Drugs and Biologics, February 1987 (new draft proposed July 1997)
- Guideline for Submitting Documentation for the Stability of Human Drugs and Biologics, February 1987

4.2 Assembling Applications for Submission

The FDA requires drug sponsors to submit multiple copies of the NDA (see Figure 4.1).

The *archival copy* contains all sections of the NDA, including the cover letter, Form FDA-356h (Application to Market a New Drug, Biologic, or an Antibiotic for Human Use), the administrative sections, a comprehensive NDA index, and all technical sections. It must contain four copies of the Labeling section. It must contain three additional copies of the CMC and Methods Validation Package in a separate binder. The archival copy is the only copy that contains the Case Report Tabulation and Case Report Forms.

The *review copy* contains the NDA's technical sections, each packaged for reviewers in the corresponding technical disciplines. In addition to the appropriate technical section, each review copy also includes the cover letter, Form FDA-356h, the administrative sections, and the comprehensive NDA index as well as an individual table of contents, the Labeling section, and the Application Summary.

The *field copy* has been required since 1993 for use by FDA inspectors during preapproval facilities inspections. It includes the cover letter and Form FDA-356h, the administrative sections, and the comprehensive NDA index as well as an individual table of contents, the Labeling section, the Application Summary, and the CMC and Methods Validation Package.

In 1997 the FDA's Center for Drug Evaluation and Research (CDER) published guidelines that allow sponsors to submit NDAs electronically instead of on paper. Guidelines for electronic submission of CTDs are still under development.

ASSEMBLING AND BINDING APPLICATIONS FOR SUBMISSION

NDA Section	Folder Color/Area To Which Section Must Be Submitted								
	Archival	Field Copy	Chemistry	Non-Clinical	Human PK and BioAval.	Micro-biology	Clinical	Statistical	Total Copies
Cover letter, 356h form, Sections 13-20 (∗)						*			7 (8*)
1. Index						*			7 (8*)
2. Labeling (±)	±					*			7 (8*)
3. Application Summary						*			7 (8*)
4. CMC and Methods Validation Package ( )									3
5. Nonclinical Pharmacology and Toxicology									2
6. Human Pharmacokinetics and Bioavailability									2
7. Microbiology (*)	★					*			2*
8. Clinical									2
9. Safety Updates (**)	★ ★			*			★		2**
10. Statistical									2
11. Case Report Tabulation									1
12. Case Report Forms									1

(∗) Sections 13. Patent Information, 14. Patent Certification, 15. Establishment Description, 16. Debarment Certification, 17. Field Copy Certification, 18. User Fee Cover Sheet, 19. Financial Disclosure, 20. Other/Pediatric

(±) Archival-4 copies, Other Sections-1 copy

( ) Methods Validation Package: 3 additional copies in separate binder

(*) Only applicable for anti-infective drugs

(**) Safety updates: 120 day report and subsequent updates

PAREXEL International Corporation

FIGURE 4.1

This table shows which NDA sections must be included in the archival, field, and technical review copies of the NDA submission. The column at far right indicates the total number of copies necessary for each section.

4.3   NDA Contents

The NDA may have as many as 20 different sections in addition to the Form FDA-356h itself. To a certain degree, the specific contents of the NDA will depend on the nature of the drug and the information available at the time of submission. The components of the application, however, are uniform (see Figure 4.2).

Application: The application itself consists of a cover letter and a completed Form FDA-356h (see Figures 4.3a and 4.3b), along with several other supporting items as appropriate (see Figure 4.4, Figure 4.5). These documents include:

- Item 13: Patent Information
- Item 14: Patent Certification
- Item 15: Establishment Description (if applicable)
- Item 16: Debarment Certification

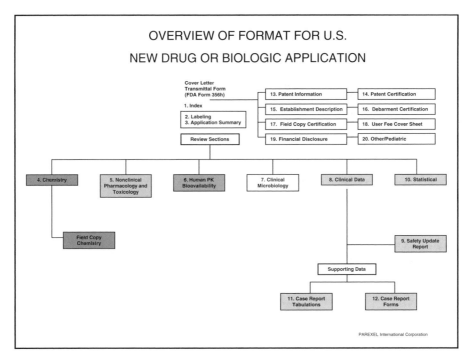

OVERVIEW OF FORMAT FOR U.S.

NEW DRUG OR BIOLOGIC APPLICATION

FIGURE 4.2
This chart provides an overview of how the various sections of the NDA are organized.

- Item 17: Field Copy Certification
- Item 18: User Fee Cover Sheet (Form FDA-3397)
- Item 19: Financial Disclosure (Form FDA-3454, Form FDA-3455)
- Item 20: Other/Pediatric Use

The application Form FDA-356h serves as a checklist as well as a certification that the sponsor agrees to comply with a range of legal and regulatory requirements. The applicant must sign the form and include a U.S. address. If the applicant does not reside or maintain a place of business in the U.S., the form must also include the signature, name, and address of the applicant's authorized U.S. agent.

4.3.1 NDA Section 1: Index

The NDA index is a comprehensive table of contents that enables the reviewers to find specific information in this massive document quickly. The NDA index should follow immediately after the Form FDA-356h and the administrative items. It must show the location of every section in the archival NDA by volume and by page number (see Figure 4.6). It should guide reviewers to data in the technical sections, the summary, and the supporting documents.

DEPARTMENT OF HEALTH AND HUMAN SERVICES
FOOD AND DRUG ADMINISTRATION

APPLICATION TO MARKET A NEW DRUG, BIOLOGIC, OR AN ANTIBIOTIC DRUG FOR HUMAN USE
(Title 21, Code of Federal Regulations, Parts 314 & 601)

Form Approved: OMB No. 0910-0338
Expiration Date: August 31, 2005
See OMB Statement on page 2.

FOR FDA USE ONLY
APPLICATION NUMBER

APPLICANT INFORMATION

NAME OF APPLICANT

DATE OF SUBMISSION

TELEPHONE NO. *(Include Area Code)*

FACSIMILE (FAX) Number *(Include Area Code)*

APPLICANT ADDRESS *(Number, Street, City, State, Country, ZIP Code or Mail Code, and U.S. License number if previously issued):*

AUTHORIZED U.S. AGENT NAME & ADDRESS *(Number, Street, City, State, ZIP Code, telephone & FAX number)* IF APPLICABLE

PRODUCT DESCRIPTION

NEW DRUG OR ANTIBIOTIC APPLICATION NUMBER, OR BIOLOGICS LICENSE APPLICATION NUMBER *(If previously issued)*

ESTABLISHED NAME *(e.g., Proper name, USP/USAN name)*

PROPRIETARY NAME *(trade name)* IF ANY

CHEMICAL/BIOCHEMICAL/BLOOD PRODUCT NAME *(If any)*

CODE NAME *(If any)*

DOSAGE FORM:

STRENGTHS:

ROUTE OF ADMINISTRATION:

(PROPOSED) INDICATION(S) FOR USE:

APPLICATION INFORMATION

APPLICATION TYPE
(check one) ☐ NEW DRUG APPLICATION (21 CFR 314.50) ☐ ABBREVIATED NEW DRUG APPLICATION (ANDA, 21 CFR 314.94)
☐ BIOLOGICS LICENSE APPLICATION (21 CFR Part 601)

IF AN NDA, IDENTIFY THE APPROPRIATE TYPE ☐ 505 (b)(1) ☐ 505 (b)(2)

IF AN ANDA, OR 505(b)(2), IDENTIFY THE REFERENCE LISTED DRUG PRODUCT THAT IS THE BASIS FOR THE SUBMISSION
Name of Drug   Holder of Approved Application

TYPE OF SUBMISSION *(check one)* ☐ ORIGINAL APPLICATION ☐ AMENDMENT TO A PENDING APPLICATION ☐ RESUBMISSION
☐ PRESUBMISSION ☐ ANNUAL REPORT ☐ ESTABLISHMENT DESCRIPTION SUPPLEMENT ☐ EFFICACY SUPPLEMENT
☐ LABELING SUPPLEMENT ☐ CHEMISTRY MANUFACTURING AND CONTROLS SUPPLEMENT ☐ OTHER

IF A SUBMISSION OF PARTIAL APPLICATION, PROVIDE LETTER DATE OF AGREEMENT TO PARTIAL SUBMISSION: _____

IF A SUPPLEMENT, IDENTIFY THE APPROPRIATE CATEGORY ☐ CBE ☐ CBE-30 ☐ Prior Approval (PA)

REASON FOR SUBMISSION

PROPOSED MARKETING STATUS *(check one)* ☐ PRESCRIPTION PRODUCT (Rx) ☐ OVER THE COUNTER PRODUCT (OTC)

NUMBER OF VOLUMES SUBMITTED _____ THIS APPLICATION IS ☐ PAPER ☐ PAPER AND ELECTRONIC ☐ ELECTRONIC

ESTABLISHMENT INFORMATION (Full establishment information should be provided in the body of the Application.)
Provide locations of all manufacturing, packaging and control sites for drug substance and drug product (continuation sheets may be used if necessary). Include name, address, contact, telephone number, registration number (CFN), DMF number, and manufacturing steps and/or type of testing (e.g. Final dosage form, Stability testing) conducted at the site. Please indicate whether the site is ready for inspection or, if not, when it will be ready.

Cross References (list related License Applications, INDs, NDAs, PMAs, 510(k)s, IDEs, BMFs, and DMFs referenced in the current application)

FORM FDA 356h (9/02)

PSC Media Arts (301) 443-1090 EF

PAGE 1

FIGURE 4.3a
Form FDA-356h (front (A) and back (B)) provides a checklist of all the elements that the NDA should include.

This application contains the following items: *(Check all that apply)*		
1. Index		
2. Labeling *(check one)*	☐ Draft Labeling	☐ Final Printed Labeling
3. Summary (21 CFR 314.50 (c))		
4. Chemistry section		
A. Chemistry, manufacturing, and controls information (e.g., 21 CFR 314.50(d)(1); 21 CFR 601.2)		
B. Samples (21 CFR 314.50 (e)(1); 21 CFR 601.2 (a)) (Submit only upon FDA's request)		
C. Methods validation package (e.g., 21 CFR 314.50(e)(2)(i); 21 CFR 601.2)		
5. Nonclinical pharmacology and toxicology section (e.g., 21 CFR 314.50(d)(2); 21 CFR 601.2)		
6. Human pharmacokinetics and bioavailability section (e.g., 21 CFR 314.50(d)(3); 21 CFR 601.2)		
7. Clinical Microbiology (e.g., 21 CFR 314.50(d)(4))		
8. Clinical data section (e.g., 21 CFR 314.50(d)(5); 21 CFR 601.2)		
9. Safety update report (e.g., 21 CFR 314.50(d)(5)(vi)(b); 21 CFR 601.2)		
10. Statistical section (e.g., 21 CFR 314.50(d)(6); 21 CFR 601.2)		
11. Case report tabulations (e.g., 21 CFR 314.50(f)(1); 21 CFR 601.2)		
12. Case report forms (e.g., 21 CFR 314.50 (f)(2); 21 CFR 601.2)		
13. Patent information on any patent which claims the drug (21 U.S.C. 355(b) or (c))		
14. A patent certification with respect to any patent which claims the drug (21 U.S.C. 355 (b)(2) or (j)(2)(A))		
15. Establishment description (21 CFR Part 600, if applicable)		
16. Debarment certification (FD&C Act 306 (k)(1))		
17. Field copy certification (21 CFR 314.50 (l)(3))		
18. User Fee Cover Sheet (Form FDA 3397)		
19. Financial Information (21 CFR Part 54)		
20. OTHER *(Specify)*		

CERTIFICATION

I agree to update this application with new safety information about the product that may reasonably affect the statement of contraindications, warnings, precautions, or adverse reactions in the draft labeling. I agree to submit safety update reports as provided for by regulation or as requested by FDA. If this application is approved, I agree to comply with all applicable laws and regulations that apply to approved applications, including, but not limited to the following:

1. Good manufacturing practice regulations in 21 CFR Parts 210, 211 or applicable regulations, Parts 606, and/or 820.
2. Biological establishment standards in 21 CFR Part 600.
3. Labeling regulations in 21 CFR Parts 201, 606, 610, 660, and/or 809.
4. In the case of a prescription drug or biological product, prescription drug advertising regulations in 21 CFR Part 202.
5. Regulations on making changes in application in FD&C Act Section 506A, 21 CFR 314.71, 314.72, 314.97, 314.99, and 601.12.
6. Regulations on Reports in 21 CFR 314.80, 314.81, 600.80, and 600.81.
7. Local, state and Federal environmental impact laws.

If this application applies to a drug product that FDA has proposed for scheduling under the Controlled Substances Act, I agree not to market the product until the Drug Enforcement Administration makes a final scheduling decision.

The data and information in this submission have been reviewed and, to the best of my knowledge are certified to be true and accurate.

Warning: A willfully false statement is a criminal offense, U.S. Code, title 18, section 1001.

SIGNATURE OF RESPONSIBLE OFFICIAL OR AGENT	TYPED NAME AND TITLE	DATE
ADDRESS *(Street, City, State, and ZIP Code)*		Telephone Number ( )

Public reporting burden for this collection of information is estimated to average 24 hours per response, including the time for reviewing instructions, searching existing data sources, gathering and maintaining the data needed, and completing and reviewing the collection of information. Send comments regarding this burden estimate or any other aspect of this collection of information, including suggestions for reducing this burden to:

Department of Health and Human Services   Food and Drug Administration
Food and Drug Administration   CDER, HFD-94
CBER, HFM-99   12420 Parklawn Dr., Room 3046
1401 Rockville Pike   Rockville, MD 20852
Rockville, MD 20852-1448

An agency may not conduct or sponsor, and a person is not required to respond to, a collection of information unless it displays a currently valid OMB control number.

FORM FDA 356h (9/02)

PAGE 2

FIGURE 4.3b
Continued.

DEPARTMENT OF HEALTH AND HUMAN SERVICES Food and Drug Administration **CERTIFICATION: FINANCIAL INTERESTS AND ARRANGEMENTS OF CLINICAL INVESTIGATORS**	**Form Approved: OMB No. 0910-0396** **Expiration Date: June 30, 2002**

TO BE COMPLETED BY APPLICANT

With respect to all covered clinical studies (or specific clinical studies listed below (if appropriate)) submitted in support of this application, I certify to one of the statements below as appropriate. I understand that this certification is made in compliance with 21 CFR part 54 and that for the purposes of this statement, a clinical investigator includes the spouse and each dependent child of the investigator as defined in 21 CFR 54.2(d).

Please mark the applicable checkbox.

☐ (1) As the sponsor of the submitted studies, I certify that I have not entered into any financial arrangement with the listed clinical investigators (enter names of clinical investigators below or attach list of names to this form) whereby the value of compensation to the investigator could be affected by the outcome of the study as defined in 21 CFR 54.2(a). I also certify that each listed clinical investigator required to disclose to the sponsor whether the investigator had a proprietary interest in this product or a significant equity in the sponsor as defined in 21 CFR 54.2(b) did not disclose any such interests. I further certify that no listed investigator was the recipient of significant payments of other sorts as defined in 21 CFR 54.2(f).

Clinical Investigators		

☐ (2) As the applicant who is submitting a study or studies sponsored by a firm or party other than the applicant, I certify that based on information obtained from the sponsor or from participating clinical investigators, the listed clinical investigators (attach list of names to this form) did not participate in any financial arrangement with the sponsor of a covered study whereby the value of compensation to the investigator for conducting the study could be affected by the outcome of the study (as defined in 21 CFR 54.2(a)); had no proprietary interest in this product or significant equity interest in the sponsor of the covered study (as defined in 21 CFR 54.2(b)); and was not the recipient of significant payments of other sorts (as defined in 21 CFR 54.2(f)).

☐ (3) As the applicant who is submitting a study or studies sponsored by a firm or party other than the applicant, I certify that I have acted with due diligence to obtain from the listed clinical investigators (attach list of names) or from the sponsor the information required under 54.4 and it was not possible to do so. The reason why this information could not be obtained is attached.

NAME	TITLE
FIRM / ORGANIZATION	
SIGNATURE	DATE

Paperwork Reduction Act Statement

An agency may not conduct or sponsor, and a person is not required to respond to, a collection of information unless it displays a currently valid OMB control number. Public reporting burden for this collection of information is estimated to average 1 hour per response, including time for reviewing instructions, searching existing data sources, gathering and maintaining the necessary data, and completing and reviewing the collection of information. Send comments regarding this burden estimate or any other aspect of this collection of information to the address to the right:

Department of Health and Human Services
Food and Drug Administration
5600 Fishers Lane, Room 14C-03
Rockville, MD 20857

FORM FDA 3454 (6/02)   Created by PSC Media Arts (301) 443-2454   EF

FIGURE 4.4

Form FDA-3454 certifies that the clinical investigators listed have no financial interests or arrangements with the sponsor as defined in 21 CFR Part 54.

DEPARTMENT OF HEALTH AND HUMAN SERVICES Public Health Service Food and Drug Administration **DISCLOSURE: FINANCIAL INTERESTS AND ARRANGEMENTS OF CLINICAL INVESTIGATORS**	Form Approved: OMB No. 0910-0396 Expiration Date: 3/31/02

TO BE COMPLETED BY APPLICANT

The following information concerning _____ , who par-
Name of clinical investigator

ticipated as a clinical investigator in the submitted study _____
Name of

_____ , is submitted in accordance with 21 CFR part
clinical study

54. The named individual has participated in financial arrangements or holds financial interests that are required to be disclos ed as follows:

> *Please mark the applicable checkboxes.*

☐ any financial arrangement entered into between the sponsor of the covered study and the clinical investigator involved in the conduct of the covered study, whereby the value of the compensation to the clinical investigator for conducting the study could be influenced by the outcome of the study;

☐ any significant payments of other sorts made on or after February 2, 1999 from the sponsor of the covered study such as a grant to fund ongoing research, compensation in the form of equipment, re tainer for ongoing consultation, or honor aria;

☐ any proprietary interest in the product tested in the covered study held by the clinical investigator;

☐ any significant equity interest as defined in 21 CFR 54.2(b), held by the clinical investigator in the sponsor of the covered study.

Details of the individual's disclosable financial arrangements and interests are attached, along with a description of steps taken to minimize the potential bias of clinical study results by any of the disclosed arrangements or interests.

NAME	TITLE
FIRM / ORGANIZATION	
SIGNATURE	DATE

Paperwork Reduction Act Statement

An agency may not conduct or sponsor, and a person is not required to respond to, a collection of information unless it displays a currently valid OMB control number. Public reporting burden for this collection of information is estimated to average 4 hours per response, including time for reviewing instructions, searching existing data sources, gathering and maintaining the necessary data, and completing and reviewing the collection of information. Send comments regarding this burden estimate or any other aspect of this collection of information to:

Department of Health and Human Services
Food and Drug Administration
5600 Fishers Lane, Room 14-72
Rockville, MD 20857

FORM FDA 3455 (7/01)
Created by Electronic Document Services USDHHS (301) EF

FIGURE 4.5
A completed Form FDA-3455 describing disclosable financial interests and arrangements must be included for each clinical investigator not identified on Form FDA-3455.

SECTION 1

OVERALL NDA INDEX

	VOLUME	PAGE
Cover Letter	1	--
Form FDA 356h	1	--
Referenced Applications	1	--
Section 13: Patent Information	1	--
Section 14: Patent Certification	1	--
Section 16: Debarment Certification	1	--
Section 17: Certificate for Field Copy	1	
Section 18: User Fee Cover Sheet- Form FDA 3397	1	
Section 19: Financial Disclosure Certification	1	
Section 20: Other, Include: Pediatric Use Section or Waiver,		
FDA Correspondence	1	

		VOLUME
SECTION 1:	OVERALL NDA INDEX	1
SECTION 2 INDEX:	LABELING	1
SECTION 3 INDEX:	OVERALL SUMMARY	1
SECTION 4 INDEX:	CHEMISTRY, MANUFACTURING AND CONTROLS	1
SECTION 5 INDEX:	NONCLINICAL PHARMACOLOGY AND TOXICOLOGY	1
SECTION 6 INDEX:	HUMAN PHARMACOKINETICS AND BIOAVAILABILITY	1
SECTION 7 INDEX:	MICROBIOLOGY (IF APPLICABLE)	1
SECTION 8 INDEX:	CLINICAL DATA	1
SECTION 9 INDEX:	SAFETY UPDATE	1
SECTION 10 INDEX:	STATISTICAL DATA	1
SECTION 11 INDEX:	CASE REPORT TABULATIONS	1
SECTION 12 INDEX:	CASE REPORT FORMS	1
SECTION 13 INDEX:	PATENT INFORMATION	1
SECTION 14 INDEX:	PATENT CERTIFICATION	1

FIGURE 4.6
The NDA index should be formatted to show information by volume and by page, as shown here. A facsimile of a complete index appears at the end of this chapter.

Each separately bound technical section should also contain a copy of the overall NDA index in addition to its own table of contents based on the index.

4.3.2 NDA Section 2: Labeling

The labeling section must include all draft labeling that is intended for use on the product container, cartons or packages, including the proposed package insert.

As noted above, the NDA must have four copies of the draft labeling. One copy should be bound into the archival copy. Copies should also be placed in the review copies of the clinical, chemistry, and pharmacology sections.

4.3.3 NDA Section 3: Application Summary

The application summary is an abbreviated version of the entire application. This overview is one of the few elements of the application that all reviewers receive, and it should give them a clear idea of the drug and its application. The summary usually comprises 50 to 200 pages. It must include:

Proposed annotated package insert. Per 21 CFR § 201.57, the draft product labeling must include the following sections:

1. Description
2. Clinical Pharmacology
3. Indications and Usage
4. Contraindications
5. Warnings
6. Precautions
7. Adverse Reactions
8. Drug Abuse and Dependence
9. Overdosage
10. Dosage and Administration
11. How Supplied

For each section of the labeling, include annotations referring to information in the summary and technical sections of the application that support the inclusion of each statement in the labeling with respect to animal pharmacology and/or animal toxicology, clinical studies, and Integrated Summary of Safety (ISS) and Integrated Summary of Effectiveness (ISE) (see Figure 4.7).

Pharmacologic class, scientific rationale, intended use, and potential clinical benefits. Include one to two pages of text that give the reviewer the basic information about the drug product.

Foreign marketing history. The summary must include a list of any countries in which the drug is or was marketed, along with the dates when it was marketed, if they are known. It must also include a list of any countries in which the drug has been withdrawn from marketing for any reason relating to safety or efficacy or in which an application has been rejected. Provide specific reasons for the withdrawal or the rejection of the application.

If any related form of the drug has been marketed in another country, include its foreign marketing history as well.

Chemistry, manufacturing, and controls summary. Include an abbreviated version of the chemistry, manufacturing and controls information on the drug substance or drug product from NDA Section 4. The summary should include a tabular list of all formulations used in the important clinical studies.

Nonclinical pharmacology and toxicology summary. An abbreviated version of the NDA Section 5, this portion of the summary should include

NDA [number] [Trade Name] (generic name) Section3A – Annotated Labeling	Sample Page				
	Application Summary Vol. Page		Technical Section Vol. Page		Reference
[Trade Name] [generic name] XX mg and YY mg film-coated tablets					
DESCRIPTION [Trade Name] is the first of a new class of [therapeutic area] agents...					
[Trade Name] (generic name) belongs to a class of... It is designated chemically as [chemical name] and has the following structural formula:	2.1	177	1.1	33	Section 4
	2.1	178	1.1	34	
[Generic Name] has a molecular weight of XX and a molecular formula of XX. [Generic Name] is a white to yellowish powder. It is poorly soluble in water (0.001 g/100 mL) and in aqueous solutions at low pH (0.1 mg/100 mL at pH 1.1 and 4.0; 0.2 mg/100 mL at pH 5.0). Solubility increases at higher pH values (43 mg/100 mL at pH 7.5). In the solid state, [Generic Name] is very stable, is not hygroscopic and is not light sensitive.	2.1	178	1.1	35	
[Trade Name] is available as XX mg and YY mg tablets for oral administration containing with the following excipients: corn starch...	2.1	186	1.1	377	Section 4
CLINICAL PHARMACOLOGY **Mechanism of action**					
[Generic Name] is a dual XX Receptor Antagonist with affinity for both AA and BB receptors. [Generic Name] decreases both pulmonary and systemic vascular resistance resulting in increased cardiac output without increasing heart rate.	2.1 2.1	213	1.7 1.7	221 326	Section 5

FIGURE 4.7
This sample page shows the annotated labeling required for the application summary section.

information on pharmacology, toxicology and pharmacokinetics (PK). The FDA guidelines define specific tables for each of the following:

- Pharmacology
- Acute toxicity
- Subchronic, chronic, carcinogenicity
- Special toxicity
- Reproduction studies (segments I, II, and III)
- Mutagenicity
- Absorption, distribution, metabolism, excretion (ADME)

Human pharmacokinetics and bioavailability (HPKB) summary. Provide a summary of NDA Section 6. It should include a tabular listing and brief description of each HPKB study as well as an integrated summary including the drug product's pharmacokinetic characteristics. If pertinent, compare the drug product's bioavailability with other dosage forms. Identify differences in pharmacokinetics in various subgroups, for example, age group or renal status. Finally, include a brief discussion of the drug product's dissolution profile.

Microbiology summary. A section on microbiology is only required for antibiotic drugs. If applicable, include a summary of the results of the microbiological studies of the drug.

Clinical data summary and results of statistical analysis. Summarize NDA Sections 8 and 10. The summary must include:

Clinical pharmacology — Provide a table of clinical pharmacology studies, narrative results of each study, and an integrated conclusion.

Overview of clinical studies — Provide an overview of clinical trials conducted, a summary of any important discussions of FDA interaction on major issues, and an explanation of clinical features such as duration, study design, adverse events expected, etc.

Controlled clinical studies — Following the same format as the clinical pharmacology section, include a table of controlled clinical studies, narrative results of each study, and an integrated conclusion.

Uncontrolled clinical studies — Following the same format as the clinical pharmacology and controlled clinical studies sections, include a table of uncontrolled clinical studies, narrative results of each study, and an integrated conclusion.

Other studies and information — Provide a summary of information not covered under clinical pharmacology and controlled and uncontrolled clinical trials. This might include information on other studies, publications, and analyses of foreign marketing experience or epidemiologic data.

Safety summary (general safety conclusions) — Address the extent of exposure and adverse reactions. Include tables of the most important adverse events (AEs), such as serious and/or frequent events. Provide a separate analysis of controlled and uncontrolled studies and also integrate the safety data for controlled and uncontrolled studies. Discuss differences related to dose, duration, age and gender and provide an analysis of discontinuations.

Overdosage and drug abuse — Provide information on treatment of overdose. If the drug product has potential for abuse, provide a summary of studies performed and other relevant information. If the drug is not considered abusable but belongs to a class of drugs with potential for abuse, provide reasons why drug abuse studies were not performed.

Discussion of benefit/risk relationship. The summary must include a brief benefit/risk assessment based on ISE to ISS and results of the clinical studies. Include information on the toxicity and safety of the drug from both human and animal studies. Present the benefits and risks of alternative treatments for the population. Finally, describe any postmarketing studies that are proposed.

4.3.4   NDA Section 4: Chemistry, Manufacturing, and Controls (CMC)

The first technical section of the NDA is the chemistry section. It includes information on the composition, manufacture, and specifications of the drug substance and the drug product. The three main elements are (1) chemistry, manufacturing and controls information, (2) samples and, (3) methods validation package. Deficiencies in this section are common.

Description of the drug substance. The CMC information must include a description of the drug substance or active ingredient, including its stability and physical and chemical characteristics, and provide the *names/designations* of the drug substance, including:

- Generic/common name
- Chemical name (IUPAC/USAN/CAS)
- Code(s) (CAS/internal)

Deficiencies often arise when multiple internal code numbers do not correspond to codes used in the documents that accompany the submission. Provide a *structural overview*, including:

- Molecular structure
- Empirical formula
- Molecular weight
- Elemental composition

Be certain that chemical names and structure accurately convey stereochemistry/chirality.

The description of the drug substance's *physical and chemical characteristics* should include:

- Appearance, including color, crystalline form, and odor
- Melting/boiling point
- Refractive index, viscosity, and specific gravity
- Polymorphs, including modifications (forms) and relative kinetic/ thermodynamic stabilities

Common deficiencies in the description of physical characteristics arise when temperatures are not precisely controlled and/or specified for temperature-dependent physical and chemical criteria. Solubility studies at different pHs that are not adequately designed to differentiate from counter-ion effects can also result in a deficiency.

The physical and chemical characteristics should also include solubility, ionization constants, and partition coefficients at various pHs. Discuss solubility in common organic solvents as well as in various aqueous media:

- Water
- 0.1 N HCl
- 0.02 N HCl
- SGF without pepsin
- Water buffered to various acidic/neutral/basic pHs

The solubility data in aqueous media must correlate with the drug product dissolution characteristics. Inadequate correlation can result in a deficiency.

Other common deficiencies include partitioning studies that are not logically designed and inadequate physical or chemical data on alternative polymorphs and stereoisomers.

Provide a *reference standard* to elucidate the drug substance's chemical structure, including preparation method, test methods, and test results as shown by a certificate of analysis. Be sure to include specification for the reference standard. Provide proof that the reference standard was adequately tested and characterize the spectra completely.

Provide structural elucidation using a reference standard as applicable. Measures might include:

- X-ray (in the case of absolute configuration or polymorphism)
- UV/visible spectrum
- FTIR spectrum
- ^{1}H NMR/^{13}C NMR spectrum
- Low-resolution/high-resolution mass spectrum
- Elemental analysis

Other spectrums as appropriate (e.g., heteroatom NMR, fluorescence, raman, microwave)

The CMC information must also include the *names, addresses and functions of each site where the drug substance is manufactured or tested.* Synthesis often takes place at more than one site. If this is the case, it must be adequately represented in the submission to avoid a deficiency.

Drug Master File (DMF) authorization letters must be included. Ensure that these are current.

The description of the drug substance *manufacturing methods* must include:

- Synthesis scheme
- Synthesis description
- Typical executed manufacturing record
- Compilation of and analytical controls for starting materials; reagents, solvents and catalysts, and intermediates
- Suppliers for starting materials

Deficiencies commonly arise when synthesis descriptions are not precise, when the in-process testing for the reaction completion cited for various synthetic steps is insufficient, or when reviewers deem that the explanation provided when multiple syntheses are involved is inadequate.

Provide a description of, and specifications for, the *container and closure components* used for the bulk drug substance. Common deficiencies in this section include providing inadequate specifications and using a container-closure system that does not exactly match the one used in stability studies.

The discussion of *drug substance analytical controls* should include the following:

- Specifications
- Methods
- Rationale for methods/specifications
- Method validations
- Batch analytical data (including impurity profiles cross-referenced with toxicology studies)
- Sampling plan

An NDA may be deficient if the specifications, methods, or method validations are inadequate.

To be considered adequate, specifications should reflect more than one identification test. They should be based on batch history and scientific justification, and individual and total impurity standards must be established properly. Specification should account for all possible stereoisomers and should include proper limits on particle size.

Methods will be found inadequate if no reference standards are established for impurities when using an external standard approach for impurity testing; if the assay is performed by a nonspecific method such as titration, with no correction for the impurities that are present; and if the sampling plan does not have a statistical basis; or insufficient system suitability.

Method validations are inadequate if the method validation is performed outside the specified range or if they do not support system suitability.

Provide information on *drug substance stability*, including:

- Ambient/accelerated stability data

- Retest dating
- Highly stressed (e.g., acid, base, reflux) data

The application is deficient if it offers insufficient or marginal data for filing; this is especially the case with Investigational New Drug (IND) filings. Another common deficiency is lack of proper control over conditions — such as temperature, humidity, or high-intensity light exposure — that affect stability. Finally, if the analytical methods used do not indicate stability, the information is deficient.

Description of the drug product. The CMC technical section also includes a description of the drug product. The description will include some of the same kinds of information required in the description of the drug substance.

Information on the *drug product components/composition* should include qualitative and quantitative listings of each drug product component used in the clinical formulation or formulations (when filing IND) and marketed formulation or formulations (when filing NDA). Deficiencies result when the quantitative composition does not match the composition listed in the batch record, when component ranges are given without proper validation, or when the component ranges provided actually are specifications.

Provide a listing of all *inactive ingredients*. For compendial (e.g., UPS/NF) inactive ingredients, reference the appropriate current compendial monographs and provide more precise specifications as necessary. Be aware that misinterpretation of compendial monographs is a common deficiency.

For noncompendial ingredients that fall under 21 CFR such as D&C and FD&C dyes, reference the appropriate section of 21 CFR and provide any additional specifications beyond the scope of the CFR.

For noncompendial items that are not regulated by 21 CFR, provide appropriate analytical specifications and methods.

Provide the names, addresses, and functions of each site where the *drug product is manufactured, tested, or packaged*. If too many sites are involved, reviewers may determine that the overall manufacturing scheme is too complex.

As noted above, Drug Master File (DMF) authorization letters must be included. Ensure that these are current, that is, within the last two years.

Provide information on the *drug product manufacturing methods*:

- Summary and schematics of manufacturing procedure
- Master batch record for proposed marketed products, including actual operating conditions, type and size of equipment, and in-process controls and tests
- Executed batch record

Applications are often found deficient because the master and executed batch records that are submitted vary too much from one another. The master batch record itself is deficient when the description of equipment is too limited or restrictive or when the in-process controls are inappropriate.

Examples of the latter include controls that do not address key in-process criteria or that do not correlate with the finished process controls.

The section on *drug product packaging* must include:

- Summary of container/closure system(s)
- Listing of packaging components and component/resin suppliers
- Specifications for each packaging component
- DMF authorization letters
- Description of the packaging process
- Test methods (as appropriate)
- Developmental data that confirms the suitability of the packaging. This includes water vapor permeation data for plastic containers/closures and compatibility testing for solutions, suspensions, emulsions, etc.

Applications are often found deficient because the product packaging does not exactly match the product packaging described in the application. Be aware also that certain complex packaging components, such as bottle liners, may create difficult issues. For example, the use of certain vinyl polymers in bottle liners may necessitate a test for the corresponding vinyl monomer. Ideally, appropriate component identification testing should be performed upon receipt of packaging components.

The discussion of *drug product analytical controls* should include the same elements as the corresponding discussion of the drug substance:

- Specifications
- Methods
- Rationale for methods/specifications
- Method validations
- Batch analytical data (including impurity profiles)
- Sampling plan

As in the discussion of drug substance analytical controls, the information is deficient if the specifications, methods or method validations are inadequate. In addition to those points noted above, common reasons for deficiencies in this section include use of frequently inferior methods of impurity/degradant analyses in lieu of frequently superior methods — for example, thin layer chromatography (TLC) instead of high-pressure liquid chromatography (HPLC) as well as interference from the excipient matrix, particularly if the specific method was developed using an earlier, and therefore different, formulation.

The *drug product stability* information will differ slightly from the drug substance stability information. For the drug product, provide:

- Unstressed/stressed stability data
- Statistical analysis to establish consistency of data and expiration dating
- Expiration dating
- Postapproval stability commitment/protocol

Insufficient supporting stability data is a common deficiency, as is attempt to convert to a reduced stability protocol without a sufficient existing stability database. Another pitfall is overcommitment with regard to marketed stability studies.

For an NDA, provide a list of all *drug product investigational formulations* used in clinical studies, along with the quantitative composition of each formulation. Include references to each pivotal clinical and bioavailability study and to the batch used.

Every NDA must include either an *environmental assessment* (EA) or a claim for an exemption to the EA submission requirement. The regulation applies regardless of whether the product is manufactured in the U.S. or overseas. The EA, also called the environmental impact analysis report, includes an analysis of the manufacturing process and ultimate use of the drug product as well as a discussion of how the process and the drug product may affect the environment.

Under current regulations, the FDA grants categorical exclusions to most drugs and biologics, as long as the application's approval will not increase the use of the active moiety, or if the active moiety at the point of entry into the aquatic environment due to use at the 5th year of marketing will be below 1 part per billion (PPB) (see Figure 4.8).

Samples. In addition to the chemistry, manufacturing and controls information, the CMC technical section must include a commitment to submit samples to FDA laboratories for testing and validation of analytical methods. Actual samples are submitted only upon FDA request. If samples are requested, submit the drug product, the drug substance, and the reference standards.

Methods validation package. The final component of the CMC technical section is the methods validation package. The package must comprise:

- Specifications and test methods for each component used in the drug product
- Specifications and methods for the drug product
- Validation of test methods
- Names and addresses of component suppliers
- Names and addresses of the suppliers of the container closure system

Environmental Assessment

In accordance with 21 CFR 25.31(b), **COMPANY NAME** claims categorical exclusion based on the calculation which shows that the estimated concentration of the active moiety, **NAME OF DRUG SUBSTANCE**, at the point of entry into the aquatic environment due to use at the fifth-year of marketing will be below 1 part per billion (ppb).

The calculation was based on the assumptions and equation as stated in the FDA Guidance for Industry, *Environmental Assessment of Human Drug and Biologics Applications* (July 1998).

The expected introduction concentration (EIC) of an active moiety into the aquatic environment was calculated as follows:

EIC-Aquatic (ppb) = $A \times B \times C \times D$ where

A = kg/year produced for direct use (as active moiety). Current marketing projections anticipate **XX** Kg of **NAME** active moiety to be produced in the fifth-year of marketing

B = 1/liters per day entering publicly owned treatment works. Which according to 1996 Needs Survey, Report to Congress, is 1.214×10^{11} liters per day

C = year/365 days

D = 10^9 µg/kg (conversion factor)

Thus
   (EXAMPLE CALCULATION IF A = 300 KG)

$$\text{EIC-Aquatic} = \frac{3.00 \times 10^2 \text{ kg} \times 10^9 \text{ µg/kg}}{1.214 \times 10^{11} \text{ l/d} \times 365} = 0.0068 \text{ ppb}$$

Furthermore, with respect to compliance with the categorical exclusion criteria to the best of our knowledge, no extraordinary circumstances exist.

FIGURE 4.8
The NDA must include an environmental assessment or a claim for categorical exclusion, as shown here.

- Names and addresses of contract facilities for manufacturing or testing
- Batch analyses of testing of inactive ingredients and drug product

4.3.5   NDA Section 5: Nonclinical Pharmacology and Toxicology

The second technical section of the NDA provides a description or summary of all animal and *in vitro* studies with the drug.

The *table of contents* should clearly identify all studies not previously submitted to the IND.

Include a narrative *summary* of notable findings in all studies and a discussion of notable findings across the various studies. This discussion might include intra- and interspecies differences or similarities. Provide a tabular display of data, and cross-references to individual study reports.

Provide *individual study reports*, including pharmacology, toxicology, and ADME studies. For the pharmacology studies, present data as follows:

1. Effects related to the therapeutic indication, such as the pharmaco-dynamic ED_{50} in dose-ranging studies and the mechanism of action (if known)
2. Secondary pharmacological actions in order of clinical importance as possible adverse effects or as ancillary therapeutic effects
3. Interactions with other drugs (or cross-reference the location of the information in any of the above subsections)

The toxicology information must include information on acute toxicity, multidose toxicity (including subchronic, chronic, and carcinogenicity) and special toxicity studies, as well as reproduction studies and mutagenicity studies.

Present toxicology data by intended route of administration in the following order:

1. Oral
2. Intravenous
3. Intramuscular
4. Interperitoneal
5. Subcutaneous
6. Inhalation
7. Topical
8. Other *in vivo*
9. *In vitro*

Provide data for males first, followed by females, then groups.

For acute toxicity studies, present the animal study data in the following order:

1. Mouse
2. Rat
3. Hamster
4. Other rodent(s)
5. Rabbit
6. Dog
7. Monkey
8. Other nonrodent mammal(s)
9. Nonmammals

Present the ADME data in the following order:

1. Absorption
2. Distribution (protein binding, tissue distribution, accumulation)
3. Metabolism (enzyme induction or inhibition)
4. Excretion (serum half-life)

When compiling the Nonclinical Pharmacology section, be sure to identify the structural formula for all names by which the compound is referred. Identify all metabolites and reference compounds by chemical name or structural formula. Include batch or lot numbers of the test substance and specify all animal suppliers and animal strains used in the studies. Reports of any studies used to determine safety should include Good Laboratory Practice (GLP) statements per 314.50 (d) (2) (v) and 21 CFR Part 58.

4.3.6 NDA Section 6: Human Pharmacokinetics and Bioavailability

This technical section includes data from Phase I safety and tolerance studies in healthy volunteers and ADME studies.

The first element in this section is a *tabulated summary of studies* showing all *in vivo* biopharmaceutic studies performed. List them in descending order of importance.

Include a *summary of data and overall conclusions*. This summary should address all bioavailability and pharmacokinetic data and conclusions. It should include a table of PK parameters, giving the values for the major parameters (mean and % cv) such as:

- Peak concentration (Cmax)
- Area under the curve (AUC)
- Time to reach peak concentration (tmax)
- Elimination constant
- Distribution volume (Vd)
- Plasma and renal clearance
- Urinary excretion

Drug formulation information should include a list of all formulations used in clinical trials and in *in vivo* bioavailability and PK studies (see Figure 4.9). Identify the studies in which each formulation was used. In addition, note any significant manufacturing and formulation changes for the drug product that affected those batches used in bioavailability and PK studies (see Figure 4.10).

Summarize the *analytical methods* used in each *in vivo* biopharmaceutic study. Include detailed information, such as sensitivity, linearity, specificity,

Firm _____

Drug _____

NDA/ANDA _____

IN VIVO STUDY DATA SUMMARY

Study Number	Route of Administration Dosage Form	Dose	Cmax	Tmax	Vd	AuC	$t_{1/2}$	Urinary Excretion	CLp	CLr	Comments

FIGURE 4.9
Use this format to summarize *in vivo* study data for the Human Pharmacokinetics and Bioavailability technical section.

Firm _____

Drug _____

NDA/ANDA _____

DRUG FORMULATION DEVELOPMENT SUMMARY

Study Number	Lot No.	Dosage Form and Strength	Batch Size	Formulation or significant Manufacturing Change (if any) and reason for change	Effect of change

FIGURE 4.10
Use this format to summarize drug formulation development information for the Human Pharmacokinetics and Bioavailability technical section.

and reproducibility of the analytical test methods used in each study (see Figure 4.11).

Provide *dissolution* data on each strength and dosage form for which an approval is sought. Include a comparative dissolution study with the lot in the *in vivo* biopharmaceutic study. Include a summary of the product's dissolution performance, dissolution method, and specifications (see Figure 4.12 and.Figure 4.13).

This technical section must include *individual study reports* from any of five types of biopharmaceutic studies as described below:

Firm _____

Drug _____

NDA/ANDA _____

IN VIVO ANALYTICAL METHODS SUMMARY

Study Number	Submission Date	Type of Biol. Fluid	Method	Sensitivity of Method/Range	Specificity (Parent/ Metabolites)

FIGURE 4.11
Use this format to summarize *in vivo* analytical methods for the Human Pharmacokinetics and Bioavailability technical section.

Firm _____

Drug _____

NDA/ANDA _____

DRUG PRODUCT DISSOLUTION TESTING

Date of Test	Dosage Form and Strength	Lot Number	Dissolution Apparatus	Media/ Temperature	Speed of Rotation/Flow	Collection Times	Units Tested Range/Mean % Dissolved /% C.V.

FIGURE 4.12
Provide drug product dissolution data for each strength and dosage form submitted for approval in a table like the one shown here.

Pilot or background studies are carried out in a small number of subjects to provide preliminary assessment of ADME information as a guide to the design of early clinical trials and definitive kinetic studies.

Bioavailability/bioequivalence studies include several types of studies. Bioavailability studies define the rate and extent of absorption relative to a reference dosage form, such as IV, solution, or suspension. Bioequivalence studies compare pharmaceutical alternatives to establish equivalent extents and, where necessary, equivalent rates of absorption. Dosage strength equivalence studies show that equivalent doses of different dosage forms deliver the same amount of drug. For example, three doses of 100 milligrams (mg) is equivalent to a single 300 mg tablet.

Firm _____

Drug _____

NDA/ANDA _____

PROPOSED PRODUCT DISSOLUTION METHOD
AND SPECIFICATION

(1) Dosage Form

(2) Strength(s)

(3) Apparatus Type

(4) Media

(5) Volume

(6) Speed of Rotation (Rate of Flow for Flow-through Apparatus)

(7) Sampling Time(s)

(8) Brief Description of Dissolution Analytical Method

(9) Recommended Dissolution Specification

FIGURE 4.13
Include a summary of the drug product's dissolution performance, dissolution method, and specifications.

Pharmacokinetic studies are designed to define the drug's time course and, where appropriate, major metabolite concentrations in the blood and other body compartments. With this type of study, it is critical to demonstrate the rate of drug absorption and delivery to systemic circulation and the rate of elimination of the drug through metabolic or excretory processes. Dose-dependent changes in kinetic parameters are of particular interest. Other information from PK studies may include the influence of demographic characteristics such as age, gender, or race; certain disease states (e.g., cirrhosis); or external factors such as meals or other drugs. Include information on studies that show drug binding to biological constituents such as plasma protein or red blood cells; studies performed in special patient populations (e.g., steroid-dependent patients), and studies performed under conditions of therapeutic use.

Other in vivo studies include any bioavailability studies that employ pharmacological or clinical measurements or endpoints in humans or animals. In addition, chemical analysis of body fluids in animals may be used when appropriate.

In vitro studies should include studies designed to define the release rate of a drug substance from the dosage form. Such studies are conducted in order to characterize a dosage form and to assure consistent batch-to-batch behavior. Other *in vitro* studies may be conducted for further characterization of the drug moiety (e.g., protein binding).

4.3.7   NDA Section 7: Microbiology

The microbiology technical section is only required for antiinfective drug products.

Antimicrobial drugs differ from other classes of drugs in that they are designed to affect microbial physiology rather than patient physiology. *In vitro* and *in vivo* studies on the effects of the antimicrobial drug on the microorganism are critical in establishing the new drug's effectiveness, especially if the microorganism has the potential to develop, or has developed, resistance to other antimicrobial drugs. It is usually necessary to compare the microbiological testing of the new drug to other closely related antimicrobial products.

This section requires the following technical information and data:

1. A complete description of the biochemical basis of the drug's action on microbial physiology.

2. The drug's antimicrobial spectrum. Include results of *in vitro* studies demonstrating the concentrations of the drug that are required for effective use.

3. Describe any known mechanisms of resistance to the drug and provide information or data of any known epidemiologic studies demonstrating prevalence to resistance factors.

4. Clinical microbiology laboratory methods, such as *in vitro* sensitivity discs, necessary to evaluate effective use of the drug.

4.3.8   NDA Section 8: Clinical Data

This technical section of the NDA comprises ten elements. The document's largest and most complex section, the clinical data and analyses are key to the FDA's understanding of the new drug's safety and effectiveness.

The first element in this section is a *list of investigators and list of INDs and NDAs*. The list of investigators should include all investigators who have used any dosage form. Alphabetize the list and note each investigator's address, the type of study, the study identifier, and its location in the NDA. Provide a list of all known INDs under which the drug, in any dosage form, has been studied. Also include any relevant NDA of which the applicant is aware.

The next element is the *background/overview of clinical investigations*. This narrative should describe the general approach and rationale used in developing the clinical data. It should explain how information about the drug derived from clinical pharmacology studies led to critical features of the clinical studies. The narrative should support the basis for the design features of the clinical trials, such as number of patients, duration, selection criteria, and controls. The overview should provide references to FDA clinical guidelines, explaining any deviations from them, and reference any discussions between the FDA and the drug sponsor. Address the reason for selecting areas of special interest, such as demographics, gender or drug interactions, and discuss any effectiveness or safety issues raised by other drugs in the same pharmacologic or therapeutic class. Finally, answer any specific questions raised by the clinical trials for the study drug or by other similar drugs that were not answered in the clinical program.

The *clinical pharmacology* section should include ADME studies, pharmacodynamic dose range, and dose response studies, and any other studies of the drug's action. The format and order of presentation is as follows:

1. A table of all studies grouped by study type. Provide the investigators, study numbers, start date, and location of the report in the NDA.

2. For each group of studies, a brief synopsis of each study

3. An overall summary of the clinical pharmacology data

For the *controlled clinical trials* section, provide the following material in the order presented below:

1. A table of all studies

2. Full clinical trial reports of all controlled studies in the following order:

   a. Completed studies (U.S. studies followed by non-U.S. studies and any published trials)

   b. Ongoing studies with interim results (same order as above)

   c. Incomplete or discontinued studies (same order as above)

3. Full reports of dose-comparison concurrent control studies, followed by those for "no-treatment" concurrent control, active control studies, and historical control studies

The above material may be followed by an optional summary of all of the controlled clinical studies, but it is preferable to include the results in the integrated summaries elsewhere at the end of the clinical data section.

Uncontrolled clinical trials generally do not contribute substantial evidence for the effectiveness of a drug. They may be used to provide support for controlled studies and to provide critical safety information. This section should include a table of all studies. Group full reports of studies according to completeness and availability of Case Report Forms (CRFs). Incorporate the summary of these studies into the integrated summaries.

The *other studies and information* section should include a description and analysis of any additional information that the applicant has obtained from any source, foreign or domestic, that is relevant to evaluating the product's safety and effectiveness. It should include a table of all studies followed by reports of other controlled and uncontrolled studies. These should be followed by information on commercial marketing experience and foreign regulatory actions, including:

- List of countries in which the drug has been approved
- Details of any rejected registrations
- Copies of approved labeling (package inserts) from major regions such as Europe, Canada, Australia, New Zealand, and Japan
- Any other reports from the literature not provided elsewhere in the NDA

The purpose of the *integrated summary of effectiveness data* is to demonstrate substantial evidence of effectiveness for each claimed indication. It should also include a summary of evidence supporting the dosage and administration section of the labeling, including the dosage and dose interval recommended, and evidence regarding individualization of dosing and any need for dosage modifications for specific subgroups. Include a table of all studies.

The narrative should first identify the adequate and well-controlled studies. Next, compare and analyze the results of all controlled trials. Only pool data across similar studies. If the studies did not support the anticipated conclusions, explain the discrepancy. Discuss uncontrolled studies to the extent that they contribute supportive evidence of effectiveness.

Provide an integrated summary and analysis of all data relevant to the relationship of dose response or blood level response to effectiveness. Include data from animal, pharmacokinetic, pharmacodynamic, and controlled and uncontrolled studies. Explain how this information comes to bear on dose selection, dose interval, starting and maximal dosing, method of dose titration, and any other instructions in the proposed labeling. The effectiveness summary should also include an analysis of responses in subsets of patients. Address drug/demographic, drug/drug, and drug/disease interactions. Describe any evidence of long-term effectiveness, tolerance, and withdrawal effects.

The *integrated summary of safety information* should incorporate safety data from all sources, including pertinent animal data, clinical studies, and foreign marketing experience. The database from which every analysis is derived must be carefully defined.

This section requires a table of all studies and extent-of-exposure tables. The latter must include patient exposure by time period, by gender, by other subgroups, and by dose.

Describe the demographics and other characteristics of the entire drug-exposed population and also of logical groups of studies.

Provide a narrative discussion of adverse events in all studies and support it with tabulations and analyses. Group studies (i.e., controlled, similar duration, foreign/domestic) to determine event rates. Additionally, group adverse events by body system. Analyze the adverse events to compare treatment and control rates, relationship to the study drug, dose, duration of treatment, cumulative dose, demographics, and other variables. Display and analyze deaths and dropouts due to adverse events and other serious events. Evaluate them in terms of their relationship to the study drug.

Present an analysis of clinical laboratory data, evaluating clinically significant abnormalities. Summarize adverse events and laboratory abnormalities from sources other than clinical trials.

Summarize any animal data pertinent to human safety, emphasizing carcinogenicity and reproductive toxicology results. Include an integrated analysis of data from animal and human studies that show any relationship between dose response and adverse events.

Include a discussion of drug/drug interactions, include any potential interactions, from any source. Summarize any drug/demographic or drug/disease interactions.

Any pharmacologic effects of the drug other than the property of principal interest must be discussed, as should long-term effects and data from any long-term studies. Summarize specific studies regarding or any evidence of withdrawal effects.

Drug abuse and overdosage information is required if the drug has potential for abuse. Describe and analyze studies or information related to abuse of the drug. Include a proposal for scheduling under the Controlled Substances Act.

Ordinarily the *integrated summary of benefits and risks of the drug* recapitulates the evidence for effectiveness and safety. This section can also include information on the presence of a particularly severe known or potential human toxicity as well as a positive, or possibly positive, carcinogenicity finding. It may include information that indicates marginal or inconsistent effectiveness. It may also point to a particularly limited database or the use of surrogate endpoints.

4.3.9   NDA Section 9: Safety Update Reports

A pending application must be updated when new safety data becomes available that could affect any of the following:

- Statements in draft labeling
- Contraindications
- Warnings
- Precautions
- Adverse events

Safety update reports are not to be used to submit any new final reports that may impact FDA review time unless the FDA agrees at the pre-NDA meeting that it will accept the reports in this manner.

Safety updates are submitted 4 months (120 days) after the initial application, following the receipt of an approval letter and at any other time that the FDA requests such an update.

4.3.10   NDA Section 10: Statistics

This technical section includes descriptions and documentation of the statistical analyses performed to evaluation the controlled clinical trials and other safety information. It must include copies of:

- All controlled clinical trial reports
- Integrated efficacy and safety summaries
- Integrated summary of risks and benefits

4.3.11   NDA Section 11: Case Report Form Tabulations

This section must include complete tabulations for each patient from every adequately or well-controlled Phase II and Phase III efficacy study, and from every Phase I clinical pharmacology study. It also must include tabulations of safety data from *all* clinical studies. Routine submission of data from uncontrolled studies is not required.

Note that data listings are most often placed with the final reports in each section rather than with the CRF tabulations.

4.3.12   NDA Section 12: Case Report Forms (CRFs)

It is necessary to include the complete CRF for each patient who died during a clinical study and for any patients who were dropped from the study due to an adverse event, regardless of whether the AE is considered to be related to the study drug, even if the patient was receiving a placebo or comparative drug.

Additional CRFs must be provided at the request of the FDA.

4.4   The NDA in CTD Format

As noted above, ICH has developed a Common Technical Document to streamline regulatory submissions in Europe, the U.S. and Japan. CTD is an information format that contains clinical, nonclinical, and manufacturing technical data (see Figure 4.14).

The CTD format features well-defined modules, with a highly specific structure and numbering of sections within the modules. It makes a clear distinction between subjective information sections and objective information sections. It allows for some flexibility within the modules, particularly at the lower levels. Module 1 is not harmonized; that is, it includes documents specific to each region, such as application forms and proposed labeling. This content is specific to each of the three ICH regions (see Figure 4.15, Figure 4.16).

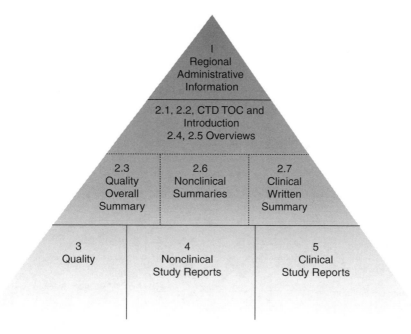

FIGURE 4.14
The Common Technical Document developed by ICH is organized into well-defined modules.

CTD	NDA: 314.50	
Module 1	(a)	Application Form
	(c)(2)(i)	Annotated Text of Proposed Labeling
	(d)(1)(v)	Statement of Field Copy
	(e)	Samples and Labeling
	(h)	Patent Information
	(i)	Patent Certification
	(j)	Claimed Exclusivity
	(k)	Financial Certification or Disclosure
Module 2	(b)	Comprehensive Table of Contents
	(c)	Summaries
	(d)(5)(vii)	Abuse Potential
Module 3	(d)(1)	CMC
Module 4	(d)(2)	Nonclinical Pharmtox
Module 5	(d)(3)	Human Pharmacokinetics
	(d)(4)	Microbiology
	(d)(5)	Clinical Data
	(d)(6)	Statistical Section
	(d)(7)	Pediatric Use
	(f)	CRF and CRT

FIGURE 4.15
This table shows which sections of the NDA, numbered per 314.50, are included in each of the five CTD modules.

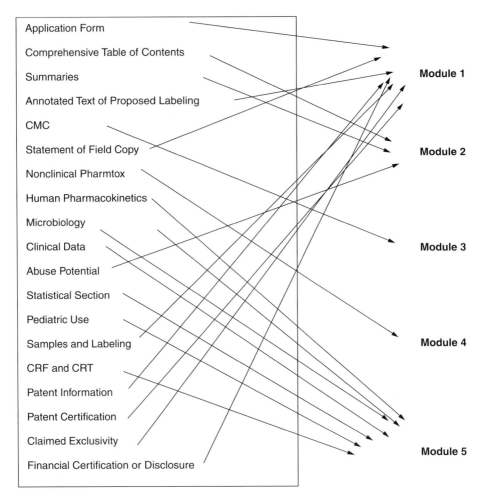

FIGURE 4.16
This listing shows where each section of the NDA is included in the CTD format.

The CTD guidance addresses format, not technical or scientific content. Content and requirement are covered in the ICH Technical Guidelines sections Quality (Q), Safety (S), and Efficacy (E.) The CTD format can be applied to the NDA content, as a comparison of the tables of contents of the two documents shows.

Use of the CTD format benefits both regulatory agencies and the pharmaceutical industry. In addition to enhancing reviews, the CTD's use of common elements facilitates communications between the agencies and the applicants and simplifies the exchange of information between regulatory authorities. The document also provides a common basis for continuous improvement of Good Regulatory Practices.

Using the CTD significantly reduces the time and resources necessary for sponsors to compile global registration applications. It provides a consistent order for data presentation and allows more flexible utilization of multiregional resources.

As of July 2003, Europe and Japan implemented the CTD, and the format is accepted, but not required, in the U.S. The FDA will accept the CTD format for NDAs and biologics license applications (BLAs), amendments, and supplements. If traditional NDA/BLA and CTD formats are to be placed in the same submission, however, prior FDA agreement is required. Any deviations from the guidance should be discussed at the pre-NDA/BLA meeting. Presubmission meetings will continue to be essential while the industry transitions to the CTD format and regulatory authorities become more familiar with CTD reviews.

5

Meeting with the FDA

Alberto Grignolo

CONTENTS

Face-to-face meetings with the FDA are a critical component of the regulatory review and approval process for new prescription drugs, biologics, and medical devices. These direct exchanges between Agency personnel and company scientists provide a forum for the sharing of information that is essential to demonstrating the safety, efficacy, and quality of a product to the FDA's satisfaction. The purpose of this chapter is to illustrate the types and objectives of various meetings with the FDA and to highlight some of the pitfalls and critical success factors associated with Agency interactions. While the main focus of the chapter is on drugs, the principles apply broadly to all meetings with the FDA.

Successful meetings with the FDA depend on three key factors: good science and good medicine; regulatory knowledge; and sound management of the meeting process. While a pharmaceutical product's approval is ultimately determined by the strength and adequacy of its scientific data, the way a sponsor interacts with the FDA throughout the lengthy drug development and regulatory review process can spell the difference between a relatively smooth, timely approval and a costly delay or rejection of an application. A product's chances for approval can be substantially increased if the sponsor manages the meeting process in a way that presents the scientific data effectively and facilitates reaching consensus on key issues.

If handled properly, these meetings can actually reduce the approval time for a new product. A study by the Tufts Center for the Study of Drug Development indicated that companies that hold effective pre-IND and end-of-Phase-II meetings with the FDA achieve shorter clinical development times.[1] This is a significant finding for the highly competitive pharmaceutical industry, where time-to-market is a crucial success factor. By employing the right resources and the right approach — and avoiding some common pitfalls — sponsors can take full advantage of the opportunities presented by FDA meetings to expedite the review process and help their products reach the market more quickly.

5.1   Types of FDA Meetings

The purpose of meeting with the FDA and its Review Divisions is to present proposals, provide answers, and resolve scientific and technical issues that arise concerning the development of a pharmaceutical product at various stages of the regulatory review process. These meetings also mark major development milestones, helping to determine if a product will be able to move forward to the next stage. Some of the most important types of FDA meetings are:

- **Pre-IND meetings**, where a sponsor presents characterization, manufacturing, nonclinical test data, and other information, and discusses the initial plan and protocols for clinical trials. The goal of these meetings is to receive FDA feedback on the proposed studies and to reach agreement on what information the sponsor needs to submit in the IND application so that it is likely to be placed on active status by the FDA (rather than being placed on hold due to safety concerns on the part of the Agency).

- **End-of-Phase-II meetings**, which are, perhaps, the most critical regulatory meetings during the development process. The sponsor is expected to provide proof of concept for the product through early efficacy data and other information demonstrating that the drug is performing a desired function. Equally important, Phase III trial

---

[1] DiMasi, J.A. and Manocchia, M., Initiatives to speed new drug development and regulatory review: The impact of FDA-Sponsor conferences, *Drug Inf. J.*, 31, 771–788, 1997.

designs are discussed during these meetings, including the types of information on indications, dosing, safety, and manufacturing that the FDA would expect to see in a strong NDA or BLA.

- **Special Protocol and *Ad Hoc* Technical meetings**, which are held to discuss and resolve specific technical issues that arise during drug development, including detailed review of key clinical protocols, discussion of challenging manufacturing issues, or review of carcinogenicity study protocols.

- **Pre-NDA/BLA meetings**, where a sponsor and the FDA typically discuss process-oriented issues concerning an upcoming application — how the data will be presented and how the application will be organized.

- **Advisory Committee meetings**, which take place as a public forum after an NDA/BLA submission, are conducted for certain products when the FDA wants to obtain the advice of academic, medical, and other external experts about the approvability of an application. The FDA names a panel of experts to hold public meetings about the submission.

- **Labeling meetings**, where the negotiations take place between the FDA and the sponsor on the specific language of the product labeling (prescribing information). These meetings are held after an NDA/ BLA is submitted and are the final and critical stage in drug development prior to FDA approval of a drug.

There are some variations among the three FDA Centers focused on drugs, biologics, and medical devices for human use — CDER, CBER, and CDRH — concerning the different types of meetings, as well as differences among the divisions within the each center. A guidance document — Guidance for Industry: Formal Meetings with Sponsors and Applicants for PDUFA Products — is available from the FDA that details the regulations covering these meetings. Meeting guidelines are also published by each of the Centers (see Table 5.1 for information about obtaining these documents).

In addition, meetings with the FDA are classified as one of three different types — Type A, B, or C — for the purpose of setting priorities and timelines for action, based on their urgency. A Type A meeting is one that is immediately necessary to resolve an issue that is preventing a drug development program from moving forward — a high priority or "critical path" meeting. An example is a Phase III study in which the dosage specified in the trial protocol is not effective, requiring a new study design or protocol. Type B meetings are those with normal priorities, including pre-IND, end-of-Phase-II, and pre-NDA meetings. Type C meetings, with the lowest priority, encompass any other type of meeting. Meetings involving issues with a submitted NDA/BLA take priority over other meetings because of performance targets established by PDUFA for FDA for processing submissions. A meeting's classification determines its

TABLE 5.1

How to Obtain Meeting Guidance Information from the FDA

Guidance Document	Web Site Address
Guidance for Industry: Formal Meetings With Sponsors and Applicants for PDUFA Products	http://www.fda.gov/cder/guidance/2125fnl.pdf
Formal Meetings Between CDER and CDER's External Constituents	http://www.fda.gov/cder/mapp/4512-1.pdf
Guidance for Industry: IND Meetings for Human Drugs and Biologics; Chemistry, Manufacturing and Controls Information	http://www.fda.gov/cber/gdlns/ind052501.pdf
Disclosure of Materials Provided to Advisory Committees in Connection with Open Advisory Committee Meetings Convened by the Center for Drug Evaluation and Research Beginning on January 1, 2000	http://www.fda.gov/cder/guidance/3431fnl.pdf
Draft Guidance for Industry: Disclosing Information Provided to Advisory Committees in Connection with Open Advisory Committee Meetings Related to the Testing or Approval of Biologic Products and Convened by the Center for Biologics Evaluation and Research	http://www.fda.gov/cber/gdlns/advguid0201.htm
Early Collaboration Meetings Under the FDA Modernization Act (FDAMA), Final Guidance for Industry and CDRH Staff	http://www.fda.gov/cdrh/ode/guidance/310.htm
Special Protocol Assessment	http://www.fda.gov/cder/guidance/3764fnl.pdf

scheduling: Type A meetings should occur within 30 calendar days of the FDA receiving the request; Type B, within 60 days; and Type C, within 75 days. While the sponsor makes the request for a certain meeting classification, it is the FDA that makes the final classification and determination of a meeting's priority.

5.2   FDA Expectations

In addition to the FDA's formal regulations covering these different types of meetings, an informal "FDA meetings way" has evolved over time with common criteria and characteristics about how the Agency generally expects its interactions with the pharmaceutical industry to be conducted in any type of meeting. Understanding and abiding by these expectations is just as important as following the formal regulations.

The most important characteristic to remember is that all FDA meetings are *serious and formal*. The main order of business in every meeting is a discussion of science and medicine, and the orientation of that discussion is scientist-to-scientist. A typical FDA meeting might be compared to a scientific "summit," with chief negotiators, numerous people in attendance, a limited timeframe, a very specific agenda, and minute-takers. Consistent with their scientific orientation, the emphasis at FDA meetings is on building consensus based on sound scientific data. That also means that the attendees representing the sponsor should mostly be scientists who are prepared to discuss the relevant data. Financial and product promotional discussions are seldom, if ever, appropriate at FDA meetings.

What does the FDA expect from a sponsor during these meetings? First and foremost, the Agency expects discussion of a product to be supported by good science and good medicine. All meetings should be focused on scientific or medical issues that directly relate to the product and FDA regulations. Every meeting should also have a clear purpose. Sponsors must know what they want to accomplish, develop a meeting agenda that helps answer the key questions, then stick to that agenda. In addition, the sponsor is expected to be well prepared — to bring the right people who understand the issues involved. Sponsors must be knowledgeable about the applicable regulations and guidelines for their products as well, so that they are speaking the same language as the FDA. A sponsor should also be careful to schedule meetings with the FDA at the appropriate times, when useful discussions are possible and the company is truly seeking Agency input.

Another important characteristic of FDA meetings is that sponsors are expected to present positions for discussion, rather than ask the Agency open-ended questions about what should be done. The FDA is not in the business of developing drugs or designing sponsors' drug development plans. What the Agency will do is comment on a sponsor's plans, provide input, voice objections, and give advice based on its broad experience with other sponsors and drugs (within the bounds of maintaining confidentiality on sponsor-proprietary information, of course). Instead of asking FDA personnel to suggest a course of action, a sponsor should tell them about the company's plans, then seek the Agency's scientific input and concurrence.

5.3 Preparing for FDA Meetings

Because preparation is essential for a successful FDA meeting, sponsors should allow plenty of time in advance of any meeting to strategize, organize materials, select attendees, and rehearse key discussions. This preparation begins with scheduling the meetings. As discussed above, every meeting is classified as Type A, B, or C, and each classification carries its own timeline for scheduling and the premeeting submission of documentation. If a Type

A meeting is requested, the FDA will expect the sponsor to provide justification for the high priority and will make the final decision about the classification. It is also important to request the meeting through the proper person in the Review Division (usually the Project Manager assigned to the product or sometimes a Meeting Coordinator) to avoid confusion or delay.

Once a meeting has been scheduled, the sponsor must submit supporting documentation at least 2 weeks in advance of Type A and C meetings, and at least 1 month in advance of a Type B meeting. This documentation, called a Briefing Package or Briefing Document, is the most critical part of the premeeting preparations, because it sets the agenda for the meeting and defines the issues to be discussed. To have a successful meeting, it is essential for the sponsor to provide a strong, focused Briefing Document that clearly states the purpose of the meeting and the issues upon which the sponsor seeks consensus. The documents must also provide sufficient background information on the drug (including chemistry, manufacturing, nonclinical and clinical summaries and data tables) to orient the FDA attendees to those issues. In recent years, the Briefing Document has completely replaced the sponsor's opening presentations at meetings with FDA. Meetings now begin with an immediate discussion of the issues raised in the Briefing Document, which the FDA personnel have read and analyzed in advance of the meeting. In that context, a sponsor presentation of the same information is superfluous and a poor use of the limited time made available by FDA for the meeting (usually 1 hour).

When planning a meeting with the FDA, the sponsor will be faced with the important decision of selecting the right people to attend the meeting. This decision can present significant internal challenges for the sponsor when dealing with corporate politics, organizational issues, and egos. However, the selection criteria should always be focused on choosing those who can contribute to the *scientific and technical* discussions, because that is what is important to the FDA. Depending on the stage of product development, a sponsor might draw on internal (or external consultant) expertise in areas such as pharmacology, toxicology, pharmacokinetics, chemistry, manufacturing, clinical development, and biostatistics, as well as regulatory affairs.

While marketing personnel are always interested in the timelines for drug approval, they should be "silent partners" at most FDA meetings (if they attend at all) except when the negotiation of the final product labeling occurs. Because the sponsor's marketing and promotional activities will be directly affected by the FDA-approved language of the product labeling, it is appropriate for marketing personnel to participate in the labeling negotiation process.

In general, company lawyers and CEOs should not attend typical FDA meetings unless there are legal issues to be discussed (which would be unusual at scientific meetings with the Agency) or unless the CEO is also the sponsor's chief scientist, with intimate knowledge of the science behind the drug. Expert consultants can play a role if they can help a sponsor articulate particular scientific or regulatory positions.

In preparing for an FDA meeting, it is also important to recognize the decision-making authority of the people who will be attending for the Agency, so that the issues being debated are commensurate with the authority of the attendees. For example, technical commitments can only be made by a therapeutic area Division Director or higher, not by the Division Project Manager, who is a sponsor's usual day-to-day contact. Drug approval decisions can only be made by Division Directors and Office Directors. Policy decisions can only come from a Center Director or the FDA Commissioner's Office. It is not appropriate for the sponsor to discuss high-level FDA policy (e.g., "Why do INDs exist?") with a Division Director.

Rehearsals are the final ingredient in good meeting preparation. A team leader should be appointed to coordinate the company's responses during the meeting with the FDA. The role of each team member at the meeting should be discussed and decided in advance, and all attendees should practice what they are going to say — although formal presentations are not typically made. Emphasis should be placed on keeping all attendees focused on the crucial issues to be discussed at the meeting and the outcomes desired by the sponsor. It is often useful to ask the regulatory affairs professional on the team to "role play" the FDA during rehearsals — asking tough questions and challenging the sponsor's positions to help the team members think through their answers carefully and thoroughly.

5.4   Conduct at FDA Meetings

How should attendees conduct themselves during an FDA meeting? The most important thing to remember is to *listen*. Introductory remarks should be brief and confined to introducing the sponsor team and stating briefly the purpose of the meeting from the sponsor's point of view. Also, the sponsor's team should not plan to make a formal presentation to convey the company's case — although it is always a good idea to have back-up material (e.g., in the form of transparencies) ready to present in case questions arise. A properly prepared Briefing Document will present the company's case in advance and spell out the issues to be discussed during the meeting.

In fact, most FDA meetings now begin with the Agency providing its input and reaction to the Briefing Document submitted by the sponsor. Attendees should listen carefully to what the FDA personnel say, take extensive notes and, most important, *should not interrupt*. Once the discussions begin, let the sponsor team leader orchestrate the team's responses to FDA questions, and stay focused on the agenda and objectives of the meeting. It is essential that the sponsor's team avoid being aggressive, arrogant, condescending, or confrontational. Keep in mind that the goal of every FDA meeting — both for the sponsor and the Agency — is to seek consensus and resolve all issues professionally and scientifically so that the drug development effort can proceed. At the end of the meeting, be sure there is a clear understanding about any decisions that have been made, as well as any actions that need to be taken — and by whom. If there are action items to be addressed after the meeting, be sure to follow up promptly with the FDA.

According to its own guidelines, the Agency is expected to provide the official minutes of the meeting within 4 weeks. Delays are common, but the Agency is trying to improve its performance in this regard. A sponsor can request changes to the minutes, but should not expect to make wholesale alterations. The sponsor can also provide the company's own minutes of the meeting, which should be delivered to the FDA within 2 to 3 days to maximize the possibility that the sponsor's input will be considered in the FDA's minutes. It must be remembered that the FDA will consider its own minutes to be the only official record of the meeting.

5.5   Avoiding the Pitfalls

By understanding the FDA's expectations and following the above guidelines for a successful meeting, most sponsors should be able to avoid the common pitfalls that can slow the regulatory approval process and delay a product's progress toward the market. But because these mistakes continue to occur regularly, it is worthwhile to reiterate some of the more frequent slips that sponsors make during their encounters with the Agency.

One of the most common errors is to present the Agency with open-ended questions rather than reasoned proposals based on science. Here are some examples that illustrate the difference:

Open-Ended Questions

1. The Phase II trials showed that several different dosages were effective for this condition. What would you recommend as the dosage for the Phase III trials?
2. How many patients should be included in the Phase III trials?
3. This drug has shown efficacy against several diseases. Which one should be selected for development first?

Reasoned Proposals

1. Several dosages were tried, and the 5 mg and 10 mg doses seem to be the most promising for the Phase III trials (as shown in the Briefing Document). Do you agree?

2. A statistical power calculation shows that a Phase III study with 1,000 patients will provide valid results. Do you agree that 1,000 will be sufficient?

3. This drug has shown efficacy against several diseases. Condition X has been chosen for the first Phase III studies because there is no therapeutic alternative and enrollment can be completed rapidly. Do you concur?

Remember that it is not the role of the FDA to make scientific, marketing, or drug development decisions for sponsors, but to provide insight and guidance, based on the regulations and the Agency's expertise.

Here are some other important "Do's" and "Don'ts" for FDA meetings:

Do	Don't
Be prepared	Waste time
Be polite	Be aggressive or rude
Reach consensus	Argue or be confrontational
Meet at the appropriate time	Meet when discussion is not useful
Discuss key product issues	Socialize or make a sales pitch
Focus on the agenda	Bring up side issues or complaints
Bring scientists and technical experts	Bring lawyers and CEOs
Present strong data	Try to rely on charm or hype
Be open and truthful	Lie or stonewall
Be clear	Obfuscate
Know key contacts	Go "blind" into the meeting
Rely on the data	Rely on political clout
Be reliable	Fail to follow through on commitments

Avoiding these meeting pitfalls can spell the difference between a successful, productive relationship with the FDA and a contentious relationship that slows the regulatory process for everyone.

5.6 Specific Meeting Objectives

In addition to understanding the characteristics and approaches that are common to all FDA meetings, it is worthwhile to note the specific purposes and objectives of the major FDA meeting categories mentioned earlier in this chapter. It is also important to keep in mind that, while most are not mandatory, these meetings play a significant role in the successful development of any new drug.

5.6.1 Pre-IND Meetings

The pre-IND meeting has several important purposes — all of which are designed to prepare the FDA for the submission of the IND application for a new drug. If the sponsor is a small company or one that is not well known to the FDA, the pre-IND meeting presents an opportunity to discuss the company's background and qualifications. The most important objective of these meetings is to introduce the new drug to the FDA, including the presentation and discussion of the entity's characterization, manufacturing process, and other nonclinical data collected in the lab.

At this meeting, the sponsor will typically present the overall clinical investigational plan for the drug and relate that plan to the targeted labeling or prescribing information. The initial clinical protocol might also be discussed, and there could be agreement on some of the details of the protocol. If the sponsor is aware of any critical scientific or technical issues concerning the drug (e.g., nonclinical safety data showing slight liver enzyme elevations in an animal species), they would be introduced — and sometimes even resolved — in this meeting. The ultimate goal of the pre-IND meeting is for the sponsor to reach an agreement with the FDA that an IND can be submitted. It should be noted, however, that a successful pre-IND meeting does not guarantee that the FDA will activate the IND application after it is reviewed in detail. The agreement only means that there is no compelling reason why the IND should not be submitted for review.

5.6.2   End-Of-Phase-II Meetings

Sponsors should *always* have an end-of-Phase-II meeting before beginning Phase III clinical trials. The end-of-Phase-II meeting is an indispensable step in the drug development process. With the pivotal importance — and significant cost — of Phase III trials for new drugs, the end-of-Phase-II meeting is a vital opportunity to obtain the FDA's commitment on Phase III study designs and key trial endpoints. This meeting also gives the sponsor a chance to solicit FDA input on the final development plan, which can help "fine-tune" the approaches for CMC, toxicology, and other key data, as well as help shape the anticipated labeling language and claims.

When should an end-of-Phase-II meeting be held? It should be scheduled once the Phase II trials have produced the key data needed to support expanded trials. This means that an effective dose has been established, and the pharmacokinetic/pharmacodynamic understanding of the drug is well advanced. It also means that the earlier trials have produced the information needed to solidify the proposed labeling, and that the design for the Phase III trials is essentially complete. As the name implies, it should be held *before* the sponsor has made a commitment to the significant financial investment required for Phase III trials.

The Briefing Document for these meetings must be thorough and informative in order to solicit the most helpful feedback from the FDA, with detailed discussions of pertinent clinical and nonclinical data. A typical briefing package would include elements such as:

- Overview/development history to date
- Meeting agenda and participants
- Key outstanding issues and questions
- Draft prescribing (labeling) information
- Detailed Phase III clinical plan
- Nonclinical pharmacology and toxicology data
- Chemistry, manufacturing, and controls information
- Clinical pharmacology data
- Statistical analysis of early clinical trials

The best way for a sponsor to ensure a successful end-of-Phase-II meeting — in addition to having strong scientific data — is to present all of the relevant information about the drug openly and completely. Sponsors should state their positions about the compound and the trials clearly, and present a strong, well-designed Phase III development plan. There should be no attempt to hide any shortcomings of the early clinical data or to postpone difficult decisions. Any issues or problems will be even more difficult — and costly — if they are brought to the surface later in the development process. The sponsor's credibility can also be significantly damaged. Being forthright and working together with the FDA in a spirit of teamwork to resolve any issues will greatly increase the likelihood that this vital part of the regulatory process will reach a satisfactory conclusion.

5.6.3 Special Protocol Meetings

This is a fairly new category of meetings, which the FDA grants in connection with three specific aspects of the drug development process: carcinogenicity studies, stability studies, and Phase III trials that will support an efficacy claim. The FDA grants these meetings because regulators understand that these types of studies are costly and time-consuming. The meetings allow both parties to agree on study designs and end-points in advance, with the agreement being documented by a binding written document.

5.6.4 Pre-NDA Meetings

Before submitting an NDA, sponsors should *always* schedule a pre-NDA meeting with the FDA. These meetings will uncover any unresolved issues that might delay the review of the submission, orient the reviewers about the content and format of the NDA, and help sponsors understand key FDA expectations about the NDA contents — such as identifying critical studies and discussing proposed analyses.

From the FDA's point of view, the pre-NDA meeting provides an important opportunity to review the NDA plan and understand its content, which will facilitate the Agency's processing of the document. The FDA will want to review any issues that were raised at the End-of-Phase-II meeting to ensure that they have been addressed. The actual submission process will also be discussed, including its timing, format (electronic vs. paper, the organization of tables, etc.), and, increasingly, agreement on the Common Technical Document (CTD) format of the NDA. A successful pre-NDA meeting will produce a consensus that makes it likely the FDA will accept the NDA for review if the agreements reached at the meeting have been satisfied.

5.6.5   Advisory Committee Meetings

In some cases, the FDA may want to obtain outside expert opinions about an NDA and the approvability of a new drug. In those circumstances, the Agency has the authority to ask an official Advisory Committee to review the NDA and hold public meetings about whether the product should be approved for sale. The FDA maintains a number of standing Advisory Committees, each with a specific therapeutic focus (for the list of standing Advisory Committees, visit www.fda.gov/oc/advisory/default.htm). These Advisory Committee meetings are unique to the FDA (compared to its counterpart agencies in other countries) and also uniquely stressful for the sponsor — primarily because they are open to the public, including competitors, financial analysts, the media, patients, patient advocates, and other consumers. Regulations require that the sponsor's presentation materials to the Advisory Committee be made available to the public no later than 1 day before the meeting. At these meetings, the sponsor and the FDA have the opportunity to present key findings about the safety and efficacy of the product to the Committee. The Advisory Committee members offer their own views, discuss the benefits and risk of the drug and, at the end of the meeting, take a vote on whether to recommend it for FDA approval. The FDA is not obligated to follow the recommendations of its Advisory Committees, but it usually does.

Advisory Committee meetings are recorded on audio and videotape, and broadcast on the web. This unusual public forum is particularly risky for the sponsor because years of development and investment are at stake. Extensive preparation by the sponsor is essential to ensure that the company's position is presented thoroughly, concisely, and professionally. Many sponsors utilize both in-house and external consultant resources, and prepare hundreds or even thousands of back-up slides that can be used to respond to detailed questions by Advisory Committee members. It is not uncommon for sponsors to hold six to ten rehearsals in the weeks leading up to an Advisory Committee presentation. The main goal of the sponsor is to present the "case for approval" by demonstrating a favorable benefit–risk profile of the drug based on clinical and nonclinical data.

5.6.6 Labeling Meetings

Labeling meetings are the final link in the long chain of drug development. They occur at the end of the NDA review process, when the FDA and the sponsor meet to negotiate the formal language that describes to physicians what specific indications a product has been approved for, the recommended dosages, the side effects, and other specific information that physicians and patients need to know about a new prescription drug. This prescribing information is known as the product labeling.

All the effort that goes into developing a new drug begins with the goal to achieve a certain target labeling, because it is this prescribing information that determines how the product will be used and, ultimately, how successful it will be on the market. This approach is commonly known as "beginning with the end in mind," and it helps sponsors focus on a specific, achievable objective for a drug at an early stage of the development process.

With so much riding on the outcome, labeling meetings can sometimes involve very difficult negotiations to reach agreement on the final language. Several rounds of meetings may be required, and extensive internal consultations within the sponsor organization (e.g., with the Marketing Department) occur. It is increasingly common to hold labeling meetings via teleconference; this enables both the Agency and the sponsor to put the conversation on "mute" and work out their respective positions in private before resuming negotiations. While this removes the advantage of observing each other's body language, it usually accelerates the negotiation process. The importance of the outcome makes it even more vital to maintain a spirit of cooperation and consensus during this process. The fundamental goal of both the FDA and the sponsor is to bring a useful new medicine to the market; finding labeling language that satisfies both parties benefits everyone. Once the final language has been approved, the product can be launched.

5.7 Conclusion

While the information in this chapter should provide some guidance about the best way to approach meetings with the FDA, it also illustrates how complex and demanding the regulatory review process can be. How the sponsor works with the FDA throughout the approval process can have a substantial impact on the approval time for a new product. The best way to approach this process is to assemble the right resources with the knowledge and experience to manage your meeting strategy efficiently — allowing the scientific data to be presented effectively and promoting consensus on key product issues. By applying sufficient resources with the proper background to manage FDA meetings, a sponsor can substantially increase a product's chances for approval and significantly reduce time to market.

6

Biologics

James G. Kenimer and John J. Jessop

CONTENTS

6.1 Definition of a Biologic Product

Unfortunately, there is no precise definition that clearly delineates a biologic product from other drugs regulated by the FDA. The classification of a particular product as a "biologic" is the result of over 100 years of interaction between science and legislation. When viewed from today's perspective, some of the resultant classifications seem inconsistent and even confusing (for example, all hormones are regulated as drugs and all vaccines are regulated as biologics — regardless of their method of manufacture).

To understand the evolution requires a brief trip through history — back to St. Louis, MO, in 1901 (refer to CBER Website[1,2] for excellent reviews of biologic product regulatory history). At this time in American history the FDA did not exist, and there were no laws regulating the safety, efficacy, and purity of drug products. There was, however, significant advancement underway in the scientific community in the areas of vaccinology and immunology, resulting in vaccines for smallpox, rabies, cholera, typhoid, and plague as well as antitoxins for diphtheria and tetanus. The public health effect of these products was often dramatic, resulting in significant pressure for wide utilization. Unfortunately, there was not a similar level of pressure to ensure that the products were safe — not until 13 children died in St. Louis in October 1901 after receiving a diphtheria antitoxin preparation that was contaminated with tetanus toxin.

This tragedy resulted in the immediate passage by Congress, with virtually no debate or opposition, of the Biologics Control Act of 1902. Biologic products were defined as "… any virus, serum, toxin, antitoxin, therapeutic serum, vaccine, blood, blood component or derivative, allergenic product, or analogous products, or trivalent arsenic compound such as arsphenamine applicable to the prevention, treatment, or cure of diseases or injuries in man." Provisions of the Act included licensure requirements for both establishments and products, labeling requirements, facility inspection requirements, and penalties for violations including suspension and revocation of licenses. In 1944 the Biologics Control Act was incorporated with only minor changes into section 351 of the Public Health Service (PHS) Act, which forms the current legal basis for the FDA regulations covering biologic products as published in the Code of Federal Regulations (CFR) Title 21, Parts 600–680.

The Biologics Control Act authorized the Hygienic Laboratory (a laboratory of the Public Health and Marine Hospital Service) to issue regulations implementing the provisions of the Act. By 1904, 13 establishments had been inspected and licensed. Products were tested by the Hygienic Laboratory for purity and potency on a monthly basis. By 1921, the number of products monitored grew to 102, and by the 1930s, vaccines had been licensed for 30 bacterial species.

In 1934, the Hygienic Laboratory was renamed the National Institute of Health (the first institute in our current National Institutes of Health (NIH)) and by 1948 was known as the Division of Biologics Control within the

---

[1] Commemorating 100 Years of Biologics Regulation: Science and the Regulation of Biological Products — From a Rich History to a Challenging Future. CBER website at www.fda.gov/cber/inside/centscireg.htm

[2] Harry Meyer Jr. Memorial Lecture presented by Dr. Paul Parkman at the CBER Centennial, September 23–24, 2002. (See www.fda.gov/cber/inside/centscireg.htm)

National Microbiological Institute (later renamed the National Institute of Allergy and Infectious Diseases).

In the early 1940s the focus of biologic product development and regulation was on products, especially blood products and certain vaccines, which were needed by U.S. military personnel in World War II.

The next tragedy to affect the course of biologics regulations occurred in 1955, when several batches of Salk polio vaccine (a "killed" vaccine given by injection) produced by Cutter Laboratories were shown to have caused almost 200 cases of paralytic polio in vaccine recipients and close vaccine contacts. Examination of the vaccine demonstrated that procedures used for inactivation were not sufficiently rigorous. Congress again decided there was a need to strengthen the regulation of biologics, and transferred these functions to a newly created Division of Biologics Standards, an independent entity within the NIH. (Note that although the predecessor to the current FDA was established in 1906 with the passage of the Federal Food and Drugs Act, regulation of biologic products remained a function affiliated with the NIH, not the FDA, until 1972 — 70 years after the initial law was passed regulating these products).

In 1972, Congress again decided to reorganize the regulation of biologic products and transferred the staff and resources of the Division of Biologic Standards from the NIH to the FDA as the renamed Bureau of Biologics (the research and testing labs remained on the NIH campus in Bethesda, MD).

In 1982, the Bureau of Biologics was merged with the Bureau of Drugs to form the National Center for Drugs and Biologics. In 1988, the regulation of drugs and biologics were again separated within the FDA, and the current Center for Biologics Evaluation and Research (CBER) and the Center for Drugs Evaluation and Research (CDER) were created.

6.2   The Center for Biologics Evaluation and Research (CBER)

In 1993, CBER was reorganized into separate program offices for vaccines, blood, and therapeutic products. In 2002, a new Office of Cell and Gene Therapy Products was created within CBER, and in 2003, the Office of Therapeutic Products (with associated staff and products) was transferred to CDER (more on this in Section V), resulting in the current organization shown in Figure 6.1.

6.2.1   Biologic Products

Although many of the products formerly regulated by the Office of Therapeutic Research and Review (OTRR), including monoclonal antibodies and other "well-characterized" biologics, have been transferred to CDER, CBER still regulates a wide-range of complex products (see Table 6.1).

CENTER FOR BIOLOGICS EVALUATION AND RESEARCH

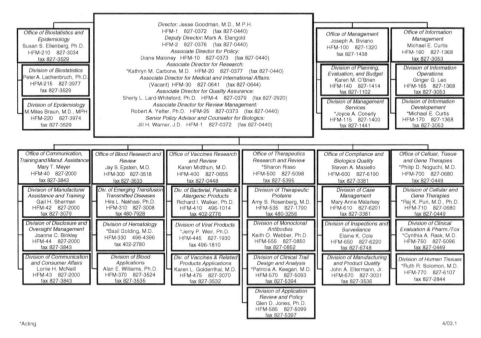

*Acting

4/03.1

FIGURE 6.1

Current CBER organizational chart.

TABLE 6.1

Products Regulated By CBER

OVRR (Office of Vaccines Research and Review)	Allergenic products
	Prophylactic Vaccines
	Various Antitoxins, Antivenins, Enzymes, and Venoms
	Various In-Vivo Diagnostic Products
OBRR (Office of Blood Research and Review)	Blood or blood products used for transfusion
	Pharmaceuticals manufactured from blood or blood products (ex., clotting factors)
	Medical devices used in the preparation or testing of blood products (ex., cell sorters, HIV test kits)
OCTGT (Office of Cellular, Tissue and Gene Therapies)	Human gene therapy products
	Various tissues intended for transplantation
	Various cellular products including stem cells
	Xenotransplantation products

TABLE 6.2

21 CFR Parts 600–680

Part 600	Biological Products: General
Part 601	Licensing
Part 606	Current Good Manufacturing Practice for Blood and Blood Components
Part 607	Establishment Registration and Product Listing for Manufacturers of Human Blood and Blood Products
Part 610	General Biological Products Standards
Part 640	Additional Standards for Human Blood and Blood Products
Part 660	Additional Standards for Diagnostic Substances for Laboratory Tests
Part 680	Additional Standards for Miscellaneous Products

Note that although most of the therapeutic protein products formerly regulated by OTRR at CBER have been transferred to CDER, they will continue (at least until the publication of this book) to be regulated as biologic products under the authority of the PHS Act.

6.2.2 Biologic Product Regulations

As mentioned in Section 6.1, the specific regulations governing market approval of biologic products are published in 21 CFR Part 600 thru Part 680 (Table 6.2). The Investigational New Drug (IND) regulations for biologic products are the same as for drugs regulated under the Federal Food, Drug, and Cosmetics (FD&C) Act, and are published in 21 CFR 312.

For certain unique medical devices and drugs CBER has the authority to issue approvals under the authority of the FD&C Act rather than the PHS Act. For medical devices CBER can approve products using either the 510k approval process or the Premarket Approval Application (PMA) process (21 CFR 814) [see www.fda.gov/cber/efoi/510k.htm or www.fda.gov/cber/efoi/pma.htm for listing of CBER-approved medical devices]. A listing of drugs approved by CBER using the New Drug Approval (NDA) regulations (21 CFR 314) can be found at www.fda.gov/cber/efoi/nda.htm.

6.2.3 Biologic Product Guidance Documents

The FDA makes extensive use of "guidance documents" to convey the agency's current thinking on the various topics and to provide clarification of how the various regulations should be interpreted. Although these documents are not legally binding to the FDA or to the public, they have become essential pieces in the regulatory information puzzle. Guidance documents dealing with various biologic product issues can be found at http://www.fda.gov/cber/guidelines.htm.

6.3   Preclinical Issues Unique to Biological Products

6.3.1   Introduction

Preclinical animal studies play an integral role in the development of a biological product. Preclinical pharmacology studies (*in vitro* and *in vivo* proof-of-concept studies) are required to demonstrate that there is a potential benefit for administration of a given biological product to humans for a proposed indication and are often useful in determining an appropriate starting dose for the clinic. Preclinical pharmacokinetics studies provide critical information on the bioavailability and systemic exposure of biological products administered by various routes of administration and certain dosing regimens while preclinical biodistribution studies offer information that can be used to identify potential target organs of toxicity. Toxicology studies (and to some extent safety pharmacology studies) are utilized to demonstrate that it is safe to administer a biological product to humans for the first time in a Phase I clinical trial. Toxicology studies continue to be utilized throughout biological product development to examine the safety of repeat dose administration of products for varying lengths of time as dictated by the Phase II and Phase III study protocols, to evaluate the effects of product administration on reproduction, to evaluate, in some limited circumstances, the mutagenic and carcinogenic potential of the product and, at times, as part of a comparability study, to demonstrate that significant manufacturing changes have not introduced new safety risks to the product.

Most importantly, due to the vast array of different biological product classes (vaccines, blood products, therapeutic proteins, monoclonal antibodies, cytokines, enzymes, gene therapy products, etc.) and the differences in chemical composition with respect to drugs (new chemical entities), the preclinical/nonclinical requirements for development of a given biological product can vary considerably from that for a drug. Furthermore, the diversity of biological product classes makes "one toxicology program fits all" a scientific impossibility. Therefore, many biological products raise safety issues that are unique to either the specific product or product class and the preclinical pharmacology and toxicology programs often need to be designed on a case-by-case basis.

6.3.2   Products and Regulatory Authority

The FDA has gone to great lengths to ensure that the preclinical pharmacology and toxicology study requirements for the various biological products (and drugs as well) in the U.S. are as consistent as possible. They have done so through publication of various guidance documents and participation in the International Conference on Harmonization (ICH) process. However, due to the diverse nature of the various biological product classes, the preclinical/nonclinical requirements are often somewhat different for each product class and are determined by the responsible FDA Office (OVRR, OBRR, and OCTGT).

The OVRR is responsible for the regulation of prophylactic vaccine development and is currently in the process of writing a guidance document for preclinical testing of vaccines. Up until now, preclinical requirements for prophylactic vaccines have been provided through the use of sound scientific principles and discussions with the OVRR staff. Current vaccine guidance documents that contain recommendations for preclinical testing include the Points to Consider on Plasmid DNA Vaccines for Preventive Infectious Disease Indications (1996) and Guidance for Industry: Considerations for Reproductive Toxicity Studies for Preventive Vaccines for Infectious Disease Indications (2000). There is also a joint FDA/NIH document available on the NIH website (www.niaid.nih.gov/daids/vaccine/Science) titled Vaccine Preclinical Toxicology Testing[3] that offers some useful guidance on the development of a preclinical toxicology program for a vaccine. This particular document is intended to provide HIV researchers with general advice on preclinical toxicology testing and preclinical product development and includes the disclaimer "The recommendations provided in this document do not reflect official U.S. Food and Drug Administration (FDA) policy. A FDA guidance in this area is under development ... "

The ICH S6 document Guidance for Industry: S6 Preclinical Safety Evaluation of Biotechnology-Derived Pharmaceuticals (1997) provides general guidance as to the preclinical/nonclinical toxicology testing for cytokines, plasminogen activators, recombinant plasma factors, growth factors, fusion proteins, enzymes, receptors, hormones, and monoclonal antibodies in addition to some recombinant DNA protein vaccines, chemically synthesized peptides, plasma derived products, endogenous proteins extracted from human tissue, and oligonucleotide drugs. This ICH S6 document should be used in conjunction with the ICH Guidance for Industry: M3 Nonclinical Safety Studies for the Conduct of Human Clinical Trials for Pharmaceuticals (1997) document that provides the appropriate timing and duration of toxicology studies as they relate to the proposed clinical trials. Other pertinent guidance documents providing recommendations for preclinical toxicology testing of biological products include Points to Consider in the Manufacture and Testing of Monoclonal Antibody Products for Human Use (1997) and Guidance for Industry: Guidance for Human Somatic Cell Therapy and Gene Therapy (1998). This latter document applies to preclinical testing of cellular and gene therapy products regulated by CBER/OCTGT.

There are a number of additional ICH and FDA guidance documents related to preclinical/nonclinical testing that can also apply to biological products under certain limited circumstances. These include the following:

---

[3] Vaccine Pre-clinical Toxicology Testing. P.Y. Chang, Ph.D., CDR Rebessa Sheets, Ph.D., Stuart Shapiro, M.D., Ph.D., Sally Hargus, Ph.D., and Marion Gruber, Ph.D. NIAID Division of HIV Vaccine Website at (www.niaid.nih.gov/daids/vaccine/Science/VRTT/00_Main.htm).

- Joint CDER/CBER document Guidance for Industry and Reviewers: Estimating the safe Starting Dose in Clinical Trials for Therapeutics in Adult Healthy Volunteers (December 2002)
- Joint CDER/CBER document Guidance for Industry: Nonclinical Studies for Development of Pharmaceutical Excipients (September 2002)
- FDA/CDER document Guidance for Industry: Single Dose Acute Toxicity Testing for Pharmaceuticals (August 1996)
- ICH S1A document Guideline on the Need for Carcinogenicity Studies of Pharmaceuticals (November 1995)
- ICH S1B document Testing for Carcinogenicity in Pharmaceuticals (July 1997)
- ICH S1C document Dose Selection for Carcinogenicity Studies in Pharmaceuticals (October 1994)
- ICH S2A document Genotoxicity: Specific Aspects of Regulatory Tests (July 1995)
- ICH S2B document Genotoxicity: Standard Battery Tests (July 1997)
- ICH S3A document entitled Toxicokinetics: Guidance on the Assessment of Systemic Exposure in Toxicity Studies (October 1994)
- ICH S3B document Pharmacokinetics: Guidance for Repeated Dose Tissue Distribution Studies (October 1994)
- ICH S4A document Duration of Chronic Toxicity Testing in Animals (Rodent and Non-Rodent) (September 1998)
- ICH S5A document Detection of Toxicity to Reproduction for Medicinal Products (June 1993)
- ICH S5B(M) document Reproductive Toxicology: Male Fertility Studies (November 1995)
- ICH S7A document Safety Pharmacology Studies for Human Pharmaceuticals (November 2000)

Please note that this list of guidance documents is not intended to be all-inclusive, but it does cover most of the major FDA and ICH documents that pertain to preclinical/nonclinical testing of biological products from IND through marketing approval.

6.3.3   The Biologics Development Process

For the FDA to become involved in the development of a biological product, a company must first demonstrate that it has a viable product to develop. This involves a demonstration of the ability to manufacture the product consistently. From a preclinical standpoint it involves a demonstration that there is a potential benefit for administration of the product to humans for a given indication. This is accomplished through completion of a number of *in vitro* and *in vivo* animal pharmacology (proof-of-concept) studies.

The next step in development is to show that it is safe to administer the product to humans for the first time (Phase I clinical trial). This evidence is provided from a well-designed program of appropriate preclinical studies, including safety pharmacology and general toxicology studies. Local tolerance studies and immunogenicity studies can also be required at this stage of development. This stage may also require completion of a single genetic toxicology study (Ames test) if appropriate to the specific product class and completion of reproductive toxicology studies if the drug is proposed for administration to pregnant women in the Phase I clinical trial. This preclinical information is submitted to the FDA in the form of an IND application proposing the initiation of a specific clinical trial.[4,5]

Once the biological product has been administered to humans in a Phase I clinical trial, additional nonclinical studies are required as the product development process proceeds. Additional general toxicology studies can be required to support clinical trials (Phase I, II, or III) that include dosing regimens with repeat dosing of longer duration than the initial Phase I trial. Additional general toxicology studies can also be requested in the event of an adverse finding in the ongoing clinical trials, in an attempt to better understand what is happening in the clinic (especially in the case of a vaccine). While genetic toxicology studies and carcinogenicity studies are usually inappropriate for biological products, there are a few situations in which these can apply. For example, genetic toxicology studies might be required for a conjugated protein product because of the presence of an organic linker molecule. Also, products that have the ability to support or induce proliferation of transformed cells and clonal expansion (e.g., growth factors, immunosuppressive agents) should be examined for the ability to stimulate growth of normal or malignant cells expressing the receptor. When *in vitro* data give cause for concern regarding carcinogenic potential, further studies in a relevant animal model may be required. Completion of reproductive toxicology studies is required in some form for the majority of the biological products that are proposed for administration to women of childbearing age. However, the degree of reproductive toxicology testing and the stage of development at which completion of these studies is required vary with biological product class. The entire pharmacology–toxicology package is included in the Biologics Licensing Application (BLA). The final step in the preclinical/nonclinical development process is the incorporation of the results of the various studies into the product labeling.

---

[4] Safety Evaluation of Vaccine Adjuvants: National Cooperative Vaccine Development Meeting Working Group. K.L. Goldenthal, J.A. Cavagnaro, C.R. Alving, and F.R. Vogel. AIDS Research and Human Retroviruses, Vol. 9, Suppl. 1, 1993.

[5] IND Submission for Vaccines: Perspective of IND Reviewers. D.K.F. Chandler, L.D. McVittie, and J.M. Novak. In: *Vaccines: Technologies and Practical Techniques*, L.C. Paoletti and P. McInnes, Eds. Ann Arbor Press, Chelsea, MI, 1998.

Therefore, the completion of the preclinical/nonclinical pharmacology and toxicology studies is crucial to the development of a biological product. It is imperative that the appropriate studies be completed at the right time in development in order to allow for the development process to flow smoothly, and it is very important to understand that while certain general principles do apply, an adequate pharmacology/toxicology study for a biological product needs to be designed on a case-by-case basis.

6.3.4　Pharmacology

Preclinical pharmacology studies are important to the biological products development process, especially at the pre-IND and Phase I stage of development. The pharmacology studies include primary pharmacodynamics studies (*in vitro* and *in vivo*), secondary pharmacodynamics studies, and safety pharmacology studies. Primary pharmacodynamics studies include demonstration of the biological activity of the product as related to the mechanism of action through which the product is thought to treat the proposed indication. These studies can include *in vitro* binding studies (e.g., monoclonal antibodies, receptors, cytokines) and functional assays as well as *in vivo* studies carried out in animal disease models that mimic the proposed clinical indication (proof-of-concept studies). Requirements for appropriate animal models differ with product class. For example, to demonstrate that a human recombinant cytokine is effective in an animal model of disease, the cytokine must express biological activity in the chosen animal model. Or to show that a given monoclonal antibody mediates a desired therapeutic effect in a given animal model of disease might require that the appropriate antigenic epitope is expressed in the chosen animal model. Similar principles can apply to blood products, vaccines, enzymes, gene therapy products, etc.

The purpose of these primary pharmacodynamics studies is to demonstrate that there is a potential benefit associated with administration of the biological product in the clinic for the proposed indication. These studies are important to the overall risk/benefit analysis process that is used to determine whether or not a biological product should be administered to humans for the first time. While products are seldom placed on clinical hold based upon inadequate proof-of-concept information, some FDA offices place more emphasis on potential benefit than others. Results of these studies can also be used to determine a starting dose and appropriate dosing regimen for the clinic.

Secondary pharmacodynamics studies include a study of the pharmacological activity of a biological product that is not directly related to the proposed indication. These studies are often completed in an attempt to identify additional potential indications for a given biological product.

Safety pharmacology studies are defined in the ICH Guidance for Industry: S7A Safety Pharmacology Studies for Human Pharmaceuticals (July 2001) document as those studies that investigate the potential undesirable pharmacodynamic effects of a substance on physiological functions in relation to exposure in the therapeutic range and above. That document includes the FDA's current recommendations regarding safety pharmacology studies and describes a core battery of studies (CNS, cardiovascular, and respiratory systems) that can be included in an IND submission to add valuable information to the safety profile for the product. For biotechnology-derived products there are certain conditions described in which the safety pharmacology studies can be reduced in number or eliminated. For example, for biotechnology-derived products that achieve highly specific receptor targeting, this guidance states that it is often sufficient to evaluate safety pharmacology endpoints as part of toxicology and/or pharmacodynamics studies. However, for biotechnology-derived products that represent a novel therapeutic class and/or those products that do not achieve highly specific receptor targeting, a more extensive evaluation by safety pharmacology studies should be considered. While the completion of a battery of safety pharmacology studies is currently recommended by the FDA, it is unlikely that a biotechnology-derived product would be placed on clinical hold solely on the basis of an inadequate safety pharmacology program. This guidance also includes a recommendation that the core battery of safety pharmacology studies be completed in compliance with Good Laboratory Practices (GLP). In the event that GLP compliance is not possible, FDA recommends that study reconstruction should be ensured through adequate documentation of study conduct and archiving of data. Any study or study component not conducted in compliance with GLP should be adequately justified and the potential impact on the study results should be explained.

6.3.5 Pharmacokinetics, Toxicokinetics, and Tissue Distribution

Pharmacokinetics studies examine the systemic exposure (Area Under the Curve — AUC) to the biological product when administered by the route of administration proposed for the clinic. A comparison of systemic exposure by the proposed clinical route vs. systemic exposure by the intravenous route reveals the bioavailability (F) of the product when administered by the proposed clinical route. Other pharmacokinetics parameters include $t_{1/2}$, Tmax, and Cmax, parameters that are useful in determining the appropriate dosing regimen. Toxicokinetics data evaluate the systemic exposure to the product as administered in the animal toxicology studies, and for repeat dose studies toxicokinetics data can reveal such processes as accumulation of the product over time or decreased systemic exposure over time, perhaps due to the production of a neutralizing antibody (immunogenicity). Tissue distribution studies identify tissue/organ systems in addition to the desired target site where the biological product in question might concentrate and are thus useful for the identification of potential target organs of toxicity.

Pharmacokinetics and single and multiple dose toxicokinetics studies as well as tissue distribution studies are recommended for the development of many, but not all, biological products. The importance of these studies can again vary with product class. These data are important for most of the therapeutic products, including monoclonal antibodies, cytokines, growth factors, enzymes, and most recombinant therapeutic proteins. However, these studies are not as important for the development of many prophylactic vaccines. In addition to the therapeutic products, tissue biodistribution studies are also important for gene therapy products and nucleic acid and virus-vector based vaccines to determine if the construct has distributed to tissues other than those at the injection site, perhaps resulting in protein expression there. In addition, these product classes also often require completion of integration studies to determine whether or not the DNA sequences have integrated into the genome. There are numerous examples of important pharmacokinetics effects related to various biological product classes. For example, administration of a monoclonal antibody or other immunogenic therapeutic product can result in the production of neutralizing antibodies, and these neutralizing antibodies can increase clearance of the therapeutic product to the point where further administrations provide no additional efficacious effect. Alternatively, certain pharmacokinetics effects can result in delays in or enhanced expression of pharmacodynamic effects.

Recommendations for pharmacokinetics, toxicokinetics, and tissue biodistribution studies for the various biological products are outlined in the ICH M3 document Guidance for Industry: M3 Nonclinical Safety Studies for the Conduct of Human Clinical Trials for Pharmaceuticals (1997), the ICH S6 document Guidance for Industry: S6 Preclinical Safety Evaluation of Biotechnology-Derived Pharmaceuticals (1997) and the Guidance for Industry: Guidance for Human Somatic Cell Therapy and GeneTherapy (1998). The ICH M3 document states that PK and ADME data should be available prior to human clinical trials. The ICH S6 document also states, "Some information on absorption, disposition, and clearance in relevant animal models should be available prior to clinical studies in order to predict margins of safety based upon exposure and dose." Vector distribution studies for gene therapy products should also be completed prior to clinical trials for the purpose of identifying potential target organs of toxicity.

According to the ICH S6 document one would expect the metabolism of biotechnology-derived products to include degradation to small peptides and individual amino acids, and therefore the metabolic pathways are already generally understood. As a result, classical biotransformation studies as performed for pharmaceuticals are not necessary. However, some understanding of the behavior of the biopharmaceutical in the biological matrix (e.g., plasma, cerebrospinal fluid), and possible effects of binding proteins is useful for the understanding of pharmacodynamic effects.

6.3.6 Toxicology

While preclinical pharmacodynamic (proof-of-concept) studies provide the "benefit" half of the risk/benefit equation required to determine whether or not to administer a biological product to humans for the first time, the toxicology study results provide the "risk" half of the equation. Once a company has a viable product (demonstrated the ability to manufacture consistently and shown potential benefit through completion of appropriate pharmacodynamics studies), the next step in development is to provide evidence in an IND that it is safe to administer the product to humans for the first time. It is at the IND stage where the preclinical toxicology studies play perhaps their most important role. In lieu of previous human experience, it is at this point that the evaluation of risk of administration of the product to humans is based solely on animal data in the form of preclinical toxicology (and perhaps safety pharmacology) studies. Therefore, it is imperative to plan an appropriate toxicology program to support a given Phase I clinical trial, and this requires careful consideration of a number of factors, including the FDA regulatory process, the appropriate FDA and ICH guidance/points-to-consider documents, general principles related to the design of a toxicology program, safety issues specific to a product class, a scientific evaluation of any risk inherent in a specific product on a case-by-case basis, and finally an overall risk/benefit analysis.

Although CBER has attempted to harmonize the preclinical toxicology study requirements throughout the biological product classes, each CBER Office has a slightly different perspective on the appropriate manner in which to evaluate the safety of the product class that falls under their regulatory responsibility. Considering the diversity of the products involved, this is not particularly surprising. However, there are a number of general principles that apply to the toxicology studies recommended to support a Phase I clinical trial as well as the various other stages of product development (Phase II, Phase III, BLA submission).

Guidance regarding preclinical/nonclinical toxicology testing for the biological products are included mainly in the ICH M3 document, the ICH S6 document, the Points to Consider for Monoclonal Antibodies document, and the Human Somatic Cell and Gene Therapy document previously discussed in this chapter. The types of toxicology studies required for development of a biological product are generally similar, with a few exceptions. For the most part, to support the safety of a Phase I clinical trial, general toxicology studies including acute (single dose) studies and repeat dose studies are required for a biological product. However, for development of a vaccine, a single toxicology study of a slightly different design may suffice. Gene therapy products also do not adhere strictly to the acute and repeat dose paradigm. Completion of a single genetic toxicology study can be required for a biological product for Phase I in the few cases where genetic toxicology studies are appropriate. For the majority of the products, if the proposed Phase I clinical trial includes administration to pregnant women then completion of a reproductive toxicology study or studies is required before initiation of the Phase I clinical trial.

Once the product has been administered to humans for the first time (Phase I), additional nonclinical general toxicology studies of increasing duration can be required to support Phase II and/or Phase III clinical trials that include repeat dosing for longer periods of time. In some cases, and especially in the case of vaccine development, the occurrence of adverse events in the clinic can result in a request by the FDA for completion of additional nonclinical toxicology studies to further examine the mechanism of action of the product and clarify what is happening in the clinic. Unlike the case with drugs, genetic toxicology and carcinogenicity studies seldom apply to biological products, with a few exceptions. Completion of reproductive toxicology studies is required in some form for the majority of the biological products that are proposed for administration to women of child-bearing age. The degree of reproductive toxicology testing and the timing for requirement for submission of these study results to the FDA varies with product class. Ultimately, the results of the preclinical/nonclinical toxicology studies must be incorporated into the product labeling.

While it is true that there are several general principles that apply to a toxicology study program for development of a biological product, there are often numerous exceptions to each of these principles. Two principles that consistently apply to all such toxicology studies are that the studies should be completed in compliance with the GLP requirements and that the study design should be based on the proposed clinical protocol. The studies to support Phase I usually include acute (single dose) studies and repeat dose studies, in addition to a single genetic toxicology study and reproductive studies if the product is indicated for administration to pregnant women. While acute toxicology studies in two mammalian species (one rodent, one nonrodent, if feasible) and repeat dose studies in two species (one rodent, one nonrodent) are often recommended, many variations on this theme are possible depending on product class, the seriousness of proposed indication and the availability of "relevant" animal toxicology models, among others. Requirements can also be altered if a product development program has a fast-track designation. Doses should include the Maximum Proposed Human Dose (MPHD) and additional doses with an eye toward determining a No Observed Adverse Effect Level (NOAEL) in the repeat dose study, but the number and magnitude of the doses can vary with product class. In some cases, it is appropriate to scale the dose on a weight-to-weight or surface area basis. The route of administration should mimic the clinic. The dosing regimen and study duration vary with product class and are outlined in the appropriate guidance documents previously discussed. The toxicology study parameters to be evaluated generally include mortality, clinical signs, body weight, food consumption, clinical chemistry, hematology, urinalysis, organ weights, gross pathology, and histopathology. Additional signals can be included in the toxicology study design such as ECG, ophthalmologic evaluation, certain behavioral tests, etc. in lieu of completion of a "core battery" of safety pharmacology studies specified in the ICH S7A document. Local tolerance at the site of administration should also be evaluated (gross pathology and histopathology).

Some consideration needs to be given to the choice of a "relevant" animal toxicology model, one that has the best chance of providing the most accurate prediction of toxicity to humans possible. For a vaccine, a relevant animal model is one in which the vaccine is immunogenic with some consideration as to whether or not the animals have been preexposed to the relevant pathogenic organism. For a monoclonal antibody, a relevant animal model is one in which the appropriate antigenic epitope is expressed in a similar manner to humans, as determined by human and animal tissue binding and cross-reactivity studies. For a cytokine, a relevant animal model is one in which the cytokine demonstrates biological activity. In the absence of an available relevant animal toxicology model, the ICH S6 guidance includes a recommendation for the use of transgenic animals expressing the appropriate human receptor or the use of homologous proteins to examine the potential effects of certain biotechnology-derived products. As a final alternative in the absence of a relevant species, an appropriate transgenic animal model, or an appropriate animal model in which to study a homologous protein, the ICH S6 guidance document indicates that it may still be advisable to assess some aspects of potential toxicity in a limited toxicity study evaluation in a single species, e.g., a repeat dose toxicity study of ≤14 days duration that includes an evaluation of important functional endpoints (e.g., cardiovascular and respiratory). This guidance also includes a discussion of the use of certain animal models of disease as animal toxicology models, especially to evaluate whether or not the proposed treatment might result in undesirable promotion of disease progression. However, these animal models of disease have limited usefulness as indicators of toxicity, and may be more useful for defining toxicity endpoints, selection of clinical indications, and determination of appropriate formulations, route of administration and treatment regimen. It should be remembered that there are usually little or no historical data available for these animal models of disease, and therefore the inclusion of concurrent control and baseline data are critical to the evaluation of the study results.

Consideration must also be given to the immunogenicity of the product. Induction of a specific immune response is inherent in the mechanism of action of an effective vaccine, while induction of an immune response to a monoclonal antibody, for example, can result in local injection site inflammation, increased clearance of the monoclonal antibody with repeat administration, and formation and deposition of immune complex in various tissue sites such as the kidney.

Specific safety considerations for each product class are also important to the overall design of a toxicology program. For example, concerns regarding the prophylactic vaccines include induction of "nonspecific" antibodies, local injection site reactions, induction of undesirable cytokine production, IgE induction, inflammatory response, autoimmunity, and toxicity of a novel adjuvant, among others. Cytokines include the possibility of an exaggerated pharmacological response, immunogenicity, inflammation, and hematological effects and flu-like symptoms, among others. Monoclonal antibodies can include nonspecific binding to tissues other than the target tissue, immuno-genicity issues, and instability of the conjugate in the case of conjugation to toxins or radionuclides. Concerns related to gene therapy products include distribution to tissues other than the desired target tissue and toxicity due to expression of the intended protein there as well as the concern that the DNA sequences might become integrated into the genome. Concerns with respect to blood products such as tissue sealants, for example, include the formation of adhesions and intravascular clotting. And these are just a few of the many examples.

And to further complicate matters, each individual biological product within a given product class can include additional safety concerns based on the specific scientific properties of that product that require consideration on a case-by-case basis. For example, a hypothetical monoclonal antibody indicated for colon cancer might be designed to bind specifically to an antigenic epitope that is over expressed on colon tumors, but that epitope might also be expressed in normal cardiovascular tissue. Therefore, specific consideration would have to be given to the potential for cardiotoxic effects. Another hypothetical example would be a gene therapy vector, administered by the intramuscular route, that was found to distribute to the lung. If the corresponding protein were expressed in the lung, a local inflammatory response or other toxic effect could occur and therefore special attention would need to be given to potential respiratory toxicity. One final hypothet-ical example would be a recombinant therapeutic protein construct consist-ing in part of a cytokine receptor(s). Such a construct could theoretically bind up the cytokine and act as a cytokine pool that might later be released, resulting in an increased pharmacodynamic effect and/or toxicity. Therefore, an appropriate toxicology study program would have to be designed on a case-by-case basis for each of these theoretical products based on sound scientific principles.

6.3.7   Risk-Benefit Analysis

With respect to preclinical testing, perhaps the most important role of these studies in the analysis of risk-benefit occurs at the IND (Phase I) stage of product development. At this stage a complete IND submission contains pharmacodynamics data to demonstrate that there is some potential benefit to administration of the product to humans and toxicology data that indi-cate the potential risks associated with administration of the product to humans. At this point, the risks as indicated by the toxicology study results must be weighed against the potential benefit for administration of the product to humans, the seriousness of the proposed indication, the avail-ability of other effective treatments, and the proposed patient population. The overall principle here is that more risk is acceptable in the case of serious and life-threatening disease, especially when there is no other effec-tive treatment available.

Once the product has been administered to humans in a Phase I clinical trial, then much of the safety information from that point forward is taken from clinical data. However, repeat dose toxicology studies of longer duration are often required to evaluate potential toxicity related to repeat administration of a given biological product over a long period of time, as determined by the dosing regimen in the proposed clinical trial. Clinical trial durations of 2 weeks, 1, 3, and 6 months constitute critical time points for requirement of additional general repeat dose toxicology studies, as outlined in the ICH M3 document. As previously stated, in the case of biological products, genetic toxicology and carcinogenicity studies rarely apply. Exceptions to this include protein conjugates with a linker molecule and gene therapy products. In the case of gene therapy products, some *in vitro* data might be required to examine mutagenic potential and the issue of carcinogenicity should be discussed with the FDA, as current standard carcinogenicity assays may not apply. Reproductive toxicology studies are usually completed for biological products in some form, depending on product class, to allow for an assessment of safety of administration of the product to women of child-bearing age.

6.3.8   Conclusion

Preclinical/nonclinical studies are an integral part of the biologics development process. One of the most important steps in this process is the demonstration that it is safe to administer the product to humans for the first time (Phase I). This is especially difficult because this demonstration of safety is limited to the use of preclinical *in vitro* and *in vivo* studies, including animal pharmacology, pharmacokinetics, and toxicology studies. This is accomplished by completion of a carefully planned pharm/tox program. While some of the same principles that apply to preclinical/nonclinical testing of drugs apply to biological product development, there are many exceptions based on the diversity of the biological product classes. The planning of a successful pharm/tox program requires consideration of the FDA regulatory process, the appropriate FDA and ICH guidances, general principles related to the design of a toxicology program, safety issues related to product class, a scientific evaluation of potential risk based on scientific information for a specific biological product on a case-by-case basis, and an overall risk–benefit analysis. The development process cannot proceed until the product is deemed safe for first in human administration. Once the product has been administered to humans for the first time, then additional toxicology studies including longer term repeat dose studies, and reproductive toxicology studies, and, in a few cases, genetic toxicology and/or carcinogenicity studies are required for product development to proceed to marketing approval. It is recommended that this entire preclinical/nonclinical testing process involve continuous communication with the FDA through pre-IND meetings, end-of-Phase I (if applicable) and end-of-Phase II meetings, and a pre-BLA meeting, among others. This is a time-consuming and expensive process that requires careful planning and evaluation early on and throughout product development.

6.4   The Biologics License Application (BLA)

6.4.1   Introduction

The Biologics Control Act of 1902 required licensure of both the biologic product and the establishment in which it was manufactured. Until the late 1990s, CBER (and its predecessors) required biologics manufacturers to file two separate license applications: a Product License Application (PLA) containing the required information about the manufacture and testing (preclinical and clinical) of the product, and an Establishment License Application (ELA) containing the required information about the manufacturing facility. In 1996, as part of the Reinventing Government Initiatives (REGO), the separate ELA filing for specific biologic products was eliminated and a single form (form 356h) was introduced to replace the multiple product–specific PLA forms which were then in use. In 1999, a final Federal Register notice was published which applied these changes to all biologic products. A copy of Form 356h is shown Figure 6.2. Note that this form is used for all new drug and biologics. In the "Application Information" section, the application type can be selected. When used to support licensure for a biologic product, the application is referred to as a Biologics License Application (BLA). From a product information perspective, the difference in the BLA and the PLA is primarily one of format. From a facilities perspective, the new BLA contains significantly less information that the previous ELA. Establishment compliance with Good Manufacturing Practice (GMP) is now primarily assessed during the preapproval inspection performed by the FDA prior to final approval of the BLA.

Of course, just as the biologics industry is getting familiar with the change from the PLA/ELA format to the BLA format, the international regulatory harmonization effort has proposed a market application format, the Common Technical Document (CTD), which is slated to become the standard of the future (see Chapter 13 in this book for a discussion of the International Conference on Harmonization (ICH) and the new CTD format).

In August of 2001, CBER and CDER issued a Draft Guidance Document (Guidance for Industry: Submitting Marketing Applications according to the ICH-CTD Format — General Considerations, available at www.fda.gov/cber/gdlns/mrktapich.pdf). This document, which was labeled as "Draft — Not for Implementation," contained the following guidance: "We are now able to accept and review applications organized as described in the CTD guidances. You can submit a BLA for a specified biotechnological product, and an NDA or an ANDA for all drug products, in the CTD format. You can

DEPARTMENT OF HEALTH AND HUMAN SERVICES FOOD AND DRUG ADMINISTRATION	Form Approved: OMB No. 0910-0338 Expiration Date: August 31, 2005 See OMB Statement on page 2.
APPLICATION TO MARKET A NEW DRUG, BIOLOGIC, OR AN ANTIBIOTIC DRUG FOR HUMAN USE (Title 21, Code of Federal Regulations, Parts 314 & 601)	**FOR FDA USE ONLY** APPLICATION NUMBER

APPLICANT INFORMATION

NAME OF APPLICANT	DATE OF SUBMISSION
TELEPHONE NO. *(Include Area Code)*	FACSIMILE (FAX) Number *(Include Area Code)*
APPLICANT ADDRESS *(Number, Street, City, State, Country, ZIP Code or Mail Code, and U.S. License number if previously issued):*	AUTHORIZED U.S. AGENT NAME & ADDRESS *(Number, Street, City, State, ZIP Code, telephone & FAX number)* IF APPLICABLE

PRODUCT DESCRIPTION

NEW DRUG OR ANTIBIOTIC APPLICATION NUMBER, OR BIOLOGICS LICENSE APPLICATION NUMBER *(If previously issued)*

ESTABLISHED NAME *(e.g., Proper name, USP/USAN name)*	PROPRIETARY NAME *(trade name)* IF ANY

CHEMICAL/BIOCHEMICAL/BLOOD PRODUCT NAME *(If any)*	CODE NAME *(If any)*

DOSAGE FORM:	STRENGTHS:	ROUTE OF ADMINISTRATION:

(PROPOSED) INDICATION(S) FOR USE:

APPLICATION INFORMATION

APPLICATION TYPE
(check one) ☐ NEW DRUG APPLICATION (21 CFR 314.50) ☐ ABBREVIATED NEW DRUG APPLICATION (ANDA, 21 CFR 314.94)
☐ BIOLOGICS LICENSE APPLICATION (21 CFR Part 601)

IF AN NDA, IDENTIFY THE APPROPRIATE TYPE ☐ 505 (b)(1) ☐ 505 (b)(2)

IF AN ANDA, OR 505(b)(2), IDENTIFY THE REFERENCE LISTED DRUG PRODUCT THAT IS THE BASIS FOR THE SUBMISSION
Name of Drug   Holder of Approved Application

TYPE OF SUBMISSION *(check one)* ☐ ORIGINAL APPLICATION ☐ AMENDMENT TO A PENDING APPLICATION ☐ RESUBMISSION
☐ PRESUBMISSION ☐ ANNUAL REPORT ☐ ESTABLISHMENT DESCRIPTION SUPPLEMENT ☐ EFFICACY SUPPLEMENT
☐ LABELING SUPPLEMENT ☐ CHEMISTRY MANUFACTURING AND CONTROLS SUPPLEMENT ☐ OTHER

IF A SUBMISSION OF PARTIAL APPLICATION, PROVIDE LETTER DATE OF AGREEMENT TO PARTIAL SUBMISSION: _____

IF A SUPPLEMENT, IDENTIFY THE APPROPRIATE CATEGORY ☐ CBE ☐ CBE-30 ☐ Prior Approval (PA)

REASON FOR SUBMISSION

PROPOSED MARKETING STATUS *(check one)* ☐ PRESCRIPTION PRODUCT (Rx) ☐ OVER THE COUNTER PRODUCT (OTC)

NUMBER OF VOLUMES SUBMITTED _____ | THIS APPLICATION IS ☐ PAPER ☐ PAPER AND ELECTRONIC ☐ ELECTRONIC

ESTABLISHMENT INFORMATION (Full establishment information should be provided in the body of the Application.)
Provide locations of all manufacturing, packaging and control sites for drug substance and drug product (continuation sheets may be used if necessary). Include name, address, contact, telephone number, registration number (CFN), DMF number, and manufacturing steps and/or type of testing (e.g. Final dosage form, Stability testing) conducted at the site. Please indicate whether the site is ready for inspection or, if not, when it will be ready.

Cross References (list related License Applications, INDs, NDAs, PMAs, 510(k)s, IDEs, BMFs, and DMFs referenced in the current application)

FORM FDA 356h (9/02)   PSC Media Arts (301) 443-1090 EF

PAGE 1

FIGURE 6.2
Form 356h.

This application contains the following items: *(Check all that apply)*	

1. Index	
2. Labeling *(check one)* ☐ Draft Labeling ☐ Final Printed Labeling	
3. Summary (21 CFR 314.50 (c))	
4. Chemistry section	
A. Chemistry, manufacturing, and controls information (e.g., 21 CFR 314.50(d)(1); 21 CFR 601.2)	
B. Samples (21 CFR 314.50 (e)(1); 21 CFR 601.2 (a)) (Submit only upon FDA's request)	
C. Methods validation package (e.g., 21 CFR 314.50(e)(2)(i); 21 CFR 601.2)	
5. Nonclinical pharmacology and toxicology section (e.g., 21 CFR 314.50(d)(2); 21 CFR 601.2)	
6. Human pharmacokinetics and bioavailability section (e.g., 21 CFR 314.50(d)(3); 21 CFR 601.2)	
7. Clinical Microbiology (e.g., 21 CFR 314.50(d)(4))	
8. Clinical data section (e.g., 21 CFR 314.50(d)(5); 21 CFR 601.2)	
9. Safety update report (e.g., 21 CFR 314.50(d)(5)(vi)(b); 21 CFR 601.2)	
10. Statistical section (e.g., 21 CFR 314.50(d)(6); 21 CFR 601.2)	
11. Case report tabulations (e.g., 21 CFR 314.50(f)(1); 21 CFR 601.2)	
12. Case report forms (e.g., 21 CFR 314.50 (f)(2); 21 CFR 601.2)	
13. Patent information on any patent which claims the drug (21 U.S.C. 355(b) or (c))	
14. A patent certification with respect to any patent which claims the drug (21 U.S.C. 355 (b)(2) or (j)(2)(A))	
15. Establishment description (21 CFR Part 600, if applicable)	
16. Debarment certification (FD&C Act 306 (k)(1))	
17. Field copy certification (21 CFR 314.50 (l)(3))	
18. User Fee Cover Sheet (Form FDA 3397)	
19. Financial Information (21 CFR Part 54)	
20. OTHER *(Specify)*	

CERTIFICATION

I agree to update this application with new safety information about the product that may reasonably affect the statement of contraindications, warnings, precautions, or adverse reactions in the draft labeling. I agree to submit safety update reports as provided for by regulation or as requested by FDA. If this application is approved, I agree to comply with all applicable laws and regulations that apply to approved applications, including, but not limited to the following:
1. Good manufacturing practice regulations in 21 CFR Parts 210, 211 or applicable regulations, Parts 606, and/or 820.
2. Biological establishment standards in 21 CFR Part 600.
3. Labeling regulations in 21 CFR Parts 201, 606, 610, 660, and/or 809.
4. In the case of a prescription drug or biological product, prescription drug advertising regulations in 21 CFR Part 202.
5. Regulations on making changes in application in FD&C Act Section 506A, 21 CFR 314.71, 314.72, 314.97, 314.99, and 601.12.
6. Regulations on Reports in 21 CFR 314.81, 314.81, 600.80, and 600.81.
7. Local, state and Federal environmental impact laws.
If this application applies to a drug product that FDA has proposed for scheduling under the Controlled Substances Act, I agree not to market the product until the Drug Enforcement Administration makes a final scheduling decision.
The data and information in this submission have been reviewed and, to the best of my knowledge are certified to be true and accurate.
Warning: A willfully false statement is a criminal offense, U.S. Code, title 18, section 1001.

SIGNATURE OF RESPONSIBLE OFFICIAL OR AGENT	TYPED NAME AND TITLE	DATE
ADDRESS *(Street, City, State, and ZIP Code)*	Telephone Number ( )	

Public reporting burden for this collection of information is estimated to average 24 hours per response, including the time for reviewing instructions, searching existing data sources, gathering and maintaining the data needed, and completing and reviewing the collection of information. Send comments regarding this burden estimate or any other aspect of this collection of information, including suggestions for reducing this burden to:

Department of Health and Human Services
Food and Drug Administration
CBER, HFM-99
1401 Rockville Pike
Rockville, MD 20852-1448

Food and Drug Administration
CDER, HFD-94
12420 Parklawn Dr., Room 3046
Rockville, MD 20852

An agency may not conduct or sponsor, and a person is not required to respond to, a collection of information unless it displays a currently valid OMB control number.

FORM FDA 356h (9/02)

PAGE 2

FIGURE 6.2
Form 356h Continued.

submit BLAs in the CTD format for other categories of biological products as guidance documents become available for these product categories. If you wish to submit BLAs in the CTD format for those products *prior* to the availability of guidance, you should contact CBER office with review responsibility prior to developing the submission. The Agency highly recommends that, by 2003, sponsors regularly submit BLAs for specified biotechnological products, NDAs, and ANDAs to the Agency in the CTD format."

This Guidance is of special interest to biologics manufacturers for several reasons. The first is the fact that it is labeled as not for implementation, which seems a bit like saying "here is some advice, but please don't make any decisions based on it." The second is that the BLA guidance is specifically restricted to "specified" biotechnology products. This terminology is applied to four distinct classes of products — originally termed "well-characterized biologic product" which includes (1) therapeutic DNA plasmid products, (2) therapeutic synthetic peptide products of 40 or fewer amino acids, (3) monoclonal antibody products for *in vivo* use, and (4) therapeutic recombinant DNA-derived products. All of these products, with perhaps the theoretical exception of some therapeutic vaccines which could meet these definitions, are included among products to be transferred to CDER in late 2003. No guidance documents covering other categories of biological products have been issued.

6.4.2   BLA Review Process

The current CBER BLA managed review process was developed to meet requirements of the Prescription Drug User Fee Act (PDUFA) of 1996. Simply stated, the FDA agreed to institute review standards and timelines in exchange for user fees paid by BLA sponsors. The goal was to standardize both the review *process* and the review *content*.

To facilitate the standardization effort, CBER has issued a number of guidance documents which provide information about the types of information to be included in the BLA for each biologic product class:

- Guidance for Industry for the Submission of Chemistry, Manufacturing, and Controls Information for a Therapeutic Recombinant DNA-Derived Product or a Monoclonal Antibody Product for *in vivo* Use — **August 1996**
- Guidance For the Submission of Chemistry, Manufacturing and Controls Information and Establishment Description for Autologous Somatic Cell Therapy Products — **January 10, 1997**
- Guidance for Industry — Changes to an Approved Application for Specified Biotechnology and Specified Synthetic Biological Products — **July 24, 1997**

- Guidance for Industry — Changes to an Approved Application: Biological Products — **July 24, 1997**
- Guidance for Industry for the Submission of Chemistry, Manufacturing, and Controls Information for Synthetic Peptide Substance — **January 16, 1998**
- Guidance for Industry: Content and Format of Chemistry, Manufacturing and Controls Information and Establishment Description Information for a Vaccine or Related Product — **January 5, 1999**
- Guidance for Industry: For the Submission of Chemistry, Manufacturing and Controls and Establishment Description Information for Human Plasma-Derived Biological Products, Animal Plasma or Serum-Derived Products — **February 17, 1999**
- Guidance for Industry: Content and Format of Chemistry, Manufacturing and Controls Information and Establishment Description Information for a Biological *in vitro* Diagnostic Product — **March 8, 1999**
- Guidance for Industry On the Content and Format of Chemistry, Manufacturing and Controls Information and Establishment Description Information for an Allergenic Extract or Allergen Patch Test — **April 23, 1999**
- Guidance for Industry For the Submission of Chemistry, Manufacturing and Controls and Establishment Description Information for Human Blood and Blood Components Intended for Transfusion or for Further Manufacture and For the Completion of the Form FDA 356h "Application to Market a New Drug, Biologic or an Antibiotic Drug for Human Use" — **May 10, 1999**

Administrative processing of BLAs under the new managed review process is detailed in a new CBER Standard Operating Procedure and Policy (SOPP) document (SOPP 8401 — available at http://www.fda.gov/cber/regsopp/8401.htm).

The review committee will initially review the BLA to make a refusal to file (RTF) decision within the required 60 days (see SOPP 8404 — available at http://www.fda.gov/cber/regsopp/8404.htm).

If the review committee determines that the BLA is complete for filing purpose (i.e., it contains all of the data and critical review elements necessary for initiating a meaningful review process), it will be filed and a complete review performed as outlined in SOPP 8405 (available at http://www.fda.gov/cber/regsopp/8405.htm).

Following the complete review CBER will issue either a Complete Response Letter, indicating that there are deficiencies remaining which preclude the approval of the application or the supplement at that time, or an Approval Letter, indicating that a marketing license will be granted (see SOPP 8405).

6.4.3 Electronic BLA

The FDA is encouraging the submission of BLAs (as well as other regulatory submission) in electronic format to both speed review and to eliminate the vast amounts of paper documents that have to be handled.

Several recent guidance documents have been published providing information about filing of the BLA in electronic format — with either the conventional 356h format or the new CTD format.

- REVISED Guidance for Industry: Providing Regulatory Submissions to the Center for Biologics Evaluation and Research (CBER) in Electronic Format — Biologics Marketing Applications [Biologics License Application (BLA), Product License Application (PLA)/Establishment License Application (ELA) and New Drug Application (NDA)] — **November 12, 1999**

- Draft Guidance for Industry: Providing Regulatory Submissions in Electronic Format — Prescription Drug Advertising and Promotional Labeling — **January 31, 2001**

- Draft Guidance for Industry: Providing Regulatory Submissions in Electronic Format — Postmarketing Expedited Safety Reports — **May 3, 2001**

- Draft Guidance for Industry: Submitting Marketing Applications According to the ICH-CTD Format — General Considerations — **September 5, 2001**

It is expected that within several years, the vast majority of all FDA submissions will be submitted electronically, however it is unlikely that the FDA will actually require electronic submissions for many years until the technology is readily available to all potential sponsors.

6.5 The Future of Biologics Regulation

The recent movement of the products and personnel from the previous Office of Therapeutics Research and Review (OTRR) at CBER to CDER is likely the first move in the eventual consolidation of the Drugs and Biologics regulatory oversight under common management. FDA has already announced a "comprehensive" restructuring of CDER to be completed by the spring of 2005. Whether this will also include the eventual repeal of the PHS Act and the regulation of biologic products under the authority of the FD&C Act is not clear, however that would seem to be the most probable future sequence of events. The products that are now classified as "biologics" will, of course, continue to be regulated by the FDA, however the days of the bench scientist–reviewer seem to be numbered.

7

FDA Medical Device Regulation

Barry Sall

CONTENTS

1-58716-007-2/04/$0.00+$1.50
© 2004 by CRC Press LLC

7.1 Introduction

Since the technological advances of the 1950s and 1960s, the rate of innovation in the medical device industry has greatly accelerated. These innovations have led to very substantial therapeutic, monitoring, and diagnostic benefits in all areas of medicine. Often, these innovative devices were selected and used by healthcare professionals who received their basic scientific training before these technologies were developed. By the early 1970s, many medical devices were becoming so complex that medical professionals were no longer able to fully assess their attributes. Device developers and manufacturers were also encountering situations where devices interacted with the body in unanticipated ways or deficiencies in the production process led to patient injuries and deaths. This history was the driving force behind the 1976 Medical Device Amendments to the Food Drug and Cosmetic Act of 1938. By 1978, when the regulations required by this new law came into full effect, the production and clinical testing of medical devices were subject to FDA review. Many new devices entering the U.S. market had to undergo FDA review, either through the 510(k) PreMarket Notification process, or the PMA Premarket Approval process. The 1976 Amendments have been modified several times over the years and now also cover the device development process. This chapter provides an introduction to medical device classification, the preparation of premarket submissions, medical device clinical research, and manufacturing regulations.

The regulations developed as a result of the 1976 Medical Device Amendments share a common goal with the existing pharmaceutical regulations. They both strive to protect the public health; however, they approach this goal in different ways. The device regulations recognize differences between medical devices and pharmaceuticals and between the medical device industry and the pharmaceutical industry. In general, therapeutic medical devices exert their effects locally by cutting tissue, covering a wound, or propping open a clogged artery; therefore, both preclinical and clinical testing can be simplified as compared to the pharmaceutical approach. Many diagnostic devices do not even come in contact with the patient; so, in these cases, pharmaceutical safety testing is entirely inappropriate. Differences in the structure of the medical device industry as compared to the pharmaceutical industry do not have a direct effect on regulation, but they do affect the pace of innovation. There are a relatively small number of very large pharmaceutical companies, with large experienced regulatory staffs. There are a large number of very small medical device companies with few or no dedicated regulatory staff. In addition, the product life cycle time for a medical device might be as short as two or three years, or approximately one tenth the time for pharmaceutical product. All of these factors make it essential that medical device professionals have an adequate understanding of both the technology underlying their company's products and of the applicable regulations. Development timelines in this industry are very short and inappropriate strategic decisions can generate substantial delays or even preclude the introduction of a potentially lifesaving technology.

The objective of this chapter is to provide the reader with a step-by-step introduction to the regulatory issues associated with the medical device development process. This information will enable the reader to identify the major steps in that process. References are provided, throughout the text, for more detailed information.

7.2   Is It a Device?

7.2.1   Product Jurisdiction

When preparing the regulatory strategy for a product or technology, it is important to first determine which regulations apply. Is the product a device? A drug? A biologic? Two factors must be considered in order to make this determination. First the indication for use of the product must be determined by management and clearly stated. Then the primary intended purpose of the product can be identified. And only then can the developer determine if that functionality is achieved through chemical action and metabolism (a drug) or by a physical action (device). If an alginate wound dressing contains an antibacterial agent, it is regulated as a device, so long as its primary intended purpose is to act as a (physical) barrier between the wound and the environment, and the antibacterial agent only functions to enhance that device function. On the other hand, if the indication for use is to deliver the antibacterial agent (chemical) to the wound in order to treat an existing infection, then the alginate dressing might be considered an inactive component of a drug product. In order to make this determination, one must carefully review the definition of a medical device contained in the 1976 Medical Device Amendments of the Food, Drug and Cosmetic Act:

> an instrument, apparatus, implement, machine, contrivance, implant, *in vitro* reagent, or other similar or related article, including any component, part or accessory, which is
>
> (1) recognized in the official National Formulary, or the USP, or any supplement to them,
> (2) intended for use in the diagnosis of disease or other conditions, or in the cure, mitigation, treatment, or prevention of disease, in man or other animals, or
> (3) intended to affect the structure or any function of the body of man or other animals, and which does not achieve its primary intended purposes through chemical action within or on the body of man or other animals and which is not dependent upon being metabolized for the achievement of any of its principal intended purposes

In addition to this definition, there are also Intercenter Agreements[1] between CDRH, CDER, and CBER that discuss jurisdictional issues.

The Medical Device User Fee Act of 2002 (MDUFA02) established the Office of Combination Products. This office is an excellent source of information on these issues. See: http://www.fda.gov/oc/combination/default.htm for more information on the Office of Combination Products and its functions.

---

[1] Food and Drug Administration, Intercenter Agreements, October 1991 http://www.fda.gov/oc/combination/intercenter.html

TABLE 7.1

Medical Device Types

Function	Form
Therapeutic	Durable
Monitoring	Implantable
Diagnostic	Disposable

Types of medical devices — There are a wide variety of medical devices in use today. They range from room-sized imaging systems that weigh several tons to ophthalmic implants that are less than 2 mm long and weigh only a few grams. Most *in vitro* diagnostic products (blood and urine tests) are also regulated as medical devices. Table 7.1 describes most devices using two of their characteristics.

Using this table one can easily characterize most medical devices by determining the function of the device from the left column, then its form from the right column. For instance, a lithotriptor that uses sound waves to break up kidney stones would be considered a durable therapeutic device. A pacemaker would be considered an implantable therapeutic device, and so on. Issues such as reuse, shelf life, and device tracking impact different types of devices in different ways.

7.3   Medical Device Classification

Once a determination has been made that a product is a medical device, the next issue that must be addressed is medical device classification. In simpler terms, "What kind of submission do I need in order to commercialize this device? Is it exempt from 510(k) Premarket Notification requirements, subject to those requirements or must we file a Premarket notification?" In order to answer this question, we need to know the class of the device.

There are three classes of medical devices. Class I devices are the simplest devices, posing the fewest risks and subject to general controls. Most of them are exempt from premarket notification requirements [510(k)] and some are also exempt from compliance with the Quality System Regulation. Examples of Class I devices include toothbrushes, oxygen masks, and irrigating syringes. FDA estimates that approximately half of the medical devices it regulates are Class I devices.

Class II devices include many moderate risk devices. In order to market a Class II device in the U.S., the manufacturer must submit a 510(k) Premarket Notification prior to commercialization. The purpose of this notification is to demonstrate that the new device is *substantially equivalent* to another device that has already gone through the 510(k) process or to a device that was on the market before the Medical Device Amendments were signed into law on May 28, 1976. Class II devices are subject to special controls, that is, FDA guidance documents, FDA accepted international standards, and the Quality System Regulation. Ultrasound imaging systems, Holter cardiac monitors, pregnancy test kits and central line catheters are all Class II devices. FDA estimates that slightly less than half of the medical devices it regulates are Class II devices. Approximately 4000 Class II devices are cleared on to the U.S. market each year.[2]

Most Class III devices require PMA approval prior to marketing in the U.S. These are devices that are not substantially equivalent to any Class II device. They are usually technologically innovative devices. There are a small number of Class III Preamedments 510(k) devices; however, the FDA has been working diligently to either down classify them to Class II, or, if their risk profile does not justify down-classification, call for PMAs. There are approximately 40 to 50 PMAs approved each year.

7.3.1   Determining Device Classification

If the product in development is similar to other medical devices already on the U.S. market with respect to its indication for use and its technological characteristics, then our classification determination becomes a search of the regulations. 21CFR 862–892 contains descriptions of a wide variety of medical devices arranged by medical practice area. The classifications, exemptions from 510(k) or QSR regulation, if any, are listed in this section of the regulations. The classification database in the CDRH website can also be a useful tool for determining device classification (see Figure 7.1 and Table 7.2).

If a description in the CFR is consistent with the characteristics of the new device, then the device classification listed in that section of the CFR should apply. Precedents can be identified in another manner as well. If one is aware of other competing devices that are already on the market, one can search the 510(k)[3] or PMA[4] databases within the CDRH website for those products and determine how they were classified. Figure 7.5 in Section 7.7 illustrates the process one can follow to identify possible predicate devices when only the name of a competitor is known.

7.3.2   Reclassification

Once FDA determines that a device is a Class III PMA device, that type of device will always be a Class III device, no matter how many other compet-

---

[2] Food and Drug Administration, ODE Annual Report FY 2002, http://www.fda.gov/cdrh/annual/fy2002/ode/2002.pdf

[3] Food and Drug Administration, http://www.accessdata.fda.gov/scripts/cdrh/cfdocs/cfPMN/pmn.cfm

[4] Food and Drug Administration, http://www.accessdata.fda.gov/scripts/cdrh/cfdocs/cfPMA/pma.cfm

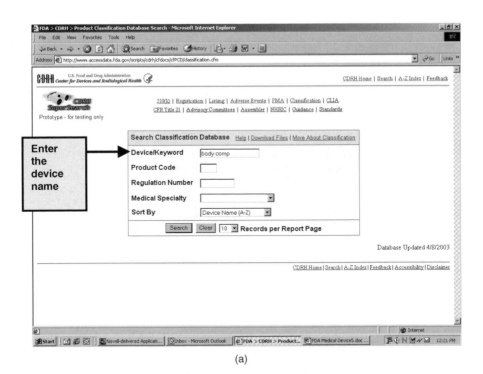

(a)

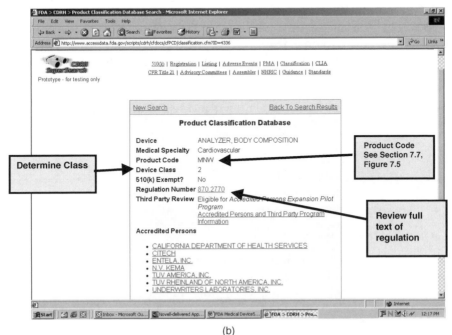

(b)

FIGURE 7.1
Device classification database search.

TABLE 7.2

Medical Device Classification

Device Classification Panel or Specialty Group	21 CFR Part
Anesthesiology	868
Cardiovascular	870
Clinical Chemistry and Clinical Toxicology	862
Dental	872
Ear, Nose, and Throat	874
Hematology and Pathology	864
Immunology and Microbiology	866
Gastroenterology and Urology	876
General and Plastic Surgery	878
General Hospital and Personal Use	880
Neurology	882
Obstetrical and Gynecological	884
Ophthalmic	886
Orthopedic	888
Physical Medicine	890
Radiology	892

itors follow with similar products. All the competitors that develop similar products will have to follow the PMA process in order to market their devices in the U.S. The only way that situation can change is if the FDA approves a reclassification petition and down-classifies the device to Class II. This type of reexamination can be initiated by either FDA or industry. In recent years, FDA has examined many device types, their overall risk, and actual frequency of problems in the field, and down-classified significant numbers of devices either from Class III to II or from Class II to I. These actions enable FDA to focus more of its resources on the higher risk products. Industry groups have also submitted their own reclassification petitions and succeeded in down-classifying devices.

7.4 An Introduction to the Medical Device Approval Process

7.4.1 Strategic Choices

Now that the classification of the device is known, we can identify an appropriate regulatory pathway. Unlike the pharmaceutical regulatory process, a medical device developer is frequently presented with more than one regulatory path to the U.S. market (see Figure 7.2). A device such as software that analyzes MRI images is designated as a Class II 510(k) product if it only measures the size or volume of anatomical structures. However, if the software detects abnormalities or provides diagnostic information, it would be considered a Class III PMA device, so the indication for use is critical to the

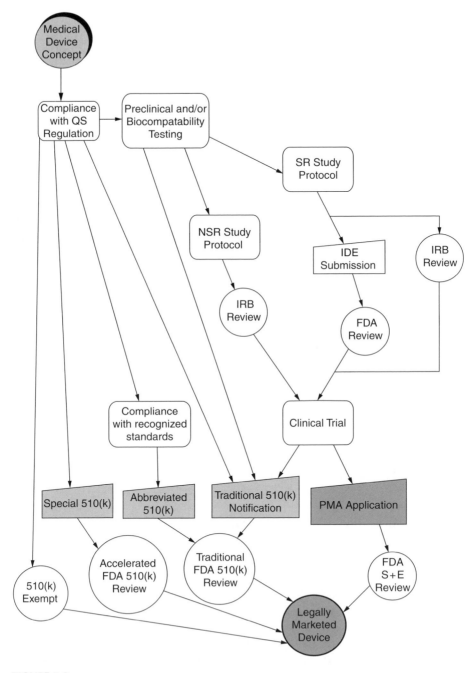

FIGURE 7.2
Selected pathways for marketing medical devices in the U.S.

TABLE 7.3

Selected MDUFMA User Fees FY04

Application Type	Fee
PMA	$206,811
Panel Track PMA Supplement	$206,811
180-Day PMA Supplement	$44,464
Real-Time PMA Supplement	$14,890
IDEs, 30-Day Notices, Special and Express PMA Supplements	No Charge
510(k) — All Types	$3,480

determination of the regulatory path. A device developer may choose to "start small" and begin FDA interactions with a simpler 510(k) and then, after gaining experience, move to the more challenging PMA. Generally, both industry and FDA would prefer to review medical devices as 510(k)s. This process provides industry with timely reviews and conserves reviewing resources for FDA. So when speed to market is the prime consideration, one always attempts to follow the 510(k) path. In some cases, device developers may choose to propose a more complex PMA indication for use, or in a situation where the device classification is not clear, suggest the more complicated Class III PMA designation. This can make sense when the developer may not have a strong intellectual property position and does have sufficient resources to conduct clinical trials. This strategy can result in the erection of a regulatory barrier of entry for other, less well funded organizations. This strategy is often called creation of a "regulatory patent." Another consideration when deciding on a regulatory path is user fees. Since October of 2002, ODE has been authorized to charge fees for reviewing 510(k)s, PMAs, and PMA supplements (see Table 7.3).

All the submission types mentioned in this section are discussed in more detail in later sections of this chapter.

7.4.2 Modification of Marketed Devices

Many changes can be made to 510(k) devices by following the design control provisions of the Quality System Regulation, rather than submit a new 510(k). Even when a new 510(k) is necessary, a sponsor may choose to submit a Special 510(k). Changes to PMA products follow a more rigid process. Most changes require advance approval via the PMA supplement process. The sponsor must also submit a PMA Annual Report that update ODE on all device changes and any new clinical data. Both the premarket and postmarket obligations must be considered when determining the preferred route to market. More information on postmarketing issues can be found in Section 10. The ease of modifying devices and other postmarket considerations also factor into the strategic regulatory planning process.

7.5   Design Controls

Once the product definition and regulatory strategy have been prepared, Class II and III device developers must work to comply with the design control provisions of the Quality System Regulation (QSR) (21CFR 820) as the device development process moves forward. The QSR is the medical device equivalent of the pharmaceutical cGMPs. The QSR, unlike cGMPs, also regulates the device development process via its design control provisions (21CFR 820.30). This section describes the device developer's obligations under the design control provisions of QSR. Other sections of the QSR are discussed in Section 7.9.

7.5.1   The Difference between Research and Development

The preamble to the QSR[5] states that research activities are not regulated by the QSR, but development activities are regulated. The regulation does not provide guidance for distinguishing between the two activities; however the preamble does add "The design control requirements are not intended to apply to the development of concepts and feasibility studies. However, once it decides that a design will be developed, a plan must be established...." Most device developers categorize investigations of a general technology as research and application of that technology to a particular product development. For example, if a device developer creates a new laser technology, that effort would be considered research. Once the developer begins to apply that technology to a particular device with specific indications for use and user requirements, then they have begun the development phase and Design Controls must be applied.

7.5.2   Design Control Components

There are eight components of Design Controls that stretch from planning for the development effort through design transfer (from development to manufacturing) and maintenance of existing designs. These controls apply to all Class II and III medical devices and a small number of Class I devices. The purpose of these controls is to ensure that devices are developed in a rational manner, in compliance with the firm's existing design control SOPs. Table 7.4 summarizes these components. If a company is just starting to develop a medical device for the first time, the design control process must be fully described in SOPs and fully implemented before the development planning begins. Design controls are closely linked to many other QSR components and the entire system must work together to produce good

---

[5] Food and Drug Administration, 1996. Final Rule. Medical Devices; Current Good Manufacturing Practice (CGMP) Final Rule; Quality System Regulation. *Fed. Regist.* 61:195, 52602–52662.

TABLE 7.4

Design Control Components

Design Activity	Personnel Involved	Examples of Issues
Design and Development Planning	Development, Management	Determine and meet the user/patients requirements Meet regulations and standards Develop specifications for the device Develop, select, and evaluate components and suppliers Develop and approve labels and user instructions Develop packaging Develop specifications for manufacturing processes Verify safety and performance of prototype and final devices Verify compatibility with the environment and other devices Develop manufacturing facilities and utilities Develop and validate manufacturing processes Train employees Document the processes and details of the device design If applicable, develop a service program
Design Input	Development, Management, Sales and Marketing, Quality, Regulatory	Determine the real need for the new device Identify users of the new device Specify where the new device will be used Determine how the new device will be used Describe the operating environment for the device Document how long the new device will be used
Design Output	Development	The design is executed
Design Review	Development, Management, and others, as needed, including one person not directly involved in the design effort	Determine that the design meets customer needs Confirm that manufacturability and reliability issues are adequately addressed Establish that human factors issues are adequately addressed
Design Verification	Development	Confirm that the design outputs meet the design input requirements by reviewing data from tests, inspections, and analysis
Design Validation	Development, Management, and Clinical	Performed under defined operating conditions on initial production units or equivalent Include software validation and risk analysis, where appropriate Ensure that devices conform to defined user needs and intended uses Include testing under actual or simulated use conditions Validation plans, methods, reports, and review must be conducted according to approved SOPs

TABLE 7.4 (Continued)

Design Control Components

Design Activity	Personnel Involved	Examples of Issues
Design Transfer	Development, Management, Quality, and Manufacturing	Prepare a plan for the transfer of all design components to Manufacturing Assure that all affected personnel are adequately trained Assure that all Manufacturing and Quality systems function according to specifications
Design Changes	Development, Management	Assure that design changes are tracked Assure that corrective actions are completed Assure that the DHF is kept current and includes all design revisions

product. Refer to Section 7.9 for discussion of the other components of the Quality System Regulation.

The Design Control regulation sets requirements for the development process. Firms must prepare and follow SOPs that comply with the regulations and that fully describe how the firm will meet all relevant regulatory requirements. All the relevant activities must be fully documented in the firm's Design History File (DHF). For example, the regulation requires device developers to prepare a list of Design Inputs. Like just about every other design control related document, this list cannot be considered a static document. As the design process progresses, inputs are modified, added, or subtracted. The design input file must be maintained as a current document throughout the development process. Another important design control function is the design review. At least once during the design process, and more frequently for a complex design effort, the design must be reviewed to ensure that the design satisfies the design input requirements for the intended use of the device and the needs of the user. All other sources of design information including design output reports, design verification documentation, and even actual prototypes should be part of this review. Most importantly, for regulatory compliance, a report must document all the design review activities, their results, and list the individuals that participated in the review. The regulation requires that at least one member of the review team be an independent reviewer that has not been directly involved with the design effort.

7.6   Medical Device Clinical Research

Once the regulatory pathway has been determined and development is underway, clinical data may be necessary. Keep in mind that the vast majority of 510(k) Notifications do not contain clinical data.

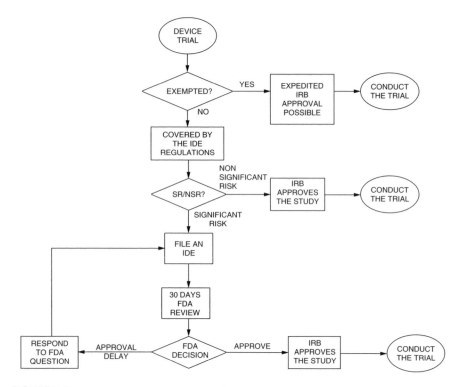

FIGURE 7.3
Regulatory paths for medical device clinical research.

Figure 7.3 graphically depicts the pathways for medical device clinical research. Unlike the pharmaceutical model, there are three levels of regulation of medical device clinical research. Some research is exempted from the Investigational Device Exemption (IDE) regulation, some is subject to just some sections of the IDE regulation, and other types of research is subject to all sections of the IDE regulation. More information on risk determinations can be found at: http://www.fda.gov/cdrh/d861.html.

7.6.1 Exempted Studies

Most exempted studies involve either previously cleared or approved devices or investigational *in vitro* diagnostic devices. If a sponsor wishes to conduct a study that, for example, compares the performance of their own previously cleared device with the performance of their competitor's previously cleared device, that study would be exempt from the IDE regulations as long as both devices are used for their cleared indications. No prior FDA review or approval of the study is necessary. Of course, due to privacy concerns and institutional regulations, any human clinical trial should utilize an informed consent form and be reviewed and approved by the appropriate IRB. Most *in vitro* diagnostic field trials are also exempt, so long as invasive means are not used to collect samples and the data obtained from the investigational assay are not used to make treatment decisions. Animal studies and custom device studies are also exempt from the IDE regulation.

7.6.2 Non-Significant Risk Studies

Many studies that do not involve highly invasive devices, risky procedures, and/or frail patients can be conducted under the Non-Significant Risk provisions of the IDE regulation. These provisions provide an intermediate level of control for the study without requiring the study sponsor to prepare and file an IDE. See Table 7.5 for a comparison of sponsor and investigator responsibilities. Areas where the requirements for NSR and SR studies differ are shaded. When a sponsor determines that a study is NSR, no FDA involvement is required, although many sponsors will consult with FDA to confirm that the study is indeed NSR and that its design is consistent with FDA expectations. Each IRB that reviews a NSR study must document three conclusions. First, that they concur with the sponsor's NSR determination, next, that the study protocol is approved, and lastly that the consent form is approved. If just one IRB formally determines that a study is not NSR, then the sponsor must report this to ODE. If all IRBs approve the study, it may proceed. In this case the local IRBs monitor the progress of the study according to their own SOPs, and FDA is not in the process.

7.6.3 Significant Risk Studies

Significant Risk studies require an approved IDE in order to treat patients in the U.S. Typical Significant Risk studies involved implantable devices or devices that introduce significant quantities of energy into the body. Studies with devices that sustain or support life are nearly always considered Significant Risk. If a study sponsor is unsure of the risk status of a study, consultation with the appropriate branch within the Office of Device Evaluation should be considered.

7.6.4 The Investigational Device Exemption (IDE)

The IDE serves the same function for a significant risk medical device clinical trial as the IND, described in Chapter 3, does for pharmaceutical clinical trials. The submission contains data that are similar, in many respects, to data contained in an IND. There are, however, some significant differences between the two submission types due to the differences in regulatory requirements between devices and drugs. First, although preclinical testing data are included in both submissions, the data in an IDE conforms to the ISO10993 biocompatability testing standard, rather than ICH guidance. Relevant FDA guidance documents (special controls) may also list additional

TABLE 7.5

NSR/SR Comparison Chart

Item	NSR Sponsor	NSR PI	SR Sponsor	SR PI
Submit an IDE to FDA	–	–	+	–
Report ADEs to sponsor	–	+	–	+
Report ADEs to reviewing IRBs	+	+	+	+
Report ADEs to FDA	–	–	+	–
Report withdrawal of IRB approval to sponsor	–	+	–	+
Submit progress reports to sponsor; monitor and review IRB	–	+	–	+
Report deviations from the investigational plan to sponsor, and review IRB	–	–*	–	+
Obtain and document informed consent from all study subjects prior to use of the investigational device	–	+	–	+
Maintain informed consent records	–	+	–	+
Report any use of the device without prior informed consent to sponsor and reviewing IRB	–	+	–	+
Compile records of all anticipated and unanticipated adverse device effects and complaints	+	–	+	–
Maintain correspondence with PIs, IRBs, monitors, and FDA	–*	–*	+	+
Maintain shipment, use, and disposal records for the investigational device	–*	–*	+	+
Document date and time of day for each use of the IDE device	–	–	–	+
Maintain signed investigator agreements for each PI	–*	–	+	+
Provide a current investigator list to FDA every 6 months	–	–	+	–
Submit progress reports to the IRB at least yearly	+	–	+	–
Submit a progress report to FDA at least yearly	–	–	+	–
Submit final study report to FDA	–	–	+	–
Submit final study report to all reviewing IRBs	+	–	+	–
Monitor the study and secure compliance with the protocol	+	–	+	–
Notify FDA and all reviewing IRBs if an investigational device has been recalled	+	–	+	–
Comply with IDE advertising, promotion, and sale regulations	+	+	+	+
Comply with IDE labeling regulations	+	+	+	+

* Compliance with IDE regulations is recommended.

data expectations. The IDE regulation requires an investigational plan, but does not specify an Investigator Brochure. The IDE regulation also requires that the sponsor include a clinical monitoring SOP in the submission. Under the cost recovery provision of the IDE regulation, the sponsor may charge for the investigational device, so long as only R&D and manufacturing costs are recovered. An investigator agreement serves the function of FDA Form 1572 used for pharmaceutical studies. More detailed information regarding IDEs can be found at http://www.fda.gov/cdrh/manual/idemanul.pdf

7.6.5 Unique Aspects of Medical Device Studies

The informed consent, financial disclosure, and IRB regulations described in Chapter 3 apply equally for medical device studies. Provisions of the IND regulation and ICH guidelines do not apply to medical device studies. This section describes some of the unique features of medical device studies. Before we consider the regulatory differences between pharmaceutical and device studies, we need to review the procedural differences. Test article administration is frequently a prime concern in trials of therapeutic devices. In most drug trials IV, IM, or PO administration of the test article is a trivial concern that is hardly discussed. The manner in which a surgical device is used or the technique by which an implantable device is placed in the body can mean the difference between success and failure in the trial. Because of this, investigator training is a critical aspect of many device trials. Protocol compliance while using the device and while recording data is also a critical issue. In addition, the Clinical Research Associate (CRA) is called upon to transmit technical data between the technical development staff and investigators. Another global issue involves overall study design. Unlike most pharmaceutical studies that are both masked and randomized, the vast majority of device studies are not masked. Most of the time, it is not possible or ethical to mask the device, especially if the device is an implant or a surgical device.

There are also several key regulatory differences between pharmaceutical clinical trials and medical device clinical trials. First, the International Conference on Harmonisation guidelines only apply to pharmaceutical studies, not to medical device studies. The greatest effect is seen on Adverse Device Effects analysis and reporting (Refer to Figure 7.4). The IDE regulations permit an investigator to analyze a potential adverse device effect for 10 days before reporting it to the local IRB and the sponsor (most sponsors impose a 24-hour reporting period). The sponsor then has another 10 days to evaluate the event to determine if it should be reported to ODE, all reviewing IRBs, and all participating investigators. The IDE regulations do require the sponsor to directly communicate this information to the IRBs. This responsibility cannot be delegated to the investigators. While other ICH guidances do not apply, some, such as those that describe format and contents of clinical study reports, may offer device companies good suggestions for organizing their study reports. The IDE regulation also does not require the preparation of an investigator brochure. In some cases, a sponsor may chose to prepare such a document, even though it is not required. (Studies conducted in the EU must have an investigator's brochure.) FDA form 1572 is another inapplicable document. It requires the investigator to comply with key provisions of the IND regulation, so it is not relevant to device studies. In its place we have the investigator agreement. It serves roughly the same purpose as form 1572. Its contents are specified in 21CFR 812.43(c). Although not required by the regulation, many sponsors ask that the principle investigator list the subinvestigators in the agreement, as this list will simplify

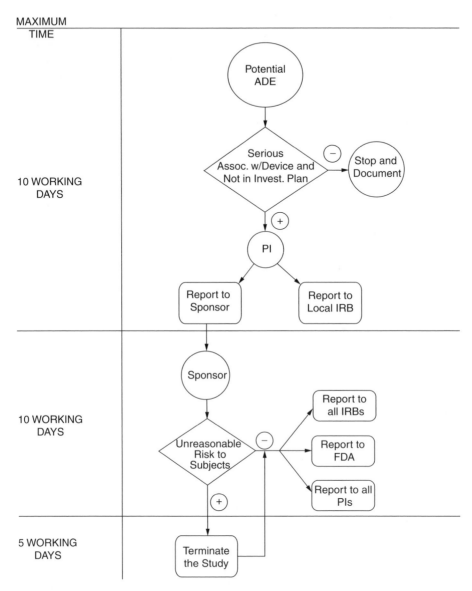

FIGURE 7.4
Adverse device effect reporting.

the gathering of financial disclosure information. There is usually a second investigator agreement, not subject to FDA review, that covers financial compensation, publishing priorities, and other unregulated activities. Lastly, the cost recovery provision of the IDE regulation [21 CFR 812.20(b)(8)] permits the sponsor to charge for the device. The sponsor can charge enough to recover research and development costs. This provision cannot be used to commercialize an investigational device.

7.7   The 510(k) Premarket Notification

More than 4000 medical devices are cleared to the U.S. market every year through the 510(k) Premarket Notification process. This represents approximately half the new devices that appear on U.S. market in a given year. The 510(k) process is relatively rapid, flexible, and adaptable to many different device types and risk levels.

The goal of the 510(k) process is:

> Demonstration of Substantial Equivalence to a device that was on the U.S. market prior to May 28, 1976, or to a device that has *already gone through the 510(k) clearance process.*

Devices that have successfully gone through the 510(k) process are described as "510(k) cleared." A distinction is made between those devices that have been reviewed according to the substantial equivalence standard and those that have been reviewed according to the Premarket Approval Application (PMA) safety and effectiveness standard. PMA devices are "approved."

The previously cleared device included for comparison purposes in a 510(k) is called the "predicate device." A 510(k) may contain multiple predicate devices that address various features of the device. The device designers should be able to provide regulatory personnel with assistance identifying key technological characteristics that demonstrate substantial equivalence. These data should already be part of the Design Inputs required as part of Design Controls. Generally, little manufacturing data are included in a 510(k). Sterile devices will include information on the sterilization process, including sterilization process validation activities and the sterilization assurance level. *In* vitro diagnostic products will frequently include data on the production of key reagents such as antibodies or nucleic acid probes. The other part of substantial equivalence relates to the indication for use. Frequently, one medical device can be used for many indications in a variety of medical specialties. When new indications are added, those indications must be cleared in a 510(k). The 510(k) must cite a predicate device with the same indication for use.

When searching for potential predicate devices, several information sources are useful. Two FDA databases, the 510(k) Database[6] and the Classification Database[7] can be very helpful. The 510(k) Database is especially useful when one knows either the name of potential predicate devices or the manufacturer of the device (see Figure 7.5). The Classification Database can be used to identify a particular device type and its corresponding Product Code. One can then transfer the Product Code to the 510(k) database and

---

[6] Food and Drug Administration   http://www.accessdata.fda.gov/scripts/cdrh/cfdocs/cfPMN/pmn.cfm
[7] Food and Drug Administration, http://www.accessdata.fda.gov/scripts/cdrh/cfdocs/cfPCD/classification.cfm

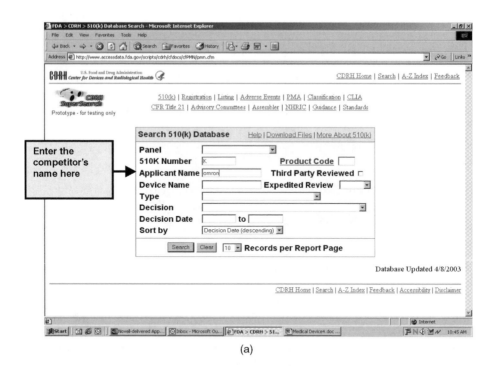

(a)

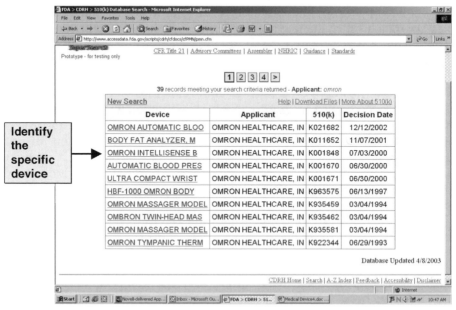

(b)

FIGURE 7.5

510(k) database search for a predicate device.

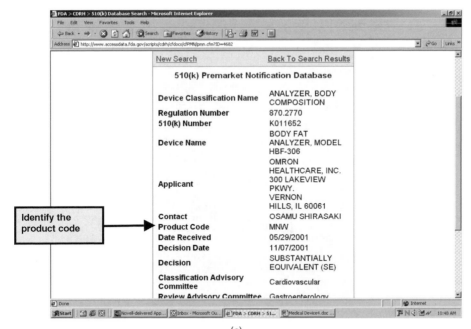

(c)

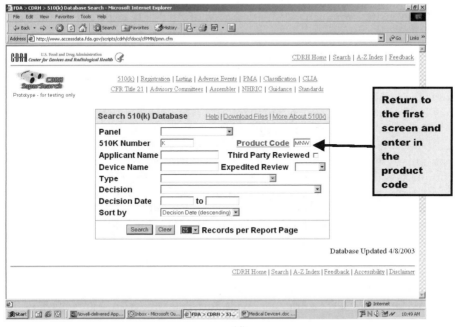

(d)

FIGURE 7.5
Continued.

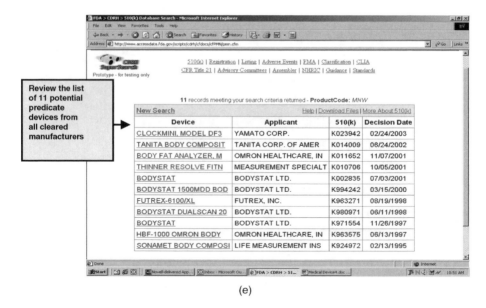

(e)

FIGURE 7.5
Continued.

generate a listing of all similar devices. Sales and Marketing staffs and competitor Websites are also excellent sources of predicate device information.

7.7.1 Substantial Equivalence

The two pillars of substantial equivalence are "intended use" **and** "technological characteristics." The sponsor must demonstrate that the new device has an intended use that is substantially equivalent to a predicate device AND that the technological characteristics of the new device are substantially equivalent to a predicate device. The predicate device must be a device that has already been cleared through the 510(k) process or a device that was in commercial distribution prior to May 28, 1976, when FDA was first able to regulate medical devices. A PMA approved device cannot serve as a 510(k) predicate device. There is some flexibility in the Office of Device Evaluation (ODE) approach to the 510(k) process, especially with respect to technology. The devices do not have to be identical. An acceptable predicate device can have different technological characteristics from the new device, so long as they do not raise new questions of safety and effectiveness, and the sponsor demonstrates that the device is as safe and as effective as the legally marketed device. Different technological characteristics might include changes in materials, control mechanisms, overall design, energy sources, and principles of operation. Safety and effectiveness can be demonstrated through engineering analysis, bench or animal testing, or human clinical testing. If it is not possible to identify a suitable predicate device or devices, the sponsor may have to consider filing a PMA.

7.7.2 Types of 510(k)s

There are four types of 510(k) Premarket Notifications. They are briefly described below. The Figure 7.6 describes the decision process used in order to determine which type of 510(k) should be submitted. Each type of 510(k) is briefly described in the following sections. For more information on these types of 510(k), see: http://www.fda.gov/cdrh/ode/parad510.pdf.

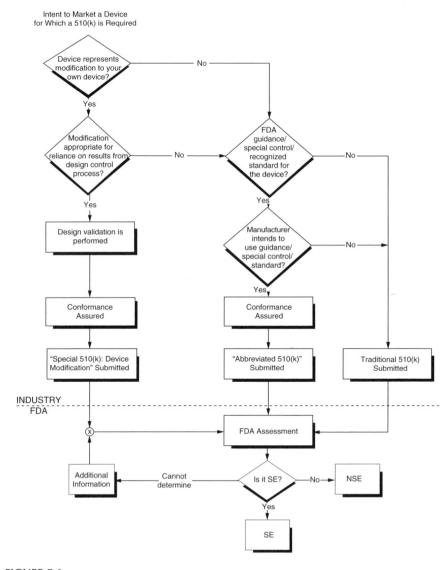

FIGURE 7.6
The new 510(k) paradigm. (From "A New 510(k) Paradigm — Alternate Approaches to Demonstrating Substantial Equivalence in Premarket Notifications" U.S. Food and Drug Administration.)

7.7.2.1   Traditional 510(k)

The traditional 510(k) is filed when the sponsor has developed a device that they believe is substantially equivalent to a device that has already been cleared through the 510(k) process, or was already on the market before the 1976 Medical Device Amendments were signed on May 26, 1976. In addition, the subject device is not a modification of one of the manufacturer's cleared devices, nor does the application contain any declarations of conformance with FDA recognized standards.[8] Once this 510(k) is submitted, ODE has 90 days to review the document.

7.7.2.2   Abbreviated 510(k)

This 510(k) is similar to the traditional 510(k) in function. A sponsor can choose to comply with FDA accepted standards during the testing process. A Declaration of Conformance is included in the 510(k), stating that the device meets the specifications in the referenced standards. Unlike a traditional 510(k), entire test reports do not need to be included. This simplifies both the 510(k) preparation and review processes. Once this 510(k) is submitted, ODE has 90 days to review the document.

7.7.2.3   Special 510(k)

A Special 510(k) is submitted when a sponsor has modified their own device, has not added a new indication for use, and has not altered the fundamental scientific technology of the device. Design controls, including a risk analysis, must be conducted. Reviews for Special 510(k)s are processed within 30 days.

7.7.2.4   De Novo 510(k)

The *de novo* 510(k) is a 510(k) without a predicate device. It is not a commonly used path (<0.5% of 510(k)s in FY02), but in some circumstances it is appropriate where the sponsor can demonstrate that the product has few risks and the extensive PMA safety and effectiveness review is not warranted. The device should be discussed with ODE in advance before embarking on this path.

7.7.3   510(k) Components

Below, the most common sections of a traditional 510(k) are described. Many of these sections are also present in the other types of 510(k)s.

---

[8] Food and Drug Administration, http://www.accessdata.fda.gov/scripts/cdrh/cfdocs/cfStandards/search.cfm.

7.7.3.1 Cover Sheet

This four-page form provides ODE with general information related to the submission in a standardized format. Completion of this document is not mandatory. Only relevant data fields should be completed. The applicant signature is not required. Indications should be taken word-for-word from the body of the 510(k). A sample cover sheet can be found at http://www.fda.gov/cdrh/manual/subcvsht.doc

7.7.3.2 Cover Letter

This letter should be no more than one or two pages long and should identify the device, very briefly summarize the contents of the application, and provide the name, address, telephone, and FAX numbers of the contact person. The type of 510(k) should also be specified.

7.7.3.3 Table of Contents

This section helps to create a "reviewer friendly" document by making it easy for the reviewer to locate each key section. Although it is not specifically required in the regulations, it is an expected component of any 510(k). Key sections of the 510(k) should be listed in the order they appear in the 510(k) along with the page number of the section. Index tabs, used selectively, can also aid the reviewer during the review process. All pages of the 510(k), beginning with general information, should be numbered consecutively. This numbering facilitates communication between the reviewer and the sponsor during the review process.

7.7.3.4 User Fee Information

A copy of the completed *Medical Device User Fee Cover Sheet* (available at: http://www.fda.gov/oc/mdufma/coversheet.html) must be included in this section. The unique Payment Identification Number present in this form enables ODE to confirm that the User Fee payment has been received. The actual user fee payment is NOT included in the 510(k). The information at the preceding URL describes the user fee payment process in detail. The FY04 user fee for a 510(k) is $3480.

7.7.3.5 Statement of Substantial Equivalence

This optional section can "sell" the 510(k) to the ODE by providing a well-reasoned rationale for a substantial equivalence determination. This section may not be necessary when there is a very simple comparison between a single predicate device and the new device. When a traditional or abbreviated 510(k) involves multiple predicate devices and complex technological comparisons, this type of statement can help communicate the sponsor's rationale. It contains a brief summary of device background information, along with a list of the predicate device(s), and most importantly, a narrative description of the sponsor's substantial equivalence claim. If appropriate, cross references to other sections of the 510(k) may be included.

7.7.3.6   Labeling

This section must provide ODE with all printed material associated with the device, including printing fixed to the outside of the device, its packaging, operator's manual, or in the case of software, controlled devices programmed into the electronics for display. Frequently, information displayed on video display screens is also reproduced in the operator's manual so it does not have to be included twice. Patient information brochures, if used, should also be included.

7.7.3.7   Advertising and Promotional Material

If provided, ODE will review the documentation and inform the sponsor of areas of noncompliance. This is optional information. If included, material should be clearly copied. Copies of actual brochures, especially if they are not on standard size paper or include fold-outs, are difficult for ODE document control personnel to handle. Advertising copy must be consistent with the indications for the use mentioned in the 510(k).

7.7.3.8   Comparative Information

This is the heart of the 510(k). This section must contain data that demonstrate that the 510(k) device is "substantially equivalent" to the predicate device(s). Careful selection of comparative parameters is essential. Comparison charts listing parameters and values for the predicate device and the 510(k) device are common. Bench and clinical testing data may also be included. Advertising for the predicate device may also be included to support statements describing the predicate device. This section must clearly demonstrate that the new device is substantially equivalent to one or more predicate devices with respect to indication for use and technological features such as materials used and operating principle.

7.7.3.9   Biocompatability Assessment (If Necessary)

Medical devices contain a wide variety of materials from stainless steel and titanium in orthopedic implants to plastics in catheters or even living cells in wound care products.[9] The data in this section must demonstrate that the device materials do not cause toxicity. Toxicity can occur through direct

---

[9] Helmus, M.N., Ed., *Biomaterials in the Design and Reliability of Medical Devices*, Kluwer Academic, Dordrecht, The Netherlands, 2003.

contact between the device and the body, such as a wound care product or an implantable device. Toxicity can also occur if materials such as plasticizers or mold release agents leach from polymers that carry blood out and back in the body, such as the tubing and components of a heart-lung bypass circuit. Adverse effects are often localized, but can be systemic, or even carcinogenic effects can occur, so the standard requires more extensive testing when the device is implanted, rather than contacting intact skin and for permanent implants, as opposed to devices that contact the body for less than 24 hours.

An FDA modified version of the international standard ISO 10993 is used to determine testing appropriate for a specific device. For more information on the use of ISO 10993 see: http://www.fda.gov/cdrh/g951.html. The FDA document includes a testing matrix that uses the length of exposure and type of exposure to determine which tests are appropriate. Before conducting recommended testing, it is advisable to confirm the testing plan with ODE, as requirements may vary for some devices.

Full reports of each required test are included in a traditional 510(k), especially if the test protocols have been modified from those specified in ISO 10993. A summary table of all biocompatibility testing and a summary of results is often useful. If the medical device does not contact the patient, biocompatibility data are generally not necessary.

7.7.3.10 Truthful and Accurate Statement

This statement identifies a person who takes legal responsibility for the accuracy of the 510(k). It follows the requirements of 21 CFR 807.87(j):

> I certify that, in my capacity as (*the position held in company*) of (*company name*), I believe to the best of my knowledge, that all data and information submitted in the premarket notification are truthful and accurate and that no material fact has been omitted.

The statement must be signed and dated by a responsible person at the submitting company. A consultant cannot sign it.

7.7.3.11 Clinical Data

ODE may request clinical data in order to demonstrate substantial equivalence to a predicate device. It may also be necessary when, as described in Section 7.7.1, the sponsor must demonstrate that the new device does not raise new questions of safety and effectiveness. At some point, ODE reviewers will become more familiar with the device and indication and require only engineering data. This often occurs once the first three or four 510(k)s for that generic type of device have successfully gone through the review process. Clinical data requirements for other 510(k) devices are specified in guidance documents and do not change over time. Generally, 510(k) clinical trials are smaller and simpler than most PMA clinical trials. Depending on the risk level of the trial, an approved IDE may be necessary in order to conduct the trial. See Section 7.6.

7.7.3.12   Shelf Life (If Necessary)

Stability of device components and packaging integrity (for sterile devices) must be demonstrated. The "Shelf Life of Medical Devices" guidance document (http://www.fda.gov/cdrh/ode/415.pdf) offers general advice. The useful life of *in vitro* diagnostic products must be determined. Accelerated data are acceptable in most cases, although sponsors should also initiate real time studies at the same time that they begin accelerated studies. A full report of real time or, where appropriate, accelerated aging studies, must be included.

7.7.3.13   Indication for Use Form

This form clarifies, for any interested party, the device's cleared indication(s) for use. The sponsor lists the indications for use on an ODE form. If the sponsor wishes to promote the device for a new indication, another traditional or abbreviated 510(k) must be cleared. Once a 510(k) is cleared, this form, the clearance letter, and the 510(k) summary are available from FDA via its Website.

7.7.3.14   510(k) Summary

Summaries are released to the public via the FDA's web site. They provide interested parties with a brief description of the device and some of the data included in the 510(k). The content of the Summary is described in 21 CFR 807.92. All relevant items must be present or ODE will request clarification, potentially delaying 510(k) clearance. When preparing summaries, regulatory professionals have to balance the regulatory requirements that mandate the inclusion of a wide variety of data describing the device and the development process with the business needs to limit disclosure of information that may benefit a competitor.

7.7.4   Practical Aspects for 510(k)s

It is important to conduct research early in the 510(k) process and become aware of the cleared indications and technologies for competitive products. It is possible to request a competitor's 510(k) under the Freedom of Information Act, although processing times can often exceed 12 months, so this is not usually a practical option. For older 510(k)s, commercial information brokers may offer considerably faster response times.

Once a 510(k) is filed, ODE will mail the sponsor a letter acknowledging receipt of the submission and including the "K" number used for internal tracking. It is important to keep a copy of every document sent to or received from the FDA. Sponsors should also designate one company FDA contact person. That individual should document all phone conversations with reviewers. FDA contact people should keep in mind that when ODE reviewers call with questions, they should listen carefully, but not leap to unsupported conclusions. If an ODE reviewer asks for specific data, confirm the data with experts in your company if you have any doubts. In most circumstances, a delay of a day or two will not be significant, compared with the risk of misstatement. Increasingly, communications with reviewers occur via e-mail. Additional data can be officially submitted via FAX or e-mail, if the reviewer concurs. Once the reviewer's questions have all been answered, the reviewer's conclusions are reviewed prior to generating a clearance letter. A copy of the clearance letter is usually FAXed to the sponsor shortly after it is signed. Commercial distribution can then begin. The official copy of the letter is mailed to the sponsor. The average review period for a traditional 510(k) was 100 days in FY02.

7.7.5 Postsubmission Considerations for 510(k)s

Manufacturers of 510(k) devices must register and list with FDA within 30 days of receiving 510(k) clearance. Detailed information on the registration and listing process can be found at: http://www.fda.gov/cdrh/devadvice/341.html and http://www.fda.gov/cdrh/devadvice/342.html. Manufacturers must also comply with the Quality System Regulation (QSR) with respect to device modifications, production, and quality operations. Injuries or deaths (to patients or medical personnel) must also be reported to FDA in accordance with the Medical Device Reporting (MDR) regulation (21CFR 803). Manufacturers are subject to inspection by FDA investigators who review QSR and MDR compliance.

7.8 The Premarket Approval Application

7.8.1 Introduction to the PMA

PMAs are necessary when the device developer wishes to market an innovative device in the U.S. that is not substantially equivalent to any other device that has been cleared through the 510(k) process. The PMA must demonstrate that the device is safe and effective. The PMA process is considerably more complex than the 510(k) process. Typical review times are approximately one year. Unlike most 510(k)s, a detailed manufacturing section describing the methods for building and testing the device must be included. Prior to final approval of the PMA, the CDRH Office of Compliance must review and approve the results of a preapproval inspection of the device manufacturing and development facilities. The sponsor of the clinical trial and two or three of the clinical investigation sites are also often subject to CDRH Bioresearch Monitoring (BIMO) inspections to confirm compliance with relevant sections of 21CFR 812. Lastly, the postmarket requirements of a PMA are considerably more complex than those related to a 510(k). Specifically, a PMA annual report must be filed with ODE each year and changes in labeling, materials, manufacturing, and quality methods, and specifications as well as changes in manufacturing location must all be reported to, and approved by, ODE, in advance. This is done through the PMA supplement process.

7.8.2   The PMA Process

PMAs are large and complex documents, often greater than 2000 pages. It can frequently take several years to obtain all the preclinical, clinical, and manufacturing data necessary for the PMA. It is essential that the PMA preparation effort be well planned, with good coordination between all functional areas involved in the development process. Advance research before a regulatory strategy is prepared and should include a wide variety of sources. Shortly after a PMA device is approved, the approval letter, Summary of Safety and Effectiveness and Official Labeling are placed on the CDRH website. These documents provide greater technical and regulatory detail than a 510(k) summary. The PMA submission itself is not available via the Freedom of Information process.

Once the indication for use and the device description have been established, it is important to confirm the key elements of the development plan with the appropriate reviewing branch within ODE. The device developer may choose to obtain this information via an informal telephone call, an informal pre-IDE meeting, a formal Designation Meeting, or a formal Agreement Meeting. See http://www.fda.gov/cdrh/ode/guidance/310.pdf for a more detailed description of these meetings. Generally, the more formal the meeting, the less interactive the discussion. Less formal meetings, while not generating binding agreements, can encourage very productive technical exchanges. The choice of meeting type involves balancing business, regulatory, and clinical needs.

Once a PMA development plan has been established and reviewed by ODE, it is time to execute it. Generally multiple activities such as manufacturing development and validation, preclinical functional and biocompatibility testing, and clinical testing proceed along parallel, often simultaneous tracks. In some cases it may be clear during the planning phase that some data, such as manufacturing process information or preclinical testing data may be available long before the clinical trial has ended. In these cases, it may be advantageous to submit the pieces of the PMA to ODE as they are completed, rather than send in all the data at the very end. This process is called a Modular PMA. If a PMA sponsor chooses to submit a Modular PMA, a PMA Shell or outline of the PMA must be prepared and approved by ODE. The shell describes the contents of each module. As the modules are submitted, ODE reviews them independently. Once review of a module has been successfully completed, ODE sends the sponsor a letter stating that the module is "locked" and will not be reopened unless some portion of data already submitted changes in later stages of the development process. When the last module is submitted, ODE considers the PMA complete.

7.8.3 Advisory Panels

When a PMA device raises questions that ODE reviewers have not previously addressed, they may choose to refer those questions to one of the advisory panels maintained for this purpose. Advisory panels are made up of experts in the field that are not FDA employees or from industry. Many panel members are in academic medicine. The panel has one non-voting industry representative and one non-voting consumer representative. An Executive Secretary, usually a senior ODE reviewer, coordinates administrative details. The conclusions of the advisor panel are not binding on FDA, although they are almost always followed. Transcripts of advisory panel meetings are available via the CDRH website. Videotapes of these meetings are also available from private sources. If competitive products have gone through the panel process these meeting minutes can provide a great deal of valuable information on the types of data and analysis expected. If such a panel meeting occurs during your development process, it is very helpful if regulatory, medical and technical development personnel attend in person. This can make preparation for your own panel meeting easier. More information on these panels can be found at: http://www.fda.gov/cdrh/panel/index.html

7.8.4 Clinical Data

According to Section 515 of the Food, Drug, and Cosmetic act, a PMA must provide valid scientific evidence that there is a "reasonable assurance" that a device is both safe and effective. Regulation 21 CFR 860.7(c)(2) states that this evidence can come from:

- Well controlled investigations
- Partially controlled investigations
- Objective trials without matched controls
- Well documented case histories conducted by qualified experts
- Reports of significant human experience with a marketed device from which it can fairly and responsibly be concluded by qualified experts that there is reasonable assurance of safety and effectiveness of a device under its conditions of use

In practice, the vast majority of PMA studies are designed as well con-trolled studies where patients are randomized to either a treatment or a control group. Less frequently, studies can be designed to compare the inves-tigational device to a historical control group, provided that the historical control group accurately reflects current U.S. medical practice and the demo-graphics of the U.S. population. Data from other types of studies must always be reported to ODE; however, they generally cannot stand as the sole source of performance data.

7.8.5   Use of International Data

Due to the international nature of the medical device industry, human clinical data may be available from non-U.S. studies before U.S. development efforts have begun. How should these data be treated? Can they be used to support the PMA? Does FDA require U.S. clinical data?

There are no FDA requirements that a PMA must contain U.S. clinical data. Good credible and ethical data will be accepted from any location. ODE suggests that sponsors planning to submit international data in a PMA discuss their plans with them early in the development process. As with any clinical study, it is critical to assure that the study meets ODE's expectations regarding medical and scientific issues such as the endpoints selected and comparators used. If all of these parameters are consistent with ODE expec-tations, then there is one last set of tests before the data can be accepted. According to 21 CFR 814.15, the study must:

- Have been conducted in accordance with the Declaration of Hels-inki, or local ethical procedures, whichever is stricter
- Utilize a patient population similar to the U.S. patient population
- Utilize a standard of care and medical practice similar to that in the U.S.
- Must be performed by competent investigators
- Generate data, including source documentation, that are available for audit by FDA

Sponsors must be especially careful that study patients are not treated with drugs or procedures that are not available in the U.S.

7.8.6   Components of the PMA

The PMA regulation (21CFR 814) contains a description of the components of a PMA. ODE has produced numerous guidance documents that describe various PMA sections. Many of these guidance documents are product-specific. Two of the more generic guidance documents can be found at: http://www.fda.gov/cdrh/manual/pmamanul.pdf and http://www.fda.gov/cdrh/blbkmem.html#pma

The items listed below include the major sections of a PMA. The length and complexity of each section will vary according to the technical details and regulatory issues associated with the product:

1. Cover page
2. Table of contents
3. Summary of safety and effectiveness
4. Device description and manufacturing data
5. Performance standards referenced
6. Technical data (nonclinical and clinical)
7. Justification for a single investigator
8. Bibliography
9. Device sample (if requested)
10. Labeling
11. Environmental assessment

7.9   The Quality System Regulation (QSR)

The QSR regulates both the device development and the manufacturing process for all Class II and Class III devices from the beginning of the development phase until the device is no longer supported by the manufacturer. It also covers the manufacturing process for many Class I devices. It does not cover the research process for any medical devices. The goal of the QSR is to create a self-correcting system that reliably produces robust device designs and production methods, ensuring that devices perform in a manner consistent with their intended use. In many ways, the QSR has evolved into the glue that holds the medical device regulatory process together from development through end of use. As discussed earlier, the existence of the QSR makes the Special 510(k) possible. Once a device is marketed, the corrective and preventive action (CAPA) provisions of the QSR are closely related to compliance with the Medical Device Reporting (MDR) regulation. An additional advantage of the QSR is that it follows the format of the international standard, ISO 9001:1994 which helps to enable device companies that sell their product internationally to maintain common systems for most design and production related activities. In most cases, the QSR requires more extensive documentation than ISO 9001:1994, or its medical device specific variant, ISO 13485.[10] The system works by requiring specific activities and documentation beginning during the development process.

---

[10] Trautman, K., "The FDA and Worldwide Quality System Requirements Guidebook for Medical Devices," ASQC Quality Press, Milwaukee, WI, 1997.

The manufacturing and quality processes also require specific evaluations and procedures, all of which must be documented. Frequently, FDA field investigators will follow the Quality System Inspection Techniques (QSIT) approach[11] when inspecting a device facility. This process breaks QSR compliance into four main modules and four satellite modules, some of which may not be applicable to all device firms. The FDA investigator will choose a subset of those modules and determine the firm's compliance with QSR. This means that not every system is reviewed during a QSIT inspection; however, this process does yield a general assessment of QSR compliance. Many firms consider the QSR requirements to be only a beginning and build on them, adding various customer-oriented feedback loops and financial accountability to the process. These integrated business systems can generate significant returns on the investment by reducing time to market, reducing the number of field corrections and recalls, increasing customer satisfaction and device safety. The remaining portions of this section describe some of the provisions of the QSR. Design Controls were already discussed in Section 7.4. Although these sections of the QSR are discussed separately, the figure below graphically demonstrates how these functions are connected to each other. Readers should refer to the regulation[12] for complete information.

7.9.1 Management Controls

Device firms need to demonstrate that they have management systems in place that can adequately control the all the processes that take place in the life cycle of their products from the development phase onwards. As Figure 7.7 illustrates, management is at the center of the Quality System. The QSR holds "management with executive responsibility" ultimately responsible for the tasks specified in the regulation. Clearly, a device manufacturer with six employees will have less complex systems than a manufacturer with 600 employees. One standard operating procedure (SOP) or a single organizational structure would not be appropriate for all device manufacturers.

One key provision of the QSR involves the controls that management places upon the regulated system. First, there must be a quality policy in place, implemented and understood by all levels of employees. A quality plan and quality system procedures must also be in place. Next, management has the responsibility to assure that there are adequate resources and organizational structure to carry out all the activities specified in the regulation. A Management Representative must be formally appointed, must be actively involved in maintaining the Quality System, and must regularly report those efforts to management with executive responsibility. Part of maintaining the quality system involves testing the system with presched-

---

[11] Food and Drug Administration, Guide To Inspections of Quality Systems, August 1999.
[12] 21CFR 820.

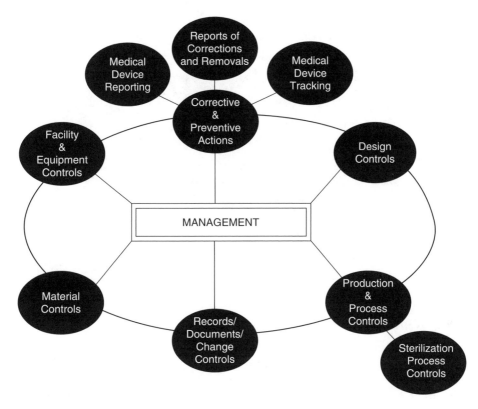

FIGURE 7.7
The seven primary QSR subsystems from FDA Guide to Inspections of Quality Systems, August 1999.

uled audits conducted by company staff that is not directly involved in the function audited. These audits must be conducted according to a SOP, recorded in an audit log, and audit results documented. (FDA investigators do not generally have the authority to request copies of these audit reports.) The function of these audits is for the company itself to identify and then correct any quality system problems detected in the audits. Management reviews of a wide variety of quality data must be conducted at regular intervals and documented. These data include, but are not limited to, audit reports. Other sources of quality data include rework records from the manufacturing floor, incoming QC testing summaries, service records, customer complaints and inquiries, and final inspection records. All of these data sources combine to paint a picture of the status of the company's products. It is critically important that the firm can demonstrate that action is taken as a result of these data. Identification of quality issues is important, but correction of problems and confirmation of the effectiveness of such corrections must also be documented.

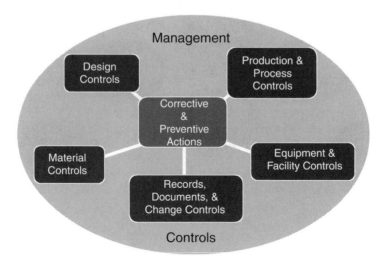

FIGURE 7.8
CAPA Diagram (from the FDA QSIT Workshop Presentation).

7.9.2   Corrective and Preventive Action

The Corrective and Preventive Action (CAPA) portion of the regulation makes the firm's quality system self-correcting and self-improving. The five functional areas depicted in the blue boxes in Figure 7.8 feed information into the CAPA system. Under the supervision of management, these data are processed and initiatives developed and executed which are intended to identify the causes of the problems and correct them. Data sources for the CAPA system include internal audits, in-coming, in-process and final QC testing results, service and repair records, and customer feedback. A variety of statistical tools may be used to better evaluate these data. Failure investigations should be conducted according to a predetermined SOP to determine the root cause of device failures. Once this has been done, a corrective action plan must be prepared and the corrective actions verified or, in appropriate instances, validated.

7.9.3   Production and Process Controls

Production and process controls are the systems at the heart of the manufacturing process. Documentation is a major part of the control process. The Device Master Record (DMR), a compilation of records containing the procedures and specifications for a finished device, is a key document for this functional area. Rather than existing as a discrete document, it is frequently an index that directs the reader to other documents where the necessary information is located. The Device History Record (DHR) is a compilation of records containing the production history of a finished device or a production run of devices. It usually contains manufacturing documentation, testing results, labeling documentation and release/approval documentation. A single DHR may be generated for a large expensive durable medical device, while another DHR may describe a production run of 10,000 disposable devices. Validation documentation, when necessary, is also a key part of Production and Process Controls. Any production process whose output cannot be 100% checked once it is completed, must be validated in order to establish, by objective evidence, that a process consistently produces a result or product meeting its predetermined specifications. Typically, processes such as sterilization or molding of plastic parts are validated. Other activities such as calibration, servicing, and maintenance of production and testing equipment and cleaning and maintenance of buildings must also be documented.

The goal of the QSR is to weave a web of systems that closely monitor development efforts to assure that a high quality design is created, that the production of that device occurs in a controlled and predictable manner, and that various streams of quality data are appropriately analyzed and used to effect corrective and preventive action, when necessary.

7.10 Postmarketing Issues

7.10.1 Medical Device Modifications

Medical device technology evolves at a very rapid rate. Often the version of the device that receives initial PMA approval is a version or two older than the one sold outside the U.S. or that is sold by the manufacturer's competitors. Also, 510(k) devices change quickly. In both cases sponsors need to understand how the FDA process will affect their product upgrade timelines and budgets. Modifications for all Class II and III devices must be developed in accordance with the Design Control provisions of the Quality System Regulation. Design Controls have added enough extra confidence to the system so that, since 1998, FDA has created new processes such as Special 510(k)s and 30-Day Notices for PMAs that permit sponsors to rapidly implement some device modifications, as long as they comply with the Design Control provisions of the QSR.

7.10.1.1 Modifications to 510(k) Devices

There are three main classifications of 510(k) device modifications (see Table 7.6). They include those that require a documented review and a determination by the company that a new 510(k) is not needed, those that require a special 510(k), and those that require a traditional or abbreviated 510(k). A useful source of more detailed information on changes to 510(k) devices can be found at: http://www.fda.gov/cdrh/ode/510kmod.pdf.

TABLE 7.6

Modifications to 510(k) Devices

Regulatory Action	Examples of Modifications
Review, document in a memo to the file	Redesigning the external case of a durable medical device so that it consists of few pieces in order to reduce production costs
File a special 510(k)	Adding a feature that has already been incorporated in another device of the same type*
File a traditional or abbreviated 510(k)	Adding a new indication, significant change in technology

* Modification to firm's own device and no change in intended use or fundamental scientific technology

TABLE 7.7

PMA Supplement Types

PMA Supplement Type	Examples of Modifications
180-Day Supplement	A major change in the design of the device or in manufacturing or quality control methods
180-Day Panel Track Supplement	Adding a new indication for use where clinical data are required to support the application
Special PMA Supplement — Changes Being Effected[a]	A change that enhances the safety of a device, such as labeling changes that add or strengthen a contraindication, warning, precaution, or information about an adverse reaction
30-d Notice[a]	A change in the type of process used, (e.g., machining a part to injection-molding the part)
Real Time Supplement[b]	Minor design modifications that would otherwise require a 180-day supplement
Annual Report	Update the microprocessor for the device, when equivalence test has previously been approved by ODE

[a] The sponsor may choose either submission type.
[b] With the prior approval of the responsible ODE Branch Chief
* Modification to firm's own device and no change in intended use or fundamental scientific technology

7.10.1.2   Modifications to PMA Devices

Modifications to PMA devices are more closely controlled than modifications to 510(k) devices. Table 7.7 briefly summarizes the various types of PMA supplements. http://www.fda.gov/cdrh/ode/pumasupp.pdf

PMA sponsors must also submit a PMA Annual Report to ODE every year. This report contains updates on ongoing clinical trials, device modifications, adverse device effects, and MDR reports. More information on PMA Annual Reports can be found at http://www.fda.gov/cdrh/devadvice/pma/post-approval.html#annual.

7.10.2 Medical Device Reporting (MDR)

Significant problems with marketed medical devices must be reported to FDA using the FDA Form 3500A (MedWatch). While this same form is used to report pharmaceutical adverse events, Section D — Suspect Medical Device, Section F — For Use by User Facility/Distributor-Devices Only, and Section H — Device Manufacturers Only are specific to devices. The process for evaluating and reporting device incidents is described in 21 CFR 803 and is not related to the ICH procedures employed for pharmaceuticals.

The MDR regulation originally implemented in 1984 and the final regulation was published in December of 1995, effective July 31, 1996. A MDR SOP must be in place for every device manufacturer, regardless of device class. This applies even if the firm has never made a MDR report. MDR reports are available on the CDRH website at: http://www.fda.gov/cdrh/mdr/mdr-file-general.html. Figure 7.9 summarizes the MDR process.

7.10.2.1 MDR Reporting Timeframes

The manufacturer must report incidents to FDA 5 working days after becoming aware of events *requiring remedial action* to prevent an unreasonable risk of substantial harm or events for which FDA has required 5-day reporting. This type of notification commonly occurs when a recall or field correction is necessary. The manufacturer must report incidents to FDA 30 working days after becoming aware of information that reasonably suggests that a device may have *caused or contributed to a death or serious injury* or if the device malfunctions in a manner likely to cause or contribute to death or serious injury. It is important to note that the regulation does not differentiate between injuries to patients, medical professionals, or family members. An injury to anyone that is caused by the device can be reportable.

7.10.2.2 Key MDR Definitions

Serious Injury: Life threatening, permanent impairment or damage, or medical/surgical intervention necessary to preclude such damage. Cosmetic or trivial irreversible damage is not serious.

Malfunction: The failure of the device to meet its performance specifications or otherwise perform as intended.

"Becomes Aware": When *any* employee at any level of the company becomes aware of a reportable event.

"Reasonably Suggests": A professional medical opinion relating to the causal relationship between the adverse event and the medical device. If a physician working for the manufacturer concludes that an event is not related to the device, no report is necessary. This decision must be documented.

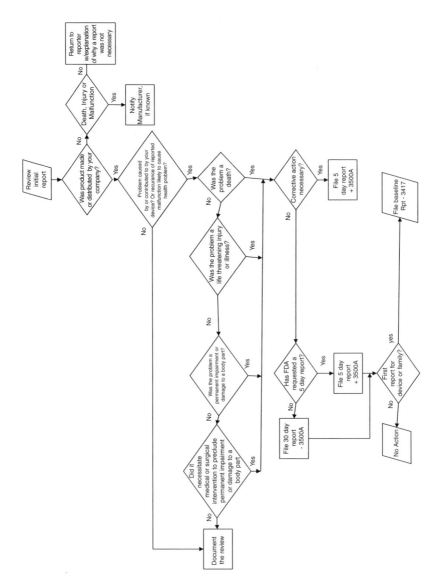

FIGURE 7.9
MDR decision tree.

"Caused or Contributed to": Causation can be attributed to device failures or malfunctions due to improper design, manufacturing methods, labeling, or operator error.

Remedial action: Any action that is not routine maintenance, routine servicing, and is intended to prevent the recurrence of the event.

7.10.2.3   Other MDR Requirements

Manufacturers must retain all MDR records for two years or for the expected life of the device, whichever is longer. The types of records that must be retained include all MDR related forms submitted to FDA, explanations why reports were not submitted for specific events that were not reported, and documentation relating to all events investigated. Written procedures must be present for identification and evaluation of events, a standardized review process to determine reportability and for procedures to assure that adequate reports are submitted to FDA in a timely manner. Additional information on the MDR regulation can be found at: http://www.fda.gov/cdrh/mdr/.

7.10.3   Advertising and Promotion

Unlike pharmaceuticals, no preclearance of ad copy is required for medical devices, even PMA devices. Promotional material must conform with cleared or approved indications for use. If a device is cleared for a general indication, more specific indications cannot be promoted unless they are specifically cleared.

8

The Development of Orphan Drugs

Marlene E. Haffner

CONTENTS

8.1 Introduction

In January 1983, when the Orphan Drug Act[1] was signed into law in the U.S. by President Ronald Reagan, incentives were for the first time provided for the pharmaceutical industry to develop drugs that otherwise have little commercial value but which are necessary, and at times life-saving, for patients with rare diseases. A 1984 amendment defined applicable rare diseases as those affecting fewer than 200,000 patients in the U.S. Products (known as orphan products) to treat these populations include drugs and biologicals which, despite potential usefulness, remain inadequately tested and/or unavailable to patients due to the limited commercial interest.

With this 1983 legislation, the Federal Government established a policy to cooperate and assist in the development of orphan products through the Food and Drug Administration (FDA). Previously, there had been drug development programs in the National Institutes of Health (NIH), the National Cancer Institute (NCI) (dedicated to the development of drugs to

[1] Public Law 97–414.

1-58716-007-2/04/$0.00+$1.50
© 2004 by CRC Press LLC

treat various cancers), and in the National Institute of Neurological Disorders and Stroke (NINDS) which is committed to drug development for epilepsy. But it was truly unique for the FDA to assume a proactive role and assist individuals needing drugs and biological products, medical devices, and medical foods for rare conditions.

The Orphan Drug Act provides assistance and numerous financial incentives for the development of orphan products: 7 years of marketing exclusivity for an orphan-designated product that receives FDA market approval for the same indication; tax credits for clinical research expenses incurred to develop orphan products; and grants to fund the investigation of rare disease treatment — studies that produce data acceptable to the agency and result in or substantially contribute to approval of these products. Of these, marketing exclusivity has proven to be the most significant incentive to orphan drug research and subsequent development because it limits competition by prohibiting the FDA from approving another version of the same drug for the same indication.

8.2   FDA Office of Orphan Products Development

Because of the FDA's own desire to find ways to bring orphan drugs to the marketplace, the Agency established its Office of Orphan Products Development (OOPD) in 1982 — nearly a year before the passage of the U.S. Orphan Drug Act. At that time, the results of legislation being considered by Congress were unclear. FDA's orphan product program relied, as it does now, upon the private sector — with the U.S. Government acting as a catalyst in bringing to the marketplace drugs for rare diseases. Attaining FDA market approval for orphan products presents multiple challenges for drug sponsors. One major difficulty is the small size of the population. Careful planning of the investigational protocol is essential since there will usually be no opportunity to go back and restudy. In 1982, the OOPD functioned mainly through communication and persuasion. There were no incentives that could be offered toward the development of such needed drugs. Today, the mission of the OOPD continues to assist and encourage the identification, development, and availability of safe and effective products for people with rare diseases or rare disorders.

The OOPD is located within the Office of the Commissioner, Food and Drug Administration (FDA), and is responsible for implementing the orphan products development program. Medical reviewers in OOPD receive and evaluate sponsors' requests for orphan product designation. The OOPD review involves verifying the scientific rationale of the proposal, confirming the rare disease prevalence, and then designating drugs and biological products that qualify as orphan products. The OOPD operates separately from the FDA drug and biologics review divisions, and instead acts as an ombudsman to assist sponsors.

The OOPD also has responsibility for administering the award of orphan grant funding to defray costs of qualified clinical testing incurred in connection with the development of drugs, biologics, medical devices, and foods for rare diseases and conditions. Although the Orphan Drug Act pertains primarily to drug and biological products, the OOPD Grants Program also includes clinical studies for medical foods and devices that meet the "orphan" criteria established by Congress.

When necessary, the OOPD expands its liaison to seek commercial sponsors for promising products to treat rare diseases. In many cases, OOPD brings together researchers and pharmaceutical companies, and identifies alternate sources of funding for the development of orphan products. Above all, the OOPD consistently applies the incentives of the Orphan Drug Act in order to fulfill FDA's mission to facilitate the availability of new therapies for serious and life-threatening illness.

8.3 The Designation Process

Orphan drug designation must be obtained before a sponsor can obtain any direct financial benefits provided by the Orphan Drug Act. A sponsor may request orphan drug designation for a previously unapproved drug or a designation for a new indication for an already marketed drug. In addition, a sponsor of a drug that is otherwise the same drug as an already approved orphan drug may seek and obtain orphan drug designation for the subsequent drug for the same rare disease or condition, if they are able to provide valid evidence that their drug may be clinically superior to the first drug. More than one sponsor may receive orphan drug designation of the same drug for the same rare disease or condition, but each sponsor seeking orphan drug designation must file a complete request for designation (21 CFR Part 316.20).

Requests for designation must be made before the submission of a marketing application.[2] The content of the sponsor's application for orphan designation should include, but is not restricted to, the following information:

1. A statement that the sponsor requests orphan drug designation for a rare disease or condition, which shall be specifically identified.

2. A description of the rare disease or condition for which the drug is being or will be investigated, the proposed indication or indications for use of the drug, and the reasons why such therapy is needed.

---

[2] 53 FR 47577; November 1998 (Public Law 100–290).

3. A description of the drug and a discussion of the scientific rationale for the use of the drug for the rare disease or condition, including all data from nonclinical laboratory studies, clinical investigations, and other relevant data that are available to the sponsor, whether positive, negative, or inconclusive. Copies of pertinent unpublished and published papers are also required. When the sponsor of a drug that is otherwise the same drug as an already approved orphan drug seeks orphan designation for the subsequent drug for the same rare disease or condition, an explanation should be included of why the proposed variation may be clinically superior to the first drug.

4. Documentation with appended authoritative references to illustrate that the disease or condition for which the drug is intended affects a population of fewer than 200,000 people in the U.S. or, for a drug intended for diseases or conditions affecting more than 200,000 people per year in the U.S., evidence to substantiate that there is no reasonable expectation that the costs of research and development of the drug for the indication can be recovered by sales of the drug in the U.S. within seven years. In either case, an estimate of the population prevalence *must* be provided in each application.

5. A summary of the regulatory status and marketing history of the drug in the U.S. and in foreign countries, e.g., Investigational New Drug (IND) and marketing application status and dispositions, identification of what uses are under investigation and in what countries; for what indication is the drug approved in foreign countries; and what adverse regulatory actions have been taken against the drug in any country.

6. Evidence to demonstrate that a proposed indication intended for a *subset* of persons with a particular disease or condition complies with the definition of "medically plausible subset" found in the 1991 Notice of Proposed Rulemaking (NPRM) (*Federal Register* Vol. 56, No. 19). The NPRM uses the following example to illustrate: "... a drug might well be too toxic for use in treating a disease or condition except in patients refractory to or intolerance of other less toxic treatments; the refractory and intolerant patients might be a reasonable orphan subset. On the other hand, choosing an arbitrary subset (e.g., people with blood pressure over a certain level), simply to qualify a drug as an orphan drug would be unacceptable." In the orphan drugs final regulations,[3] the FDA declines to provide examples of medical plausibility, or to further develop the definition of this term. Application of the concept is based on the facts of each individual case.

---

[3] 21 CFR Part 316; December 1992.

The OOPD has determined that pediatric patients constitute a "medically plausible" subset of a patient population. Based on unique pharmacokinetic properties in the pediatric population, growth and developmental changes can influence the way drugs are absorbed, distributed, metabolized, and excreted, which are vastly differently from the adult. Therefore, a sponsor of a new drug or biological product may seek orphan drug designation for treatment of a disease or condition in the relevant pediatric subset of the patient population. With regard to currently marketed drugs with no approved pediatric indication, OOPD will consider a pediatric indication a new "orphan" indication, for which the sponsor may request orphan drug designation.

The FDA has long recognized pediatric patients as "therapeutic orphans" due to the lack of adequate pediatric dosing information among drugs that are on the market. This issue has been addressed, in part, by the pediatric exclusivity provision of the Food and Drug Administration Modernization Act (FDAMA) of 1997,[4] and more recently by the mandatory Final Rule promulgated by the FDA on December 2, 1998. The pediatric exclusivity was reauthorized in 2002, and is scheduled to sunset in 2007.

Population prevalence of a disease or disorder in the U.S. is one of the primary criteria for orphan status eligibility. Prevalence is defined in the Orphan Drug Regulation as the number of persons in the U.S. who have been diagnosed as having the disease or condition at the time of the submission of the application. The OOPD receives many inquiries and comments from orphan designation applicants, asserting that determination of prevalence for rare diseases is often a difficult, if not impossible, task. Applicants seeking OOPD assistance in determining prevalence are advised that there is no standard source of data on rare disease prevalence. Each application and each indication requires independent evaluation of the best and most reliable sources available. However OOPD does follow definite principles when seeking verification of prevalence estimates submitted in applications for orphan designation. These principles indicate that population prevalence information is found in five general sources:

1. Primary medical literature (refereed journals)
2. Secondary medical/pharmaceutical literature (textbooks)
3. Federal Agencies (HCFA, NCHS, CDC, etc.)
4. Rare disease organizations (NORD, NORD subsidiaries)
5. Affidavits from experts in the specific medical specialty

Incidence (the number of new cases of a disease diagnosed in one year) may be used to calculate the patient population of diseases with duration of less than 1 year, for instance, infectious diseases, acute medical events such as myocardial infarction, and Acute Respiratory Distress Syndrome

---

[4] Public Law 105–115; November 1998.

(ARDS). On the other hand, patients with chronic rare diseases may live for many years; therefore, using a calculation of incidence would grossly underestimate the potential market for use.

Proposed indications for use of orphan drugs are subject to review by the applicable FDA center, the Center for Drug Evaluation and Research (CDER), or the Center for Biologics Evaluation and Research (CBER). These centers routinely review indications for use during the approval process. The OOPD may ask the centers for their advice about the medical plausibility of potential orphan drug designations. These reviews by the centers include consideration of the appropriateness of the request for orphan drug designation, and, in particular, consideration of whether the target populations have been artificially restricted.

8.4 Tax Credits

The Internal Revenue Service administers the tax credit provisions of the Orphan Drug Act. Final regulations on the tax credits were published in the Federal Register on October 3, 1988 (53 FR 38708) and the current version of these regulations may be found in Title 26, Code of Federal Regulations Chapter 1, Part 1, Section 1.28-1. This section allows for a credit against tax owed, up to 50% of qualified clinical testing expenses related to the investigation of a drug for a rare disease or condition that is designated as an orphan drug. Public Law 105-34 (August 5, 1997) made the tax credit provisions permanent from May 31, 1997 forward, along with the carry-back/carry-forward provision. Previously, this section required reauthorization by Congress each year. The carry-back/carry-forward of unused credit allows the manufacturer to carry the excess credit back 1 tax year if they are unable to use part or all of the credit because of the tax liability limit and to then carry any additional unused credit forward for up to 20 tax years after the year of the credit.

8.5 PDUFA and Orphan Products Development

Since 1997, the multiple economic incentives available with the orphan designation of a treatment product for a rare disease include a waiver of the Prescription Drug User Fee Act (PDUFA)[5] application fee.

---

[5] The PDUFA (Public Law 102–571).

The Prescription Drug User Fee Act (PDUFA) of 1992[6] authorized FDA to collect user fees for certain applications for approval of drug and biological products from establishments where the products are made. The PDUFA of 1992 established user fees to be assessed on (1) certain applications and supplements for approval of drug and biologic products, (2) certain establishments where such products are made, and (3) certain marketed products. Resources provided by the PDUFA have significantly helped the FDA shorten review time for drugs. With the passage of PDUFA II in 1997, Congress exempted all orphan-designated drugs from paying the new drug application ("user") fees. This exemption may save the sponsor an additional several hundred thousand dollars. Prescription Drug User Fee information is available at www.fda.gov/cder.pdufa.default.htm. Orphan product sponsors still have the option to seek waivers of the establishment and product fees on a case-by-case and year-by-year basis. PDUFA II legislation effectively rewrote OOPD's relationship with the FDA user fee program. The designation process is now a PDUFA administrative function which conveys benefits to products found to qualify for orphan designation.

The fee rates established by PDUFA for FY 2003 increased by 72%: for application fees ($533,400 for an application requiring clinical data, and $266,700 for an application not requiring clinical data or a supplement requiring clinical data); establishment fees rose by 44% ($209,900); and product fees by 48% ($32,400). These fees became effective on October 1, 2002, and remained in effect through September 30, 2003.

8.6 Orphan Product Grants Program

The FDA funds the development of orphan products through its grants program for clinical studies to investigate rare disease therapies. Section 5 of the Orphan Drug Act (P.L. 97-414, January 4, 1983) authorizes appropriations for grants or contracts to assist eligible entities to defray costs of qualified experimental expenses.

Each year, an announcement is made of the anticipated availability of funds for awarding of grants in the coming year. In response to this announcement, applicants are asked to propose one discrete clinical study that is intended to facilitate FDA approval of the product. As the goal of the grant program is to encourage the clinical development of new products or of new indications for already approved products for rare diseases or conditions, all studies that are supported by this grant program must be conducted under an investigational new drug (IND) application or an investigational device exemption (IDE). Medical foods are the only exception to this requirement. The IND/

---

[6] The PDUFA (Public Law 102–571).

IDE must be in an active status and in compliance with all regulatory requirements at the time of submission of the application.

Clinical trials in any phase of development are eligible to be awarded grants up to $150,000 per year for a maximum of three years, and clinical trials in Phase II or Phase III of development may be awarded up to $300,000 per year for a maximum of 3 years. The number of grant awards varies each year, depending on the availability of funds. Studies continuing in years 2 or 3 of original funding are funded first with the remainder of funds going to fund new studies. Continued funding is dependent upon the grantee making acceptable progress towards patient enrollment goals and/or protocol goals.

Most orphan drugs are originally studied by academic researchers, however, other organizations — foreign or domestic, public or private, nonprofit or for-profit — are eligible to apply. The early Phase I and Phase II studies by these academic investigators provide the initial data necessary to interest commercial sponsorship for further development. At the start of the program in 1983, only $500,000 was available for the grant program. The last several years have seen significant growth in the program. Currently, Congress sets aside approximately $13.5 million annually to fund the FDA orphan grant program.

Applications that are received in response to the Request for Applications (RFA) published annually in the Federal Register initially undergo an administrative review by grants management and program staff for relevance and responsiveness to the RFA. This review includes assurance that the clinical study for which the grant is being applied for will be conducted under an active IND/IDE, that the clinical trial being proposed is intended to provide safety and/or efficacy data of one therapy for one indication, that the rare disease or condition has a prevalence of 200,000 or less in the U.S., that there is reasonable assurance that the necessary number of eligible patients is available for study, and that the budget is appropriate for the phase of study being proposed.

Acceptable applications are reviewed and evaluated for scientific and technical merit by ad hoc panels of experts in the subject field of the specific application. A second level review is then conducted by a National Advisory Council to concur with the recommendations made by the initial review group. Rank ordered priority scores then determine the final awards that will be made. If an application is found to be nonresponsive to the RFA, it will be returned to the applicant without further consideration or review. The most common reasons for considering applications to be nonresponsive are that the study does not have an active IND or IDE, that the study is not a clinical trial, or that the study proposed is not for a rare disease or condition.

Each year the OOPD receives approximately 100 applications for funding, and, in recent years, has funded between 15 and 20 new awards annually. Currently, OOPD manages about 100 active grants in various phases of clinical trial status and for various rare diseases and conditions. Throughout the course of the grant, staff members serve as project officers, monitoring the progress of each grant study via telephone conversations or e-mail communication with the principle investigator. Project officers consult with principle investigators regarding patient enrollment, progress towards protocol goals, and compliance with all FDA IND/IDE regulations; communications are followed by written reports. Site visits with officials of the grantee organization are also conducted on a regular basis.

The orphan products grant program is administered by the OOPD; however, OOPD has no role in the review of a product for marketing approval. Oversight of the development and approval of the product is the responsibility of the appropriate reviewing division in the FDA. While OOPD does not review products for marketing approval, members of the review staff often act as ombudsmen, working with NDA or BLA sponsors to foster communication and assist them in meeting agency requirements for product approval.

8.7 Clinical Trial Design for Rare Disease Treatment

The limited numbers of patients available for enrollment in clinical trials to investigate rare disease treatment may make it difficult to ascertain the safety and effectiveness of the product being tested for use. It is important, therefore, that the risk/benefit ratio is carefully weighed, and that trials be designed to systematically observe patients and attempt to collect adequate data to demonstrate effectiveness as well as to determine the optimal dosage.

In open label clinical trials, also known as nonmasked drug trials, all patients receive the study drug; both the physicians and patients involved in the study are aware of which drug the patient is taking. Considered in the early 1980s to be the only design option for orphan drug studies, this type of trial is not designed to generate efficacy data and its use is therefore discouraged. An open label design was used in the investigation of cysteamine for nephropathic cystinuria.

The use of historical controls is attractive to designers of clinical trials, as it requires the enrollment of fewer patients. Patients are also easier to recruit since trials based on historical controls are not placebo controlled. Patients in the historical control group have the same disease as the active study group but were evaluated and treated at an earlier time than the study group and with a different product. It is a useful design for studies of diseases where the outcome is predictable or where it would be considered unethical to withhold treatment from some of the patients. Some difficulties may arise, however, when interpreting the results. For instance, changes in standards of care may occur over time, and information about the historical control group may be incomplete for comparison. Historical controls were used in the investigation and subsequent approval of Ceredase for Gaucher disease and Pegademase (Peg ADA) for severe combined immune deficiency (SCID).

Crossover design trials have the potential for greater patient enrollment because the participants know that they will receive the treatment drug for half of the trial. Small groups of patients may be utilized in this design since the same group serves both as treatment and as control subjects. The group receiving the treatment switches to the placebo group and vice versa with neither group knowing which is which. Crossover is done to address ethical concerns about depriving one group of a possibly beneficial treatment for the duration of the trial. However, due to variations in how the disease may affect different patients, data evaluation may be difficult. Also to be considered when evaluating whether to utilize this study design is the half-life of the study drug. In order for successful crossover to a placebo, the study drug must have a short half-life and the "wash-out" period for the patient to return to baseline must also be short.

In randomized withdrawal trials all patients enrolled receive the drug at the beginning of the trial, called the treatment period. At the end of this period, those patients that demonstrate a response to the treatment, i.e., alleviation of their symptoms, are randomized to either be withdrawn from treatment or to continue on the therapy. Those assigned to the withdrawal group are monitored closely for resumption of symptoms. This type of study design is best utilized to evaluate a drug that treats symptoms vs. one that modifies the course of the disease. The investigator looks to see clear alleviation of the progression of symptoms, followed by a subsequent regression to pretreatment status once the drug withdrawal has begun. It can also be used as a design for a confirmatory trial with a drug that appears to work well in some patients and to have no efficacy in others. Similar to a crossover trial design, the study drug must have a short half-life.

The "N of 1" or single patient clinical trial design involves the analysis of single patient's response to treatment. This design can be categorized as a cross-over trial in which the same patient is repeatedly randomized to receive either the experimental treatment or the control.[7] Various diseases may affect individuals differently and this design allows the investigator to study these individual clinical responses and to account for individual characteristics. Efficacy is determined by following the response measure over a period of time. Danazol (Danocrine®) for the treatment of hereditary angioedema was approved based on a "N of 1" trial. In this case, the dosage required was based on individual clinical response of the patient.

Under the 1997 Food and Drug Administration Modernization Act (FDAMA), FDA must accelerate the review of drugs and biologics intended to treat serious or life-threatening conditions and which demonstrate the potential to address unmet medical needs. FDA may also designate a drug "fast track" when it is deemed likely to provide significant clinical benefit. Many orphan diseases are life-threatening in nature, and have no other available therapy. Therefore, FDA often reviews New Drug Application (NDA) for Orphan Drugs within an accelerated timeframe. Nevertheless,

---

[7] Senn, S.J. *Statistical Issues in Drug Development*. John Wiley, New York, 1993.

an accelerated evaluation of *all* orphan drug marketing applications is not guaranteed.

Under an accelerated approval procedure, FDA may also approve a new drug or biologic if adequate and well-controlled trials establish that the product has an effect on a surrogate endpoint that is likely to predict clinical benefit. A good example is provided by the January 2001, imatinib mesylate capsules (Gleevec™) orphan product designation. This drug was then granted accelerated approval status for treatment of chronic myelogenous leukemia (CML) in blast crisis, accelerated phase, and chronic phase after failure of interferon treatment. Gleevec received market approval after a $2^1/_2$-month FDA review — the fastest review time ever for a cancer drug. Gleevec was granted special status due to the lack of effective treatment for CML, a life-threatening disease that affects fewer than 50,000 people in the U.S. The surrogate endpoints supporting Gleevec efficacy were hematologic and cytogenetic response rates. Of chronic phase, interferon failure CML patients, 88% had a confirmed complete hematologic response and 49% had a confirmed or unconfirmed (single determination) major cytogenetic response.

The use of surrogate endpoints in clinical trials facilitates the development of a new drug that is intended for the treatment of a serious or life-threatening condition. Such endpoints could include laboratory tests or physical signs that do not in themselves constitute a clinical effect but that are judged by qualified scientists to be reasonably likely to predict clinical benefit. Validation of a surrogate endpoint for a therapy includes the generation of clinical data demonstrating that effects of the therapy on the surrogate endpoint reliably predict effects on a clinical endpoint. Sponsors receiving approval of "fast-track" products utilizing surrogate endpoints may be required to conduct appropriate postapproval studies to validate the surrogate endpoint or other wise confirm the effect on the clinical endpoint (FDAMA Sec. 506).

8.8 Accomplishments

During the past 20 years, the Orphan Drug Act incentives have worked well, and the legislation has had a substantial impact on public health. Since 1983, the OOPD has granted orphan designation to more than 1600 products to treat rare diseases. Of these, 248 have received FDA marketing approval; 88% of the approved orphan products treat life-threatening diseases. Currently marketed orphan products are available to treat patient populations that total more than 12 million in the U.S.

9

Good Clinical Practices

Robert Buckley

CONTENTS

9.1   Introduction

Good Clinical Practices (GCPs) were created to encompass a collection of regulations, guidelines, ethical principles, and industry standards that would ensure that data derived from human clinical trials could be used to

1-58716-007-2/04/$0.00+$1.50
© 2004 by CRC Press LLC

support marketing applications made to regulatory agencies for drugs, bio-logics, or medical devices. Unlike Good Manufacturing Practices, the GMPs, which are codified in 21 CFR 211: Current Good Manufacturing Practice For Finished Pharmaceuticals, there is no single regulation entitled "Good Clinical Practice." To follow GCPs is to comply with a myriad of regulations, guidelines, and ethical standards. To conduct a clinical trial in compliance with GCPs means that the research at hand protects the safety and well-being of human subjects *and* provides that quality scientific data is derived from the research.

In the chapter the origins of GCPs will be reviewed, providing both an historical and ethical basis for today's standards. In addition, current good clinical practices will be reviewed as guiding principles, and with practical ideas and examples of implementation. Finally, a set of frequently asked questions and commonly noted issues will be discussed, and some sample forms/templates provided along with a list of good Web sites for further information.

9.2 How Research Was Done

Scientific researchers have always considered human subjects the gold standard for research in human physiology. In 1865 Claude Bernard wrote "We must always, indeed, go back to the organs to find the simplest explanations of life" in an article entitled "An Introduction to the Study of Experimental Medicine." The type of early experimentation Claude Bernard speaks to is the type conducted on criminals sentenced to death, where the human subject's rights and well-being was sacrificed for the common good. Today, we aspire to conduct such human experimentation in a way that protects the rights and well-being of experimental subjects, by employing the most basic of principles: informed consent (a concept we'll discuss in great detail later on in the chapter).

One of the earliest documented examples of the use of informed consent is attributed to Walter Reed's infectious disease research, conducted at the turn of the 20th century. Reed, a U.S. Army surgeon sent to Cuba to study infectious diseases, used "informed consent" statements when he recruited volunteer subjects from among soldiers and civilians during the occupation of Cuba at the end of the Spanish–American War. Although the use of informed consent has a documented history over a century old, it was not a required practice until the 1960s.

In 1962, congress passed the Kefauver–Harris Amendments to the Food, Drug, and Cosmetic Act. In addition to requiring FDA to evaluate new drugs for efficacy, the amendments established the requirement for obtaining the informed consent of human research subjects.

9.3   The Need for Global Standards in Research

The unfortunate history behind the development of the GCPs is highlighted by the reaction to tragedy and human rights violations. Shocking discoveries of experimental impropriety, and the subsequent media attention, have provided the catalyst to change. Ethical doctrines and subsequent regulations for the protection of human subjects in research were first formalized following the Nuremberg Trials, in which Nazi doctors were tried (and some of those convicted were sentenced to death) for the bizarre military human experimentation conducted in the name of science during World War II.

The Nuremberg Code of 1947 set the foundation for all subsequent ethical guidelines. However, here in the U.S. the Nuremberg Code was not seen as a ground-breaking ethical doctrine, but as a document created to convict those mad scientists responsible for the horrific experiments conducted by the Nazi regime. In addition, although the first of the ten principles of the Code was states that "the voluntary consent of the human subject is absolutely essential," the Code fell short, in that it only applied to nontherapeutic human research.

In 1964, the World Medical Association met in Helsinki, Finland and adopted a document developed to set forth recommendations guiding physicians in biomedical research involving human subjects. The Declaration of Helsinki, as it came to be known, made some of the principles set forth in the Nuremberg Code applicable to clinical (therapeutic) research, and thus applicable to drug development studies. The Declaration of Helsinki has been amended several times since its inception, most recently in 2000.[1]

In the decades following World War II, human experimentation continued to flourish. The research budget of the National Institutes of Health increased from $17 million to $803 million over the period 1948–1967. Revelations of research impropriety also continued to make their way to the media forefront. The *New England Journal of Medicine* published a landmark article in 1966 by Dr. Henry K. Beecher entitled, "Ethics and Clinical Research." In his article, Dr. Beecher described 22 research studies published in major medical journals which he believed were examples of "unethical or questionably ethical studies." Three of the studies most commonly referenced as having highlighted the need for legislation governing clinical research (the first two were described in Beecher's article) are briefly summarized below.

---

[1] The 2000 amendment to the Declaration has caused some controversy in clinical research as it states that "the benefits, risks, burdens and effectiveness of a new method should be tested against those of the best current prophylactic, diagnostic, and therapeutic methods. This does not exclude the use of placebo, or no treatment, in studies where no proven prophylactic, diagnostic or therapeutic method exists." Simply stated, the Declaration prohibits the use of a placebo control group when there is a treatment available (approved or unapproved) for the disease of interest. This is in direct opposition to the FDA gold standard phase III placebo-controlled trial for product approval.

The Willowbrook Hepatitis Study was conducted at an institution for mentally retarded children on Staten Island, New York in 1956. The study involved injecting institutionalized children with isolated strains of viral hepatitis to test the effects of gamma globulin and to observe the natural history of viral hepatitis. Although consent from the parents was obtained, the parents were not fully informed of the potential hazards involved in the study.

The Jewish Chronic Disease Hospital Study was also conducted in New York, in 1963. This study was conducted on patients in a chronic disease hospital. The patients were "merely told they would be receiving some cells." The patients were not told they were being injected with cancer cells and the patient's consent to participate in the study was never requested or obtained.

In 1932, the U.S. Public Health Service began the now-infamous Tuskegee syphilis study. This observational study was designed to document the natural progression of syphilis in African–American men. Poor black sharecroppers living in Macon County, Alabama were enrolled into the study when there was no effective treatment for syphilis. A decade into the study penicillin was shown to be a safe and effective treatment for syphilis. The men in the study however, were misled to believe they were receiving treatment, when in fact they were not. The study continued in this fashion until 1972 when the *New York Times* published an expose.

The Tuskegee study, and perhaps the attention Dr. Beecher commanded with the 22 other cases (Willowbrook and the Jewish Chronic Disease Hospital included) of ethically questionable studies discussed in his article, are often cited as the catalyst for the U.S. government's establishment of The National Commission for the Protection of Human Subjects of Biomedical and Behavioral Research. This Commission's primary goal was to establish the basic ethical principles and policies to conduct human subject research. The Commission was responsible for publishing a series of reports, highlighted by the 1979 publishing of the Belmont Report. The Belmont Report identifies three basic ethical principles of human subject research. These three principles being: respect for persons, beneficence, and justice. Very simply stated:

- Respect for persons: Acknowledge the subject's autonomy and protect those subjects whose autonomy is diminished.
- Beneficence: Minimize potential harm to the subject and maximize their potential benefit.
- Justice: Distribute the benefits and burdens of research fairly. Avoid exploiting a subject population who would not benefit from the research for the sake of convenience.

The Belmont Report provided the foundation for the codification of Federal regulations governing the Protection of Human Subjects published in the

Federal Register in the early 1980s. The Protection of Human Subjects regulations changed the way clinical research was conducted in the U.S. during the 1980s, and laid the foundation for future regulations and guidelines that now make up good clinical practices, the GCPs.

9.4 What are the GCPs? Regulations and Guidance

The GCPs are comprised of a collection of regulations, guidance documents, ethical principles, and industry standard practices. The U.S. regulations that cover the GCPs are located in Titles 21 and 45 of the U.S. Code of Federal Regulations (CFR).

Title 21 of the Code of Federal Regulations applies to Food and Drugs. The CFR regulations under Title 21 applicable to research involving products (drugs, devices, biologics) regulated by the FDA are contained in:

- 21 CFR Subchapter A — General; Part 50 Protection of Human Subjects
- 21 CFR Subchapter A — General; Part 54 Financial Disclosure by Clinical Investigators
- 21 CFR Subchapter A — General; Part 56 Institutional Review Boards (IRB)[2]

The general sections listed above apply equally to clinical trials conducted in drugs, biologics, and medical devices. Drug-, device-, and biologic-specific sections include:

- 21 CFR Subchapter D — Drugs for Human Use; Part 312 Investigational New Drug Application
- 21 CFR Subchapter D — Drugs for Human Use; Part 314 Applications for FDA Approval to Market a New Drug
- 21 CRF Subchapter F — Biologics; Part 601 Licensing
- 21 CFR Subchapter H — Medical Devices; Part 812 Investigational Device Exemptions
- 21 CRF Subchapter H — Medical Devices; Part 814 Premarket Approval of Medical Devices

Title 45 of the Code of Federal Regulations applies to Public Welfare. The CFR regulations under Title 45 apply to research conducted by the Depart-

---

[2] IRBs are ethical review boards mandated by institutions to provide ethical guidance for research. They are the topic of considerable scrutiny and will be described in greater detail as we proceed.

ment of Health and Human Services (HHS) or conducted or funded in whole or in part by any of the 18 governmental agencies[3] that have adopted these standards, and are contained in 45 CFR Subtitle A — Department of Health and Human Services; Part 46 Protection of Human Subjects.

45 CFR Part 46 is often called the "Common Rule," referring to its common adoption by many U.S. governmental agencies. It should be noted, however, that when research involving products regulated by the FDA is funded, supported, or conducted by FDA and/or HHS, both the HHS and FDA regulations apply.[4]

There are a number of guidance documents published by FDA that are related to GCPs, but perhaps the most comprehensive "how-to" GCP document was created by the International Conference on Harmonization in 1996. This guidance was subsequently published by FDA in the Federal Register on May 7, 1997. The ICH GCP guideline "is intended to define "Good Clinical Practice" and to provide a unified standard for designing, conducting, recording, and reporting trials that involve the participation of human subjects."[5] As a formal FDA guidance, the ICH GCP guideline represents FDA's "current thinking" on good clinical practice and, if followed, will enable the data generated from the trial to be used in marketing applications submitted to a number of regulatory agencies worldwide.

The ICH established a list of principles, which are intended to describe GCP. Although there were no historic or ground-breaking revelations brought to light in this listing of GCP principles, for the first time the ethical and regulatory requirements which were previously captured in a variety of ethical doctrines and statutory regulations were brought together in one place. The ICH principles are summarized below:

- Clinical trial should be conducted ethically, consistent with the Declaration of Helsinki and applicable regulatory requirements.
- Rights, safety and well-being of subjects are paramount.
- Benefits of study must outweigh risks.
- Study to adhere to protocol that has been reviewed and approved by an ethics committee (IRB).
- Study must be scientifically sound.
- Investigator(s) must be qualified.
- Informed consent must be obtained freely.

---

[3] Ethical and Policy Issues in Research Involving Human Participants, Volume 1, Report and Recommendations of the National Bioethics Advisory Commission, Bethesda, MD, August 2001. (see http://bioethics.georgetown.edu/nbac/human/overvol1.pdf)

[4] IRB Operations and Clinical Investigation Requirements, Appendix E, Significant Differences in FDA and HHS Regulations for Protection of Human Subjects, US Food and Drug Administration, Updated 9/98. (see http://www.fda.gov/oc/ohrt/irbs/appendixe.html)

[5] 62 FR 25692 (5/7/97) International Conference on Harmonisation; Good Clinical Practice: Consolidated Guideline; Availability.

- Records must be maintained to allow for accurate reporting, inter-pretation, and verification.
- Confidentiality of records must be assured to respect the privacy and confidentiality of study subjects
- Clinical trial supplies must meet Good Manufacturing Practices.
- Systems and procedures should be implemented to assure the quality of the trial.

The ICH GCP guideline defines the responsibilities of Institutional Review Boards (IRBs), Investigators, Sponsors (e.g., drug companies), and also defines the minimum information that should be included in a clinical pro-tocol and an investigator's brochure (IB). An additional useful tool included in the ICH GCP guideline is a list of essential documents, describing each document's purpose, at what stage of the clinical trial the document should be on file, and whether it is required to be filed at the site of the investigator, the sponsor, or both. A copy of the ICH GCP guideline is a must for every regulatory, quality, or clinical professional conducting clinical trials on reg-ulated investigational drugs, devices, or biologics.

9.5   GCP–Sponsor Obligations

9.5.1   Overview

The sponsor of a clinical trial may be an individual, a drug/device/biologic company, or a contract research organization (CRO) that has taken over specific (or all) obligations of the original sponsor for a fee. The primary responsibility of a study sponsor is to ensure trials are being conducted and that quality data are generated, documented, and recorded in compliance with the IRB-approved study protocol, GCPs, and applicable regulatory requirements. To gain assurance that the study is being conducted according to set standards, the sponsor must monitor the progress of the trial on an on-going basis. The monitoring of a clinical trial can be conducted employing different levels of oversight (e.g., frequency of study visits, depth, and detail of document review) depending on the size, duration, and complexity of the clinical trial design, and the safety risk to study subjects. The most common method of clinical trial monitoring is through on-site visits made to the clinical trial site prior to the study's beginning and on a periodic basis until the study has been completed. The monitoring of clinical trials should be described in a written standard operating procedure (SOP). In addition to monitoring, the sponsor is responsible for writing, maintaining, archiving, and following SOPs to define the systems used to ensure the quality and compliance of clinical trials conducted by, or on behalf of, the sponsor. The

SOPs that should be implemented for compliance with GCPs are dependent on the sponsor organization's function and will vary widely. A list of basic SOPs to point a sponsor in the direction of GCP compliance follows:

1. Investigator Site Selection
2. Investigator Site Initiation
3. Clinical Monitoring of Investigator Site
4. Investigator Site Close-out
5. Financial Disclosure
6. Adverse Event Reporting
7. Quality Assurance Audits
8. Required Documents for Study Master File
9. Document Retention
10. Study Master File Audit
11. FDA Inspection at Sponsor facility

It should be noted that it is *uncommon* and not required that investigators to have SOPs in place that describe all, or even any, of their research practices. A notable exception to this statement might include commercial clinical research entities — doctors who have gone into the business of conducting clinical trials instead of carrying a patient load. Such organizations may implement SOPs in order to standardize their practices as they can often have a large staff responsible for conducting many studies for many different sponsors.

Once the sponsor has put together a scientifically sound clinical protocol and any applicable waiting period or approvals have been granted after regulatory filing to allow for the study of the test article, the study may begin. In order to conduct the clinical trial the study sponsor must ensure that the investigators are qualified by education and experience and are trained on the conduct of the protocol. It is often a misconception in the popular press that investigators are somehow qualified by the FDA when, in fact, this is a sponsor responsibility, mandated by regulation.

The FDA's Guideline for the Monitoring of Clinical Investigations describes the sponsor's responsibility to assure, through personal contact, "that the investigator clearly understands and accepts the obligations incurred in undertaking a clinical investigation." The Guideline describes the need for the monitor[6] to conduct a preinvestigation visit, during which the monitor must ensure that the investigator:

---

[6] The term "monitor" is used throughout to refer to personnel responsible for the operational conduct of clinical studies, often a clinical research associate (CRA), project manager, etc. This is *not* the same as a Medical Monitor, who has specific medical/clinical responsibility in terms of subject safety and assists in key medical decisions related to the study.

1. Understands the investigational status of the test article and the need to account for it
2. Understands the protocol
3. Understands his/her regulatory obligations and requirements to conduct a well-controlled study
4. Understands his/her responsibility to freely obtain informed consent from each subject enrolled using documents which contain the required elements as detailed in 21 CFR 50
5. Understands his/her responsibility to obtain IRB (ethics board) approval for the study and to notify the sponsor of IRB actions
6. Has access to an adequate number of study subjects
7. Has adequate facilities to conduct the trial
8. Has adequate time and resources to fulfill regulatory obligations

What FDA has dubbed the "preinvestigation" visit in practice is often carried out as a two-step process commonly referred to as *investigator qualification and initiation*. Investigator qualifications may be conducted during an on-site visit to the investigator's site or as a phone interview. The purpose of the qualification is to obtain information in order to assess the investigator's appropriateness to conduct the clinical trial, i.e., experienced staff, adequate facilities, time and resources, access to appropriate subjects for recruitment, as well as getting a sense of the investigator's interest in conducting the trial. The initiation covers more protocol-specific and GCP training. The initiation is typically conducted in one of two ways. An investigator's meeting hosted by the sponsor may be held, including all investigators, during which the study protocol is reviewed and additional training regarding the details of conducting the study provided. An on-site initiation visit is the second option, where the study monitor (or team of sponsor representatives) visits the clinical trial site and trains the investigator and his/her staff on the protocol and GCPs in person. Documentation of the investigator's training on the protocol, through attendance at an investigator's meeting or an on-site initiation visit, should be maintained in the investigator site's study files as well as the sponsor's files prior to the site's enrollment of study subjects.

9.6 Sponsor Oversight of Clinical Studies

Once a trial has begun it is the sponsor's responsibility to monitor the conduct of the study at the investigator's site. Although it is dependent on the trial complexity and the sponsor's approach to GCP compliance, a typical sponsor-monitoring scenario is briefly described here. One approach to "interim visit monitoring" (during the conduct of the study) often employed by study sponsors is one where the monitor will visit the site early in the patient enrollment period to ensure that the investigator is enrolling patients that meet the protocol's inclusion/exclusion criteria. Monitoring frequency is dependent upon the size of the study, complexity of the protocol, and safety risk to the study subjects. A study monitor will often visit an investigator's site once every 4–6 weeks during the active phase of the study when subjects are being seen and patient data is being collected. Again, visit frequency is study-dependent and may vary greatly. Once the study is no longer active, the sponsor monitor will continue to visit the site until all data issues have been resolved and the monitor can conduct a "close-out visit" with the site. Periodic monitoring or interim monitoring of the study as outlined in the FDA Monitoring Guideline is required to assure that:

1. The investigator site's facilities continue to be acceptable for study purposes.

2. The investigator is following the study protocol/investigational plan.

3. Any changes to the protocol have been reported to the sponsor and approved by the IRB.

4. The investigator is maintaining accurate, complete, and current records for each study subject.

5. The investigation is making accurate, complete, and timely reports to the sponsor and IRB.

6. The investigator is carrying out the activities he/she agreed to and has not delegated responsibilities to other previously unspecified staff.

During an interim monitoring visit, the sponsor monitor is responsible for ensuring that all required documentation is maintained on site, that the protocol is being followed, the investigational product is accounted for, and that the rights, safety, and well-being of the study subjects are being protected. Since the sponsor monitor cannot personally oversee the study, the realistic and most effective way to do this is through reviewing paperwork during interim monitoring visits and conducting source data verification (a process detailed below).

The ICH GCP Guideline section 8, Essential Documents for the Conduct of a Clinical Trial, provides a quick and easy reference for required documents that need to be maintained at the study site. Monitors of studies can use section 8 of the ICH GCP guideline as a reference or a study-specific checklist to ensure the site is maintaining all required documents. To ensure the investigator is following the study protocol, the monitor must review study subject medical records, study charts, and all appropriate documentation to ensure the subjects were being treated as dictated by the approved protocol.

The monitor must review investigational product dispensing/accountability logs and conduct a physical count of all investigational product on site to ensure that the investigator is appropriately dispensing and accounting for all investigational product. All investigational product must be stored in a manner that limits its distribution to those qualified and delegated by the investigator to do so. There must be adequate documentation to verify the chain of custody, i.e., shipping records that account for every unit of investigational product received, maintained at appropriate storage conditions, dispensed only to enrolled study subjects, and an accurate inventory accounting for all investigational product received, dispensed, re-collected from study subjects, and returned to the sponsor or destroyed.

The monitor must ensure that the rights, safety and well-being of study subjects are being protected. This is done initially through review of the informed consent form before a study even starts, and on an ongoing basis via a review of patient records to ensure they are receiving quality care. Informed consent is the process by which subjects have consented to participate in the study. The monitor must review the informed consent form (ICF) to verify the document contains all the FDA required elements, was properly IRB approved, was obtained from the study subject prior to having any study related procedures performed, and that the consent process was adequately documented by the investigator. FDA regulation 21 CFR 50.25 details 8 required elements of informed consent and another 6 additional elements to be included if appropriate. A checklist of required elements of informed consent is included as an attachment at the end of this chapter.

Obtaining informed consent from a study subject or their legally authorized representative is more than securing a signature on a consent form; it is a process. The process by which the investigator approaches the potential subject, provides them information regarding the study, offers the opportunity for and answers any questions, ensures the potential subject fully understands, gives the potential subject time to think about their decision and consult with family members or friends, and finally provides them with a copy of the consent form once it is signed is all part of obtaining informed consent. The process of obtaining consent should be appropriately documented so that it is clear that the subject was recruited and enrolled appropriately and that "informed consent was obtained prior to participation in the study."[7] There are exceptions from the requirement to obtain informed consent from a research subject prior to receiving an investigational product. These exceptions include limited life-threatening emergencies, either medical or for military personnel at risk for life-threatening situations. These exceptions from FDA requirements from informed consent are detailed in 21 CFR 50.23 and 50.24.

The monitor is responsible for verifying the accuracy of study data being transferred from the investigator's site to the data management group for the sponsor's evaluation. Each data point transferred from the investigator to the study sponsor in a case report form (CRF) should be verifiable by source documentation (source data verification). Source documentation is the term used to describe where a study subject's information is first

---

[7] 21 CFR 312.62(b)

recorded. This includes hospital charts, clinic records, and study specific subject records. When multiple sources of information regarding a subject's medical history and current medical care are being maintained by a variety of caregivers, there will often be conflicting information contained in the records. It is important for these contradictions to be explained in the study documents. The sponsor monitor should call the investigator's attention to any conflicting data contained in the source documents and have the investigator document why one value was chosen over another for inclusion in the CRF for reporting to the sponsor. CRF data that is not transcribed from an original source document, but, rather, is an observation directly entered into the CRF, should be described as such in the study documents. In this case the CRF *is* the source document. Explanatory notations documented in the study documents are often referred to as a notes-to-file. Any corrections made to the study source documents or the CRF itself need to allow for the determination of the classical "what, who, when, and why." To allow someone reviewing the documentation to determine what data was changed, the original entry should not be obscured and should be lined through with a single line allowing a reviewer to read the original entry, e.g., ~~correction~~. The correction must be initialed and dated by the person making the correction, and in cases where the need for the correction is not readily obvious, a brief explanation of why the change was necessary should be made. Often data correction explanations can be coded for ease of use and to avoid extraneous information in the CRF. For example, EE = entry error, CE= calculation error, and LE = late entry; any number of two-letter acronyms can be defined and used to minimize and standardize the need for data correction explanations.

The FDA Monitoring Guideline discusses the sponsor's responsibility to "compare a representative number of subject records and other supporting documents with the investigator's reports ... " As with monitoring visit frequency, study sponsors conduct source data verification using different formulas to determine a representative sample; however, many sponsors choose to conduct 100% source data verification. Source data verification of 100% means that every data point in a CRF for every subject enrolled is compared to source data to ensure complete and accurate data is being reported and that all conflicting information is adequately documented and explained in the study records.

Source data verification is necessary to ensure that the data recorded in the subject's records is completely and accurately transcribed to the CRFs, which transfer data to the sponsor, who in turn, uses that data as the basis for submisions to the FDA or other regulatory agency. Source data verification is described in FDA's Monitoring Guideline as a means to provide assurance that:

1. Information recorded in the investigator's reports is complete, accurate, and legible.
2. There are no omissions of specific data such as concomitant medications or adverse events.

3. Any missed study visits are noted in the reports.

4. Subjects who were dropped from, or failed to complete the study are noted in the report with the reason adequately explained.

5. Informed consent was executed and adequately documented in accordance with federal regulations.

Although FDA's Guideline for the Monitoring of Clinical Investigations does not specifically mention the need for a site "close-out" visit, it is industry standard for the study monitor to visit the investigator's site at the conclusion of the study to ensure that all loose ends are tied up. The monitor at "close-out" ensures all original CRFs pulled in-house and legible copies of all CRF pages remain at the site, and that all investigational product is accounted for and packaged for return or destruction. In addition, the monitor confirms that the investigator understands his or her responsibility to notify the IRB/EC of the study completion and the need to retain all study documents. Study documents are required to be retained for a period of two years following the date on which the test article is approved by FDA for marketing or two years following the date on which the entire clinical investigation (not just the investigator's part in it) is terminated or discontinued by the sponsor.

9.7 Documentation/Reporting of Study Monitoring

Each of the monitoring visits previously described (i.e., qualification, initiation, interim, and close-out visits) must be documented in a written report. A monitoring report should be adequately detailed so that the sponsor's management can accurately assess the investigator's site performance. Detailed monitoring reports can help identify "problem" sites and provide management with enough information to assess the site's ability to conduct a study in compliance with GCPs. A sponsor is required to obtain compliance from the investigator site, and if the sponsor is unable to bring the site into compliance, the sponsor is required to terminate the investigator's site participation in the study and alert the FDA of the investigator's termination. Monitoring reports should be standardized documents used by all individual CRAs monitoring a multi-center clinical trial.

9.8 FDA's Oversight of Clinical Studies

The FDA's inspection program for clinical trials is their Bioresearch Monitoring Program, often referred to as BIMO. The Bioresearch Monitoring

Program was established in 1977 by a task force with representation from the drug, biologic, device, radiological product, veterinary drug, and food branches of FDA. This task force established an inspection program for clinical investigators, research sponsors, contract research organizations, biopharmaceutic laboratories, institutional review boards, and nonclinical (animal) laboratories.

The objective of a BIMO inspection at a clinical trial site is to assess, through audit procedures, if the clinical records adequately and accurately substantiate data submitted to the FDA to demonstrate safety and efficacy in support of an FDA regulated product marketing application and to determine that the rights and well-being of human subjects was adequately protected during the course of the research. Additionally, the BIMO inspection will look to assess the investigator's compliance with applicable FDA regulations and guidelines.[8] There are three classifications of Bioresearch Monitoring Program inspections of a clinical investigator: study-oriented inspections, investigator-oriented inspections, and bioequivalence study inspections.

The *study-oriented inspection* is conducted by FDA field office personnel and is usually assigned by FDA headquarters on the basis of a pending sponsor application to market a new drug, device, or biologic. Clinical investigators are not inspected per an FDA-defined schedule, rather, they are chosen for inspection as a result of their clinical data being submitted to the FDA as part of a marketing application. When FDA reviewers are considering a marketing application or supplement for approval, they will choose clinical trials sites for inspection. The selection of a clinical trial site(s) for a study-oriented inspection is usually based upon the amount of data contributed by the clinical trial site (the highest enrolling sites will most commonly be considered for inspection).

Once a site has been selected, the FDA field office will contact the investigator to arrange an inspection date. In general, FDA will try to schedule the inspection within 10 business days of contact. Upon arrival at the clinical site the FDA field investigator will present the investigator with a Form FDA 482 "Notice of Inspection" along with the investigator's credentials.

FDA investigators are trained to conduct the inspection using the Compliance Program Guidance Manual for Clinical Investigators, which outlines the minimal scope of the inspection.[9] The investigator will first obtain facts about the study conduct through interviews with the Investigator, study coordinator, or responsible party at the clinical site, in order to understand[10]:

- Who did what?
- The degree of delegation of authority.
- Where specific aspects of the study were performed.
- How and where data were recorded.

---

[8] http://www.fda.gov/ora/compliance_ref/bimo/7348_811/48-811-2.html
[9] http://www.fda.gov/ora/compliance_ref/bimo/7348_811/Default.htm
[10] http://www.fda.gov/oc/ohrt/irbs/operations.html#inspections

- How test article accountability was maintained.
- How the monitor communicated with the clinical investigator.
- How the monitor evaluated the study's progress.

The FDA investigator will then look to audit the study data, comparing what was submitted to the Agency with all supporting documentation. The FDA investigator will request a clinical trial subject's medical records, which may come from a doctor's office, hospital, nursing home, laboratory records, outpatient clinic records, or other sources. The investigator will review these records not only for the time frame that the subject was enrolled in the trial, but will seek to ensure that the subject's existing medical history justified their enrollment into the trial and that proper follow-up was given to the subject for a period after trial completion.

An *investigator-oriented inspection* may be conducted when a single investigator's data may prove crucial to a product's approval, if the investigator has participated in many studies, or if the investigator has conducted a study outside of his specialty. An investigator may also be targeted for a "for cause" inspection if a study sponsor, patient, or any anonymous "whistle-blower" contacts FDA with a complaint about the investigator's conduct. An investigator-oriented inspection may also be conducted to investigate any unusual findings or trends noted in the data submitted to the agency. The conduct of an investigator-oriented inspection is much the same as a study-oriented inspection with the exception that the FDA investigator may dig deeper into the data audit and may audit data from more than one study.

The *bioequivalence study inspection* may be conducted on the basis of a pending new drug application (NDA) or abbreviated NDA (ANDA) for which a bioequivalence study is critical to product approval. Bioequivalence studies often support the approval of generic versions of innovator drug products and support the approval of new formulations of marketed drugs. Bioequivalence studies have both a clinical component and an analytical component, thus bioequivalence study inspections differ from study and investigator oriented inspections in that there is often participation from an FDA chemist who can assess the validity of the analytical methods used to indicate bioequivalence.[11]

The vast majority of all BIMO inspections are study-oriented. An FDA investigator will generally take 2 to 4 days on site to conduct a study-oriented inspection. At the conclusion of the inspection, an exit interview will be held with the clinical investigator, in which all findings will be discussed and clarified. If deviations from applicable regulations have been noted during the inspection, the FDA investigator will issue a Form FDA 483 "Inspectional Observations" to the clinical investigator. Note that deviations from guidance documents are not considered inspectional observations and should not be included on a Form FDA 483, although deviations from FDA guidance

---

[11] http://www.fda.gov/ora/compliance_ref/bimo/7348_001/Default.htm#PART%20I%20-%20BACKGROUND

may be included in the FDA investigator's written report submitted to FDA headquarters for evaluation [the establishment inspection report (EIR)].[12]

After FDA headquarters evaluates the field investigator's establishment inspection report, FDA headquarters issues a letter to the clinical investigator categorizing the field investigators findings. The letter can be one of the following three types as described in FDA Information Sheets[13]:

1. A notice that no significant deviations from the regulations were observed. This letter does not require any response from the clinical investigator.

2. An informational letter that identifies deviations from regulations and good investigational practice. This letter may or may not require a response from the clinical investigator. If a response is requested, the letter will describe what is necessary and give a contact person for questions.

3. A "warning letter" identifying serious deviations from regulations requiring prompt correction by the clinical investigator. The letter will give a contact person for questions. In these cases, FDA may inform both the study sponsor and the reviewing IRB of the deficiencies. The Agency may also inform the sponsor if the clinical investigator's procedural deficiencies indicate ineffective monitoring by the sponsor. In addition to issuing these letters, FDA may take other courses of action, e.g., regulatory and/or administrative sanctions.

Establishment inspection reports (EIRs) are now routinely supplied by the FDA to the clinical investigator after the report has been evaluated by FDA headquarters. Redacted copies of EIRs are available through Freedom of Information (FOI) and should be requested by clinical investigators if not supplied by the FDA. Sponsors should also request EIRs generated as a result of a study or investigator oriented inspection applicable to them. Accessing the EIR can provide additional insight to an FDA investigator's inspection strategy and expectations and can prove a useful learning tool to design future trials to be conducted in a manner that fulfills current FDA expectations.

9.9 Sponsor's "Unbiased" Oversight of Clinical Studies

9.9.1 Clinical Quality Assurance

Study sponsors are required by regulation to monitor the conduct of a clinical trial. While not required by FDA regulation, conducting clinical quality assur-

---

[12] http://www.fda.gov/ora/compliance_ref/bimo/7348_811/48-811-3.html
[13] FDA Information Sheets — Guidance for IRBs and Clinical Investigators — FDA Operations http://www.fda.gov/oc/ohrt/irbs/operations.html#inspections

ance (CQA) audits of clinical trials has become an important oversight mechanism to ensure that there has been adequate monitoring of the study. Clinical site audits have become a standard industry practice and are recommended by ICH GCP guidelines. A CQA audit of a clinical trial can be conducted by a qualified representative of the sponsor, CRO, or an independent contract auditor. The auditor should be an independent reviewer who is removed from the actual day-to-day conduct of the study so that they can provide an unbiased opinion on the set-up and conduct of the study. Although, an unbiased, independent perspective is needed, it can also be very beneficial to have a CQA representative provide consultation and input during the planning stages of a clinical trial so that the trial meets the minimum GCP requirements as well as the company's expectations — which may go far beyond the minimum requirements. In small organizations, especially, a CQA auditor is often asked to walk a fine line between providing consultant services for the study and being an unbiased reviewer. For a CQA auditor to function effectively within such an organization, communication among the clinical, regulatory affairs, and CQA staff is key. The expectations and policies should be agreed upon by at least these three groups, as well as upper-management, and documented in SOPs or written policies. Once sponsor GCP policies are in place, the CQA auditor can then independently assess compliance with these GCP policies through investigator site audits, internal study file audits, and CRO audits. After the study is over and the data has been analyzed and compiled in a clinical study report, the CQA auditor can also audit the database and clinical study report for compliance and accuracy.

CQA audits are often conducted according to the same principles the FDA Bioresearch Monitoring Program follows. CQA audits will usually decide if a clinical trial is going to be audited based on what phase of study is being conducted, whether or not the data is intended to support a regulatory application, the complexity of the study, and the level of risk to the study subjects. The number of investigator sites to be audited for the trial is determined either by a preexisting sponsor policy, e.g., 10% of Phase II study sites are audited, 20% of Phase III study sites, etc., or based on other factors. For example, these may include the duration of the trial and the prevalence of compliance issues uncovered during planned audits may lead to additional audits being conducted. The selection of investigator sites to be audited is generally based upon enrollment (high enrollers are more likely to be audited), problems discovered by study monitors, adverse event reporting (abnormally high or low adverse event rates), the presence of an investigator's financial interest in the sponsor company, or previous experience with the investigator.

9.9.2 Conducting an Audit

Once an investigator has been identified for an audit, the CQA auditor should alert the study monitor and then contact the investigator site by phone to arrange a mutually agreeable time for the audit. Audits should be confirmed in a written letter sent to the investigator site. Once on-site, the CQA auditor should meet with the investigator and/or study coordinator to determine the monitor's involvement with the study site and to determine how the investigator has delegated authority for study-related activities to members of the study team. A tour of the facility should be conducted in order to assess the adequacy of the facilities to conduct the trial (e.g., exam rooms, pharmacy, and diagnostic and/or surgical equipment). The majority of time spent during the audit will involve a thorough review of study documents. Reviewing study documents includes ensuring that all essential documents are maintained and readily available at the investigator's site. As mentioned previously, the *ICH GCP Guideline Section 8, Essential Documents for the Conduct of a Clinical Trial*, provides a quick and easy reference for required documents that need to be maintained at the study site. The following is a brief summary of documents that a CQA auditor should ensure are maintained at the study site:

1. Form FDA 1572 and current *curriculum vitae* (CVs) for the Principal Investigator and all subinvestigators listed on the 1572[14]

2. A copy of the study protocol signed by the investigator

3. Copies of all protocol amendments signed by the investigator

4. Investigator's brochure

5. IRB [or ethics committee (EC)] approval of:

    a. Protocol

    b. Protocol amendments

    c. Informed consent form(s)

    d. Recruitment advertising, if used

6. IRB/EC membership list or letter of compliance with IRB regulations

7. IRB/EC notification of serious adverse events (SAEs) and IND Safety Reports

8. Annual or periodic reports made by the investigator to the IRB/EC

9. Laboratory Certifications/Licenses and normal ranges for clinical lab values

10. Documentation of site initiation and/or protocol training

11. Documentation of delegation of authority (site responsibility log)

12. Study personnel signature sheet (can be combined with responsibility log)

13. Study monitor visit log

14. Study subject screening and enrollment logs

---

[14] The 1572 captures information about the investigator relevant to conducting the study, and is submitted by the sponsor to FDA. When it changes at the site, the sponsor needs to know, and let FDA know, so 1572s are one of the most common submissions when studies are on-going.

15. Subject identification log (to be kept/viewed only on-site)
16. Example CRF
17. Copy of investigational product labeling
18. Financial disclosure information

The CQA auditor will review informed consent forms to ensure that study subjects were appropriately consented to participate in the study prior to undergoing any study-specific procedures. Each informed consent form will be evaluated to ensure that all required signatures, dates, and initials were appropriately obtained. Often a CQA auditor will review all informed consent forms for all study subjects at the site being audited, unless the site has enrolled a large number of patients, in which case the auditor will select a representative sample of ICFs for review.

The CQA auditor will select a certain number of study subject records to ensure the rights, safety, and well-being of the subjects were protected, the protocol was adhered to, and that the study data transcribed to CRFs for transmission to the sponsor and subsequently, submitted to the FDA or other regulatory agency is substantiated by adequate and accurate source documentation. Study subjects will typically be selected for audit based upon the following factors:

1. Issues raised in monitoring reports
2. History of a subject's noncompliance with the protocol
3. Number of visits the subject has completed
4. Number and nature of adverse events or serious adverse events
5. Whether the study monitor has reviewed the patient's CRF and sent them to data management
6. Subject enrolled or seen for study visit on a day when many other subjects seen

Additionally, the CQA auditor will assess the investigator's source documentation to ensure there is adequate and accurate source documentation to verify each study visit, procedure, and each data point being transmitted via the CRF to the sponsor. It is important to determine if electronic systems are used to document study subject data. Although many clinical researchers are not aware of the FDA regulations for electronic recordkeeping (21 CFR 11) or think that it only applies to GMP operations and not clinical research, FDA's guidance for its field investigators clearly states "records in electronic form that are that created, modified, maintained, archived, retrieved, or transmitted under any records requirement set forth in agency regulations must comply with 21 CFR 11."[15] The key elements and questions to ask while at a site where an electronic system is used include:

---

[15] http://www.fda.gov/ora/compliance_ref/bimo/7348_811/Default.htm.

- What is the source of data entered into the computer?
- Is the data directly entered (no paper)?
- Who enters the data and when?
- Who has access to the computer and what security procedures are in place (user name and password protection)?
- How are data corrections entered?
- Is the original entry maintained and is there an accurate audit trail?

During source document review and verification, particular attention should be paid to reviewing patient records to ensure that all adverse events (AEs) were captured in the CRF and if serious adverse events (SAEs) were reported to the sponsor and IRB in accordance with regulatory requirements. A good source for definitions of AEs and SAEs and related terms, is the ICH-E2A Guideline, "Clinical Safety Data Management: Definitions and Standards for Expedited Reporting," March 1995. The following are the definitions of an adverse event and serious adverse event taken from the ICH guidance document[16]:

1. An adverse event (AE) can therefore be any unfavorable and unintended sign (including an abnormal laboratory finding, for example), symptom, or disease temporally associated with the use of a medicinal product, whether or not considered related to the medicinal product.

2. A serious adverse event (experience) or reaction is any untoward medical occurrence that at any dose:
   - Results in death
   - Is life-threatening (Note: The term "life-threatening" in the definition of "serious" refers to an event in which the patient was at risk of death at the time of the event; it does not refer to an event which hypothetically might have caused death if it were more severe)
   - Requires inpatient hospitalization or prolongation of existing hospitalization
   - Results in persistent or significant disability/incapacity or
   - Is a congenital anomaly/birth defect of a medicinal product, whether or not considered related to the medicinal product

AEs usually represents any unexpected/unanticipated medical change from the subject's baseline after the subject has consented to participate in the clinical trial. In addition to reporting the SAEs, it is necessary for the

---

[16] ICH-E2A Guideline, "Clinical Safety Data Management: Definitions and Standards for Expedited Reporting," March 1995.

investigator to determine and document the medical event's relationship to the investigational product.

The CQA audit should conclude with a wrap-up meeting with the investigator and perhaps other study team members as needed. The wrap-up meeting is another opportunity for the CQA auditor to discuss the investigator's responsibility for retaining study documents for the required period. Upon returning to the sponsor, the CQA auditor then compiles all findings into an audit report which is addressed to the clinical project manager for the study and copies are circulated to the regulatory affairs project representative, clinical and CQA management. All audit reports must be responded to in writing with all issues/observations brought to resolution. The final documentation required of the CQA auditor is the creation of an audit certificate, which is simply a declaration that an appropriate audit has taken place. Audit certificates must be generated and signed-off by the responsible CQA representative and must be maintained in the study master file. Applications to the U.S. FDA and other international regulatory bodies require information about audits that have been conducted for the study. Sponsors will often include copies of the audit certificates as documentation of the audit in the application.

9.10 GCP: A Complete Sponsor Effort

While ensuring compliance with GCPs during the conduct of a clinical study is primarily the responsibility of the study monitor and ultimately the clinical group within the sponsor organization, the entire sponsor organization plays a role. The second line of defense and GCP oversight is the CQA auditor. The CQA auditor acts as regulatory's eyes and ears in the field. The regulatory department compiles and submits documents to the FDA and other regulatory agencies, and it depends on CQA verification of the accuracy and quality of the data it submits. As study sponsors, FDA has regulated our responsibilities when it comes to conducting clinical trials, the most basic of which is that the sponsor "shall monitor the progress of all clinical investigations conducted under its IND."[17] The CQA auditor acts as the sponsor's impartial evaluator of clinical's compliance with applicable regulations and the GCPs to ensure that the sponsor is meeting its regulatory obligations for GCPs.

9.11 Frequently Asked Questions

Q: Are the Protection of Human Subjects regulations in 21 CFR 56 and 45 CFR 46 the same regulations, only with a different scope?

---

[17] 21 CFR 312.56(a)

A: No. Although the intent of both sets of regulations is similar, there are several significant differences related to both Institutional Review Boards and Informed Consent. The FDA maintains a list of significant differences in FDA and HHS regulations for Protection of Human Subjects on the FDA Website.

Q: Is informed consent always required to perform human subject research?
A: No. See http://www.fda.gov/oc/ohrt/irbs/except.html to see the rare exceptions (also discussed above).

Q: How can I find out if an investigator has been inspected by the FDA before
A: FDA maintains a list at http://www.fda.gov/cder/foi/special/bmis/index.htm

Q: Do U.S. clinical trials have to be conducted in compliance with the ICH Guideline for Good Clinical Practic
A: Technically, no. The guidance is just that, a guidance and doesn't carry the "force of law." However, it does represent FDA's current thinking on the subject matter and represents the minimum level of compliance per industry standards.

Q: Do all study subjects have to resign a consent form if the protocol is amended?
A: Not always. Protocol amendments must receive IRB review and approval before they are implemented, unless an immediate change is necessary to eliminate an apparent hazard to the subjects (21 CFR 56.108(a)(4)). Those subjects who are presently enrolled and actively participating in the study should be informed of the change if it might relate to the subjects' willingness to continue their participation in the study (21 CFR 50.25(b)(5)). The FDA does not require reconsenting of subjects that have completed their active participation in the study or of subjects who are still actively participating when the change will not affect their participation, for example when the change will be implemented only for subsequently enrolled subjects.

9.12 Attachments

Attachment 1: A Sample Informed Consent Checklist
Attachment 2: Sample Audit Certificate

9.13 Web Resources

The FDA's Office of Good Clinical Practice maintains a Web page offering links to all GCP-related laws and regulations as well as proposed regulations and draft guidances. The site also houses a collection of GCP presentations given by FDA and has a helpful "In the News" section to keep you informed of upcoming events and alerted to newly proposed regulations and guidances: http://www.fda.gov/oc/gcp/

The FDA's BIMO Program has numerous links and cross-references to useful information, including internal FDA guides to investigations, etc. You'll also find links to debarred and restricted investigators (the so-called "black list"): http://www.fda.gov/ora/compliance_ref/bimo/default.htm

The Office of Regulatory Affairs (ORA) maintains a Freedom of Information (FOI) pages that shows the best (or is it worst?) of the 483s and EIRs from the bioresearch monitoring program: http://www.fda.gov/ora/frequent/default.htm

The FDA also provides a Web page to distribute the necessary forms to document clinical trial information and make regulatory filings. For example, the current version of FD1572 to capture investigator information can be found here. It is updated regularly, so you'll have to visit often to make sure your form is current (instructions can also be downloaded): http://forms.psc.gov/forms/FDAHTM/fdahtm.html

FOI Services, Inc. is a commercial firm that specializes in unique FDA-related resources. They've already gone through the hassle of ordering FOI-available information from FDA, and makes it available at a reasonable rate. You can search their document catalog at the following address, or call them for a more exhaustive search: http://www.foiservices.com

The International Conference on Harmonisation (ICH) has all of the guidelines posted on their Website. The ICH guidelines are broken out into four topic areas: Q = Quality, S = Safety, E = Efficacy, and M = Multidisciplinary: http://www.ich.org/ich5.html

The ICH guidelines related to clinical studies in humans is under the "E" for efficacy header. The ICH guideline for GCPs is the E6: http://www.ich.org/pdfICH/e6.pdf

The Office for Human Research Protections (OHRP), which falls under the Department of Health and Human Services, maintains a Website with a variety of "quick links" to documents related to protecting the rights of human research subjects: http://ohrp.osophs.dhhs.gov/index.html

Links to the Nuremberg Code, Declaration of Helsinki, and the Belmont Report can be found on the OHRP Website at: http://ohrp.osophs.dhhs.gov/irb/irb_appendices.htm

9.14   Attachment 1: A Sample Informed Consent Checklist

		Yes	No	NA

Required Elements (per 21CFR 50)

		Yes	No	NA
• Statement that study involves research	(50.25(a)(1))	___	___	___
• Explanation of purpose of research	(50.25(a)(1))	___	___	___
• Expected duration of research described	(50.25(a)(1))	___	___	___
• Description of procedures to be followed	(50.25(a)(1))	___	___	___
• Identification of experimental procedures	(50.25(a)(1))	___	___	___
• Description of foreseeable risks or discomforts	(50.25(a)(2))	___	___	___
• Description of benefits to subject or others	(50.25(a)(3))	___	___	___
• Alternative procedures/treatment disclosed	(50.25(a)(4))	___	___	___
• Patient confidentiality measures described	(50.25(a)(5))	___	___	___
• Right of FDA to inspect records described	(50.25(a)(5))	___	___	___
• Compensation and/or treatment d/t injury explained	(50.25(a)(6))	___	___	___
• Contact information for research injury	(50.25(a)(7))	___	___	___
• Contact information for study related questions and patient rights	(50.25(a)(7))	___	___	___
• Statement that participation is voluntary and patient may refuse to participate or withdraw at any time without penalty or loss of benefits	(50.25(a)(8))	___	___	___

Required Elements (per ICH GCP Guidelines)

		Yes	No	NA
• Probability of random assignment to treatment	ICH GCP Gdln	___	___	___
• Anticipated prorated payment to subject	ICH GCP Gdln	___	___	___
• Subject's responsibilities	ICH GCP Gdln	___	___	___
• Statement that subject's signing ICF authorizes study				
• Monitor(s), Auditor(s), IRB/EC, (as well as regulatory authorities) to access original medical records	ICH GCP Gdln	___	___	___
• If results are published, subject's identity will				
• remain confidential	ICH GCP Gdln	___	___	___

Additional Elements (when appropriate per 21CFR 50)

		Yes	No	NA
• Statement that study may involve unforeseeable risks	(50.25(b)(1))	___	___	___
• Anticipated circumstances when investigator may terminate subject's participation without consent	(50.25(b)(2))	___	___	___
• Statement regarding additional costs to subject	(50.25(b)(3))	___	___	___
• Description of consequences of a subject's decision to withdraw from study and procedures to do so	(50.25(b)(4))	___	___	___
• Statement that significant new findings which may relate to subject's willingness to participate will be provided	(50.25(b)(5))	___	___	___
• Statement of the approximate number of subjects	(50.25(b)(6))	___	___	___

Comments:

9.15   Attachment 2: Sample Audit Certificate

9.15.1   Certificate of Audit

This certificate acknowledges that *Sponsor Name*, or a representative thereof, has conducted a Good Clinical Practice compliance audit of the investigational site conducting the protocol listed below. This audit was conducted in accordance with the *Sponsor Name* Audit plan in order to ensure compliance with the study protocol, Good Clinical Practice, applicable SOPs and regulatory requirements.

Protocol #/Title:

Site #:

Principal Investigator(s):

Investigational site:

Auditor/Affiliation:

Date of Audit:

Signature:

Date:

10

Good Manufacturing Practices (GMPs) and Enforcement Actions

Catherine A. Hay and Florence A. Kaltovich

CONTENTS

10.1 Introduction

Legislation for Good Manufacturing Practices (GMP) was developed to ensure that producers of drugs, biologics and medical devices maintain a level of quality, safety, and consistency during manufacturing. The laws are upheld and enforced by the Food and Drug Administration (FDA). Enforcement is primarily by various types of facility inspections for drugs or devices marketed in the U.S. Failure of a producer to comply with any GMP regulation shall be subject to regulatory enforcement action. The cGMPs apply to any product intended for interstate commerce in the U.S.

10.2 Regulations

The overlying regulation for GMPs is the Food, Drug and Cosmetic Act (the Act). The Act states that a drug or device is deemed adulterated if "... the methods used in, or the facilities or controls used for, its manufacture, processing, packaging, or holding do not conform to or are not operated or administered in conformity with current good manufacturing practice to assure that such drug meets the requirements of this Act as to safety and has the identity and strength, and meets the quality and purity characteristics, which it purports or is represented to possess."[1] The requirement for drugs was added to the Act in 1962 with the Kefauver–Harris Amendments.

The drug GMP regulations were first promulgated in 1963. A major revision was performed in 1978,[2] and in 1996[3] the FDA proposed a further revision to the regulations to clarify some of the manufacturing, quality control, and documentation requirements. In addition, the requirements for process and methods validation would be updated to reflect current practice. The 1996 revision has not yet been codified into law. The regulations are published in the Code of Federal Regulations (CFR) Title 21 Part 210 and Part 211 (21 CFR 210[4] and 211[5]). Initially, the regulations applied to drugs, but now they also apply to biologics, under the Public Health Service Act. In addition, biologic products are regulated by the 21 CFR 600 series.[6]

The current good manufacturing practice (cGMP) requirement for medical devices was added to the Act in 1976 via the Medical Device Amendments. The final rule prescribing the requirements was published in the Federal Register on July 21, 1978.[7] In 1996, FDA published a final rule revising the

---

[1] Food, Drug and Cosmetic Act 501(a)(2)(B), U.S. Government Printing Office, Washington, D.C.
[2] Federal Register: 43 FR 45014, U.S. Government Printing Office, Washington, D.C., September 29, 1978.
[3] Ibid: 61 FR 20103, U.S. Government Printing Office, Washington, D.C., May 3, 1996.
[4] 21 CFR 210: *Current Good Manufacturing Practice in Manufacturing, Processing, Packing, or Holding of Drugs; General,* U.S. Government Printing Office, Washington, D.C.
[5] 21 CFR 211: *Current Good Manufacturing Practice for Finished Pharmaceuticals,* U.S. Government Printing Office, Washington, D.C.
[6] 21 CFR 600: *Biological Products: General,* U.S. Government Printing Office, Washington, D.C.
21 CFR 601: *Licensing.*
21 CFR 606: *Current Good Manufacturing Practice for Blood and Blood Components*
21 CFR 607: *Establishment Registration and Product Listing for Manufacturers of Human Blood and Blood Products*
21 CFR 610: *General Biological Products Standards*
21 CFR 630: *General Requirements for Blood, Blood Components, and Blood Derivatives*
21 CFR 640: *Additional Standards for Human Blood and Blood Products*
21 CFR 660: *Additional Standards for Diagnostic Substances for Laboratory Tests*
21 CFR 680: *Additional Standards for Miscellaneous Products*
[7] Federal Register: 43 FR 31508, U.S. Government Printing Office, Washington, D.C., July 21, 1978.

TABLE 10.1

Subparts of 21 CFR 211, 21 CFR 600 and 21 CFR 820

	Subpart Topic		
Subpart	**21 CFR 211**	**21 CFR 600**	**21 CFR 820**
A	General Provisions	General Provisions	General Provisions
B	Organization and Personnel	Establishment Standards	Quality System Requirements
C	Buildings and Facilities	Establishment Inspection	Design Controls
D	Equipment	Reporting of Adverse Events	Document Controls
E	Control of Components and Drug Product Containers and Closures		Purchasing Controls
F	Production and Process Control		Identification and Traceability
G	Packaging and Labeling Control		Production and Process Controls
H	Holding and Distribution		Acceptance Activities
I	Laboratory Controls		Nonconforming Product
J	Records and Reports		Corrective and Preventive Action
K	Returned and Salvaged Drug Products		Labeling and Packaging Control

cGMP requirements for medical devices, incorporating them into a quality system regulation (QSR).[8] The regulations are codified in 21 CFR 820.[9]

10.3 Current Good Manufacturing Practices

The basic premise for cGMP is that quality cannot be tested into a product; it must be manufactured under controlled conditions where quality is built into the process. Quality control testing of the final product is not sufficient to ensure the safety, identity, and strength of the product and its reported quality and purity characteristics. The cGMP regulations are the minimum requirements for the methods, facilities, and controls used to manufacture a product. The cGMPs tend to focus on systems as is demonstrated by the organization of the regulations. The parts are divided into subparts that cover the major systems. Table 10.1 summarizes the subparts of 21 CFR 211, 21 CFR 600, and 21 CFR 820.[5,6,9]

Each subpart is then further divided into subsections that address specific topics. The information contained in each section describes what information, actions, and documentation are required to comply with the regulations. The

---

[8] Ibid: 61 FR 52654, U.S. Government Printing Office, Washington, D.C., October 7, 1996.
[9] 21 CFR 820: *Quality System Regulation*, U.S. Government Printing Office, Washington, D.C.

complete list of GMP regulations for 21 CFR 211 is found in Table 10.2. Broadly speaking, the regulations for drugs, biologics, and devices state that:

- Facilities used to manufacture the product should be clean and well-controlled.
- Personnel should have the appropriate experience and training to perform their required tasks.
- Equipment should be qualified for use in the particular process.
- The receipt and release of all raw materials should be documented per procedure, that containers and closures are controlled.
- The method of production should be validated and in a controlled, reproducible state with in-process controls.
- Analytical methods should be validated.
- Materials should be traceable.
- Procedures should be covered by controlled standard operating procedures and activities documented at the time of performance. ("If it is not documented, it was not done.")
- There are procedures in place for making changes (change control), investigating deviations, product complaints, and adverse events.
- Records are retained for at least the minimum required time period.

In addition to the controls described above, devices are subject to design controls to ensure that performance requirements for the device are established before production, the specified design is verified and validated, and the design requirements are met.

10.4   FDA Enforcement Actions

The FDA has two types of enforcement powers available to deal with noncompliance of cGMP regulations: administrative and judicial. Administrative actions include inspections, Form FDA 483 Inspectional Observations, Warning Letters, and delay, suspension, or withdrawal of product approvals. The FDA initiates and proceeds on these actions without other government agency assistance. Judicial actions, performed by the U.S. Department of Justice, who serves as trial counsel to the FDA, filing injunctions, and moving on civil seizures and criminal prosecution.

10.4.1   Administrative Actions

FDA enforcement actions begin with an inspection in which investigators look for evidence of noncompliance to GMPs. Essentially, the Agency is

TABLE 10.2

Complete List of 21 CFR 211 GMP Requirements

Subpart A General Provisions
- 211.1 Scope
- 211.3 Definitions

Subpart B Organization and Personnel
- 211.22 Responsibilities of the quality control unit
- 211.25 Personnel qualifications
- 211.28 Personnel responsibilities
- 211.34 Consultants

Subpart C Buildings and Facilities
- 211.42 Design and construction features
- 211.44 Lighting
- 211.46 Ventilation, air filtration, air heating, and cooling
- 211.48 Plumbing
- 211.50 Sewage and refuse
- 211.52 Washing and toilet facilities
- 211.56 Sanitation
- 211.58 Maintenance

Subpart D Equipment
- 211.63 Equipment design, size and location
- 211.65 Equipment construction
- 211.67 Equipment cleaning and maintenance
- 211.68 Automatic, mechanical, electronic equipment
- 211.72 Filters

Subpart E Control of Components and Drug Product Containers and Closures
- 211.80 General requirements
- 211.82 Receipt and storage of untested components, drug product containers, and closures
- 211.84 Testing and approval or rejection of components, drug product containers, and closures
- 211.86 Use of approved components, drug product containers, and closures
- 211.87 Retesting of approved components, drug product containers, and closures
- 211.89 Rejected components, drug product containers, and closures
- 211.94 Drug product containers and closures

Subpart F Production and Process Controls
- 211.100 Written procedures; deviations
- 211.101 Charge-in of components
- 211.103 Calculation of yield
- 211.105 Equipment identification
- 211.110 Sampling and testing of in-process materials and drug products
- 211.111 Time limitations on production
- 211.113 Control of microbiological contamination
- 211.115 Reprocessing

Subpart G Packaging and Labeling Control
- 211.122 Materials examination and usage criteria
- 211.125 Labeling issuance
- 211.130 Packaging and labeling operations
- 211.132 Tamper-resistant packaging requirements for over-the-counter (OTC) human drug products
- 211.134 Drug product inspection
- 211.137 Expiration Dating

Subpart H Holding and Distribution
- 211.142 Warehousing procedures
- 211.150 Distribution procedures

Subpart I Laboratory Controls
- 211.160 General requirements
- 211.165 Testing and release for distribution
- 211.166 Stability testing
- 211.167 Special testing requirements
- 211.170 Reserve samples
- 211.173 Laboratory animals
- 211.176 Penicillin contamination

Subpart J Records and Reports
- 211.180 General requirements
- 211.182 Equipment cleaning and use log
- 211.184 Component, drug product container, closure, and labeling records
- 211.186 Master production and control records
- 211.188 Batch production and control records
- 211.192 Production record review
- 211.194 Laboratory records
- 211.196 Distribution records
- 211.198 Complaint files

Subpart K Returned and Salvaged Products
- 211.204 Returned drug products
- 211.208 Drug product salvaging

building a case against the product manufacturer. There are various types of inspections such as GMP (biennial), Pre-Approval (PAI), bioresearch monitoring (BiMo), etc. Inspectional documentation includes:

- Form FDA 482 — Notice of Inspection (officially notifies manufacturer that FDA inspection has begun)
- Form FDA 483 — Inspectional Observations (list of items that may be deemed as noncompliant with cGMPs presented to the manufacturer upon completion of the inspection.)
- Form FDA 484 — Receipt of Samples (allows the FDA to take samples as evidence of noncompliance — adulterated product)
- Establishment Inspection Report (EIR) (official document written by the FDA investigator team that clearly describes issues identified on 483 with supporting evidence)

FDA officials evaluate the EIR for further regulatory actions including no action indicated (NAI), voluntary action indicated (VAI), or official action indicated (OAI). A VAI ranking means objectionable conditions were found but the FDA is not prepared to take or recommend any administrative or regulatory action. An OAI ranking means regulatory and/or administrative sanctions will be recommended and may include voluntary recalls of product. Subsequent to an OAI ranking, the FDA may issue a Warning Letter which is an informal advisory to a firm communicating the Agency's position on a matter but does not commit the FDA to taking enforcement action. Warning letters will contain direct citations to the GMP regulations (for biologics, citations from both 21 CFR 211 and 21 CFR 600 will be acknowledged). The Agency's policy is that warning letters should be issued for violations which are of regulatory significance in that failure to adequately and promptly make corrections may be expected to result in enforcement action should the violation(s) continue. The issuance of a warning letter does not commit the FDA to take further action. The firm must respond to the warning letter within 15 working days.

Other administrative enforcement powers are delay, suspension, or withdrawal of product approvals. The FDA can delay approval of a new drug, biologic, or device through review of the information provided in the marketing application and subsequent supplements and via inspection of the company's facility. The initial marketing application, e.g., New Drug Application (NDA), Biologics License Application (BLA), or Pre-Market Approval (PMA), contains descriptions of the facility, equipment, processes, and controls used to manufacture the product. FDA subject matter experts review this information in the application and evaluate its acceptability. In addition to the review of the application, in most cases, the approval process requires a preapproval inspection (PAI) to determine the accuracy of the information included in the marketing application and compliance with cGMPs. An FDA team, consisting of subject matter experts and/or investigators, performs the inspection. Compliance is essential to obtain marketing approval of the product, otherwise delays could occur until either the objectionable conditions are corrected or the firm commits to completion of a corrective action plan.

Suspension of product approval for human drugs may be accomplished if the FDA has evidence that there is an imminent hazard to the public. For biologics, a suspension may occur if there is a danger to health. Medical device suspension can only occur after a hearing between the firm and the FDA.

The ultimate FDA administrative enforcement action is withdrawal of product approval. Regulatory requirements for withdrawal of product approval include:

- The product is no longer safe and effective.
- The application contains untrue statements.
- Manufacturing changes implemented without submitting a supplement.
- Repeat or deliberate record-keeping problems.
- Refusal to permit FDA access to records.
- Inadequate methods/controls for manufacturing and packaging.
- False and misleading labeling not corrected within a reasonable time.

For biologics, the license to ship a product can be cancelled or revoked either at the request of the manufacturer or when grounds exist for the Agency to initiate such an action.

10.4.2 Judicial Actions

The FDA can proceed with more serious judicial actions if warranted. An injunction is initiated to stop or prevent violation of the law either by stopping adulterated products from reaching the public or by requiring noncompliant conditions to be corrected. Defendants in an injunction proceeding may consent to a Decree of Permanent Injunction (Consent Decree) either after a hearing or as a result of a negotiated settlement between the firm and FDA. The settlement describes the measures that will be taken to bring the company into compliance, with a schedule for that process. If the schedule is not met, the firm incurs penalty charges. Recent consent decrees are listed in Table 10.3.

Seizure is a very effective enforcement tool; it is a civil court action used to confiscate foods, drugs, devices, or cosmetics and to remove them from the market. FDA files a complaint in federal court, which identifies the goods and lists the violations and a U.S. Marshall carries out the confiscation. FDA can seize goods without providing advance notice and goods can be seized where they are located.

TABLE 10.3

Companies, Dates, and Terms of Recent Consent Decrees

Company	Date	Terms
Schering-Plough Corporation[a]	5/17/02	Four New Jersey and Puerto Rico sites $500M payment to U.S. Treasury immediately Additional payments of up to $175M $471,500 to cover inspection costs Company agreed to suspend manufacturing of 73 products Expert consultants — yearly inspections for 3 years
Elan Pharmaceuticals[b]	5/21/01	Gainesville, GA plant Independent expert — yearly inspection for 3 years
Wyeth-Ayerst Laboratories (AHP)[c]	10/3/00	Marietta, PA and Pearl River, NY Expert consultants Pay FDA $15,000/day for failure to meet schedule ($5M cap) Pay U.S. Treasury $30M within 15 day of decree
Abbott Laboratories[d]	11/9/99	Diagnostic devices — Abbott Park, IL and North Chicago, IL Pay FDA $15,000/day for failure to meet schedule ($10M cap) Pay U.S. Treasury $100M within 10 days of decree Must be in compliance in 1 year or company must pay 16% of gross proceeds by sales of medically necessary products Independent auditors

[a] FDA News: *Schering Plough Signs Consent Decree with FDA, Agrees to Pay $500 Million*, Food and Drug Administration, Rockville, MD, May 17, 2002.
[b] FDA Talk Paper: *Elan Pharmaceuticals Subsidiary Signs Consent Decree with FDA*, Food and Drug Administration, Rockville, MD, May 21, 2001.
[c] FDA Talk Paper: *Wyeth-Ayerst Laboratories Sings Consent Decree with FDA*, Food and Drug Administration, Rockville, MD, October 3, 2000.
[d] FDA News: *Abbott Laboratories Signs Consent Decree with FDA; Agrees to Correct Manufacturing Deficiencies*, Food and Drug Administration, Rockville, MD, November 2, 1999.

In an FDA White Paper entitled *Protecting the Public Health: FDA Pursues an Aggressive Enforcement Strategy*,[10] FDA restates its commitment to pursuing violations of the Act and distinguishes various enforcement activities that have occurred during fiscal years 1998 to 2002 including injunctions, recalls, arrests, and convictions, all of which have increased. Letters to product manufacturers for misleading or untrue promotional labeling have also increased.

10.4.3   Responding to FDA Enforcement Actions

For products approved for market distribution, the FDA is mandated to perform biennial inspections of the firm to determine the ongoing compliance with cGMP. In addition, the company is required to inform the FDA of

---

[10] *Protecting the Public Health: FDA Pursues an Aggressive Enforcement Strategy*. FDA White Paper, Food and Drug Administration, Rockville, MD, June 30, 2003.

changes that affect the manufacture of the product. These include changes to the facility, equipment, process, formulation, labeling, and controls. The reporting of changes will be discussed in more detail below (see Section 10.5).

Following the biennial inspection, the FDA has a variety of approaches that it can apply to ensure a company comes into compliance with cGMP. As described above, if objectionable conditions are observed during an inspection, the investigator will issue to the company an FDA-483 form that lists the observations. The company has the opportunity to discuss the observations during the closeout meeting. If the company feels that an observation is incorrect, evidence supporting that should be presented. If the information provided satisfies the investigator, he/she probably will annotate the observation on FDA-Form 483. There is no requirement to respond in writing to FDA-483, but it is very advisable to do so. If an observation remains on FDA-483 that the company feels is incorrect, the written response should address it and provide supporting evidence. For observations that do show noncompliance with cGMP, the written response should propose corrective actions and a timeline for implementation. Corrective actions should be implemented using a company-wide, systems-oriented approach. For example, if the observation was made about a condition in one department, the organization should audit other departments to determine if the same condition exists elsewhere. If the audit findings result in confirmatory conditions, the organization should ensure that the corrective action is implemented across all departments. If the timeline for completing the corrective actions cannot be met, inform the FDA. Communication with the FDA is key; the company needs to demonstrate to the Agency that it is working to come into compliance in a timely manner.

If the firm is issued a warning letter, a written response is required within 15 days of receipt of the letter. If the company cannot send a complete response to the warning letter within the required time period, a letter stating the intent to respond should be submitted along with a date for submission. Once again, the response should contain proposed corrective actions and a timeline for implementation. As mentioned before, keeping the Agency informed of the progress is essential. If the situation warrants it, e.g., there are numerous serious observations that require a long-term corrective action plan, the company may consider informing the FDA of progress on a routine basis, e.g., send a quarterly report to the Agency. The FDA will conduct a follow-up inspection to ensure that all of the items in the warning letter have been addressed appropriately.

10.5 Reporting Changes

In order to keep the marketing application up to date, the company must inform the FDA of changes that could affect the product. These include, but

TABLE 10.4

Reporting Requirements for Changes to Drug Products

Level of Change	Impact on Quality	Reporting Requirement
1	Low impact	Annual Report
2	Significant impact	Change Being Effected (CBE) Supplement
3	Likely to impact	Prior Approval (PA) Supplement

are not limited to, changes to the facility, equipment, process, assays, formulation, specifications, packaging, and labeling. For drugs and biologics, the requirements are codified in 21 CFR 314.70, Supplements and Other Changes to an Approved Application, and 21 CFR 601.12, Changes to an Approved Application, respectively.

The RA professional plays an important role in determining the significance of the change as the reporting requirements vary depending on the potential of the change to adversely affect the product quality. In addition, the regulatory review should determine if the proposed plans to qualify/validate the change meet cGMP requirements. Each company should have a standard operating procedure defining the "change control" system, the responsibilities of the groups involved, the routing requirements for signature, and a change control request form.

The FDA has published a number of guidance documents that address the reporting of changes. There is a series of documents for drugs addressing scale-up and postapproval changes (SUPAC), changes to bulk active pharmaceuticals, and analytical testing sites.[11,12,13,14,15,16] The documents are very precise in discussing different changes, the information required for the regulatory submission, and the number of lots, if any, that should be placed on stability for the type of change. By determining the potential of the change to impact product quality, the RA professional must determine the category that the proposed change falls into. Table 10.4 summarizes the reporting requirements for changes to drug products.

Level 1 changes allow the product to be distributed immediately after the change is made and qualified appropriately. The change is reported to the

---

[11] *SUPAC-IR: Immediate Release Solid Oral Dosage Forms: Scale-up and Postapproval Changes: Chemistry Manufacturing and Controls, in vitro Dissolution Testing, and in vivo Bioequivalence Document*, Food and Drug Administration, Rockville, MD, 1997.

[12] *SUPAC-MR: Modified Release Solid Oral Dosage Forms: Scale-up and Postapproval Changes: Chemistry Manufacturing and Controls, In Vitro Dissolution Testing, and in vivo Bioequivalence Document*, Food and Drug Administration, Rockville, MD, 1997.

[13] *SUPAC-SS: Non-sterile Semisolid Dosage Forms Scale-up and Postapproval Changes: Chemistry Manufacturing and Controls, In Vitro Dissolution Testing, and in vivo Bioequivalence Document*, Food and Drug Administration, Rockville, MD, 1997.

[14] *BACPAC I: Intermediates in Drug Substance Synthesis; Bulk Actives Postapproval Changes: Chemistry, Manufacturing, and Controls Documentation*, FDA, February, 2001.

[15] *PAC-ATLS: Postapproval Changes — Analytical Testing Laboratory Sites*, Food and Drug Administration, Rockville, MD, April, 1998.

[16] *Changes to an Approved NDA or ANDA*, Food and Drug Administration, Rockville, MD, November, 1999.

TABLE 10.5

Reporting Requirements for Changes to Biologic Products or Specified
Biotechnology Products

Level of Change	Potential to Impact Quality	Reporting Requirement
Minor	Minimal	Annual Report
Moderate	Moderate	Change Being Effected in 30 d Supplement (CBE30)
		Change Being Effected (CBE) Supplement
Major	Substantial	Prior Approval (PA) Supplement

FDA in the annual report(s) of changes for the affected product(s). Level 2 changes require a Change Being Effected supplement (CBE). The firm may distribute products made using a change that requires a CBE upon FDA receipt of the supplement. The product is being distributed "at risk" as the FDA has to approve the supplement. Level 3 changes require the submission of a prior-approval supplement. That is, product made using the change cannot be distributed until the FDA has approved the supplement. It is important that these changes are identified as early as possible to minimize the amount of product that has to be placed on hold.

There are two guidance documents that apply to change to either an approved biologics application or an approved application for specified biotechnology and specified biological products (applicable products are listed in 21 CFR 601.2).[17,18] In contrast to the guidance documents that apply to changes made to drug product, the guidance document that applies to biologics is relatively vague.[17] Examples of the types of changes that would fall into the various reporting categories are given, but they are not as precise as for drugs. The plans to validate the change are heavily dependent upon the process/product as the products are not well defined and easily characterized. In addition, there is no information regarding the number of lots, if any, that should be placed on stability. As with changes to drugs, the reporting category is based upon the potential of the change to adversely affect the product. Table 10.5 summarizes the reporting requirements for changes to a biologic product.

The same distribution criteria as for drugs apply to biologic or specified biotechnology products made with changes to be reported in an annual report, as a CBE, or in a prior-approval supplement. There is an additional reporting category for biologics and specified biotechnology products (either regulated as drugs or biologics): the Change Being Effected in 30 Days (CBE-30) supplement. Products made using a change that requires a CBE-30 can be distributed, at risk, 30 days after receipt of the supplement by the FDA.

---

[17] *Guidance for Industry – Changes to an Approved Application: Biological Products*, Food and Drug Administration, Rockville, MD, July, 1997.

[18] *Guidance for Industry – Changes to an Approved Application for Specified Biotechnology and Specified Synthetic Biological Products*, Food and Drug Administration, Rockville, MD, July, 1997.

The biologics and specified biotechnology products regulations [21 CFR 601.12(e) and 314.70(g)(4), respectively] contain the provision for the use of a comparability protocol. The guidance documents[17,18] briefly address its use but the FDA needs to issue more specific guidance for industry. In short, the comparability protocol is a preapproved supplement that describes the tests and acceptable specifications to be obtained to demonstrate the acceptability of a change. The use of a preapproved comparability protocol may result in a reduction of the reporting requirement, e.g., a change that would warrant a prior approval supplement could be submitted as a CBE-30. However, due to the lack of specific guidance it appears that industry is not utilizing this option very often.

If there is a doubt about the level of supplement required for a particular change or the requirements for qualifying the change, the RA professional should contact the appropriate FDA office and request advice.

10.6 The Role of the Regulatory Affairs Professional in cGMPs

One of the responsibilities of the regulatory affairs professional is to keep the company informed of the continually evolving cGMP requirements, trends, and issues. There are several different ways that this can be accomplished, and some sources are described in the following paragraphs.

10.6.1 The Federal Register

The Federal Register (FR) is the official publication of the U.S. government and is used to inform the public of federal rule-making activities. All government agencies use this publication to make changes to regulations. The FDA must provide notice of the proposed change to the public, including GMPs. Ordinarily, the FDA will allow at least 75 days for comments about the proposed rule (change) that are submitted to the agency. The FDA reviews all of the comments, and when the final regulation is published in the Federal Register, it includes a preamble. The preamble contains a discussion of the comments received and provides an insight into the FDA's rationale for proposing the regulation, their interpretation of the regulation, and what it is expected to achieve. Thus, the pre-ambles are an invaluable resource to gain insight into the FDA's thinking.

10.6.2 FDA

Under the Freedom of Information Act (FOIA), the FDA, like any federal agency, is required to disclose records requested in writing by any person.

In addition, they are required to maintain reading rooms (both paper and electronic) that give access to records such as specific agency policy statements; certain administrative staff manuals; and, as of March 31, 1997, records disclosed in response to a FOIA request that "the agency determines have become or are likely to become the subject of subsequent requests for substantially the same records."

As a result of the FOIA requirement to have an electronic reading room, the FDA website (http://www.fda.gov) provides a wealth of information regarding the FDA's approach to cGMP. The site contains numerous documents that are prepared for FDA staff to enable them to carry out cGMP inspections and compliance reviews in addition to guidance documents prepared for industry. Table 10.6 includes a list of relevant FDA regulatory policy and guidance documents that are available on the website. These documents, prepared by the Office of Regulatory Affairs (ORA), are used to train FDA investigators on specific product issues.

In addition to providing guidance to the FDA staff, the guides also are very useful for the industry as they show where the FDA will focus resources, identify areas of specific interest or concern in the industry, and define situations that could lead to further regulatory action. The manual and related inspection guides should be used as a resource when preparing for an FDA inspection or, indeed, for performing internal audits.

In addition to the Compliance Policy Guides and the Compliance Program Guidance Manual, in the 1980s the FDA started publishing guidance documents specifically to inform industry of the FDA's interpretation of cGMP, for example the Guideline on Sterile Drug Products Produced by Aseptic Processing, and the Guideline on General Principles of Process Validation. Both documents were published in 1987 and are still in effect. FDA is in the process of revising the Guideline on Sterile Drug Products Produced by Aseptic Processing and recently published a preliminary concept paper that provides some insight into the FDA's current thinking regarding cGMP and aseptic processing.[19] A complete list of available guidance documents can be found on the FDA Website.

10.7 Risk-Based GMP Approach

The GMP regulations do not detail or instruct manufacturers of drugs and devices on how to achieve compliance with the regulations. That is, the regulations are broad in scope and are open to interpretation. There is an ongoing debate as to what constitutes "current" good manufacturing practice. For nearly 40 years, GMPs have remained relatively unchanged, inter-

---

[19] Preliminary Concept Paper: *Sterile Products Produced by Aseptic Processing Draft,* Food and Drug Administration, Rockville, MD, September 27, 2002.

TABLE 10.6

Useful Inspection and Compliance References

Inspection References

Field Management Directives
The primary vehicle for distributing procedural information/policy on the management of Office of Regulatory Affairs (ORA) field activities

Guides to Inspections of ...
Guidance documents written to assist FDA personnel in applying FDA's regulations, policies and procedures during specific types of inspection or for specific manufacturing processes

IOM: Investigations Operations Manual
Primary procedure manual for FDA personnel performing inspections and special investigations

Inspection Technical Guides
Guidance documents that provide FDA personnel with technical background on a specific piece of equipment or a specific manufacturing or laboratory procedure, or a specific inspectional technique, etc.

Medical Device GMP Reference Information

QS Regulation/Design Controls

Compliance References

Revisions
Revisions, Drafts, and Updates to ORA Compliance References

Manuals
Compliance Program Guidance Manual (CPGM)
Compliance programs and program circulars (program plans and instructions) directed to field personnel for project implementation

Compliance Policy Guides (CPG)
Contains FDA compliance policy and regulatory action guidance for FDA staff

Regulatory Procedures Manual (RPM)
Contains FDA regulatory procedures for use by FDA personnel. A reference document for enforcement procedures, practices and policy guidance

Other Compliance Documents
Application Integrity Policy
Regarding the integrity of data and information in applications submitted for FDA review and approval

Bioresearch Monitoring Program
(BIMO) of on-site inspections and data audits designed to monitor all aspects of the conduct and reporting of FDA regulated research. The BIMO Program was established to assure the quality and integrity of data submitted to the agency in support of new product approvals, as well as to provide for protection of the rights and welfare of the thousands of human subjects involved in FDA regulated research

Disqualified/Restricted/Assurance List for Clinical Investigators
Restricted from receiving investigational drugs, biologics, or devices if FDA determines that the investigator has repeatedly or deliberately failed to comply with regulatory requirements for studies or has submitted false information to the study's sponsor.

TABLE 10.6 (Continued)

Useful Inspection and Compliance References

Electronic Records; Electronic Signatures, 21 CFR Part 11
Background information and updates on the rule that allows the use of electronic records and
  electronic signatures for any record that is required to be kept and maintained by other FDA
  regulations

FDA Debarment List
Firms or individuals convicted of a felony under Federal law for conduct (by a firm) relating
  to the development or approval, including the process for development or approval, of any
  abbreviated drug application or (an individual convicted) for conduct relating to development
  or approval of any drug product, or otherwise relating to any drug product under the Federal
  Food, Drug, and Cosmetic Act

Public Health Service (PHS) Administrative Actions Listings
Of certain individuals who have had administrative actions imposed against them. The list is
  maintained by the PHS Office of Research Integrity (ORI)

Reading Room (Electronic Freedom of Information Act)
ORA documents frequently requested by the public through the Freedom of Information Act

---

pretation aside. Many purport that the "current" in cGMPs raises the level
of compliance expected by regulators without revision of the regulations.
Both FDA and industry may have their own interpretation and often industry standards are the more current interpretation. This situation has the
potential to lead to problems when the company's interpretation of cGMP
does not meet that of the FDA. Recently, however, in it's ongoing initiative
to modernize the regulation of drug manufacturing and product quality, the
FDA announced a major, agency-wide initiative on Pharmaceutical Current
Good Manufacturing Practices (cGMPs) for the 21st Century: A Risk Based
Approach in August 2002.[20,21] This 2-year program applies to pharmaceuticals, including biologics and veterinary drugs. The objective of the initiative
is to evaluate and improve the FDA's approach to reviews and inspections
related to the manufacturing of regulated products. The major goals of the
initiative include:

- Ensuring that state-of-the-art pharmaceutical science is utilized in
  the regulatory review and inspection policies

- Encouraging the adoption of new technological advances in high
  quality and efficient manufacturing by the pharmaceutical industry

- Assessing the applicable cGMP requirements relative to the best
  quality management practices

---

[20] FDA News Release: *FDA Unveils New Initiative to Enhance Pharmaceutical Good Manufacturing
Practices,* Food and Drug Administration, Rockville, MD, August 21, 2002.
[21] FDA News Release: *FDA Completes First Steps of Its Broad Initiative to Improve Regulation of Pharmaceutical Manufacturing,* Food and Drug Administration, Rockville, MD, February 20, 2003.

- Strengthening public health protection by implementing risk-based approaches that focus both industry and FDA attention on critical areas for improving product safety and quality
- Enhancing the consistency and coordination of FDA's drug quality oversight activities[11]

The implications for industry are significant and warrant close attention and communication with the FDA regarding the proposals that result from the evaluation. Further information can be found online at http://www.fda.gov/cder/gmp/index.htm.

10.8 Summary

The Regulatory Affairs professional plays an important role in ensuring that the company is compliant with the cGMP requirements by ensuring the integrity of the information included in the marketing application, maintaining the information flow to the Agency, and by monitoring the FDA and industry for evolving requirements and standards. The RA professional should endeavor to use all information sources available to maintain and increase his/her knowledge and understanding of the ever-changing cGMP requirements. Evidence and past experience shows that maintaining a state of compliance with the cGMPs is a serious and important responsibility. Failure to do so can result in the FDA taking regulatory action against a company — a situation that can, and should, be avoided.

11

Electronic Submissions: A Guide for
Electronic Regulatory Submissions to the FDA

Shylendra Kumar and Vahé Ghahraman

CONTENTS

1-58716-007-2/04/$0.00+$1.50
© 2004 by CRC Press LLC

11.1 Introduction

The documentation required in an application for marketing approval of a new drug is intended to accurately present the drug's whole story, including what happened during the clinical tests; how the drug is formulated (its components and composition); results of animal studies; how the drug behaves in the human body; and how it is synthesized, processed, manufactured, and packaged. The Food and Drug Administration (FDA) requires samples of the drug that represent the different levels of dosage available to the public, along with associated labeling. Full reports of a drug's studies must be submitted so that the FDA can evaluate the data. The review team at the Agency — chemists, pharmacologists, physicians, pharmacokineticists, statisticians, and microbiologists — need access to this information in order to evaluate the safety, efficacy, benefits, and risks of the drug in order to complete the approval process.

Until recently, most of the new drug/biologic applications were submitted to the Agency in paper form and commonly ran into thousands of pages. In order to accommodate copies required for all review team members, for archiving, and for internal record keeping, the sponsor had to create multiple copies of the dossier. After shipping to the Agency, these documents needed to be recorded, archived, and sent to the appropriate divisions for review. The handling of such enormous volumes of documents was at best a formidable and time-consuming task, and often resulted in delays in the review process. As one FDA official stated "A typical drug application has so much paper that we need a forklift to transfer it."[1]

After more than 15 years of collaborations with the industry and experiencing the potential benefits of the computer-assisted marketing applications, in 1999, the FDA released several guidance and specification documents on full electronic submissions related to New Drug Application (NDA) and Biologics License Application (BLA).[2,3,4] In November 2001, the FDA released the draft guidelines for an electronic Abbreviated New Drug Application (ANDA).[5] Subsequently, in February 2002, CBER released a new guidance document for electronic Investigational New Drug Application

---

[1] Trenter, M.L., Ed., Food and Drug Administration, From Test Tube to Patient: Improving Health Through Human Drugs, *FDA Center for Drug Evaluation and Research* Special Report, 1999.

[2] Food and Drug Administration, Regulatory Submissions in Electronic Format; General Considerations (issued January 1999; posted January 27, 1999).

[3] Food and Drug Administration, Regulatory Submissions in Electronic Format; New Drug Applications (issued January 1999; posted January 27, 1999).

[4] Food and Drug Administration, Guidance for Industry — Providing Regulatory Submissions to the Center for Biologics Evaluation and Research (CBER) in Electronic Format — Biologics Marketing Applications, November 1999.

[5] Food and Drug Administration, Providing Regulatory Submissions in Electronic Format — ANDAs Draft Guidance (issued November 2001).

(IND)[6] where pilot submissions by sponsors were strongly encouraged. In November 2000, another milestone for electronic submission was reached by the finalization of the common technical document (CTD), which aimed at harmonizing the global dossier submissions in different regions. In February 2002, the final guidelines[7] for an electronic CTD were published.

Some of the most important advantages of a complete electronic submission, compared to a paper or partial electronic submission include:

- Enhanced quality and organization of the dossier
- Expedited review process by providing
  - Easy access to documents and data
  - Faster navigation
  - Flexibility
  - Capability to copy and paste information
- Improved and more efficient communication and correspondences between the Agency and the sponsor, especially when there are questions and inquiries
- Elimination of the need for compiling and shipping of thousands upon thousands pages of documents
- Reduction and often elimination the need for storage and archiving of huge volumes of paper

The process of regulatory electronic submission is a dynamic one, and it is still in its evolving stages. New concepts for streamlining and expediting the drug development process, along with advancing technological tools and the establishment of new regulations and requirements, are among a variety of factors that contribute to the evolution of this fast changing field.

This chapter presents an overview of the regulatory process that started over two decades ago, and led to the introduction of electronic submissions as an alternative to the paper format for submitting a new drug application. The chapter also presents a brief history and background of the electronic submissions activities within the different divisions of the FDA. Furthermore, the type of submissions for which currently FDA accepts marketing applications in electronic format have been described. Finally, the specific requirements for the planning of an electronic submission to regulatory agencies have been outlined and the process for electronic regulatory submission has been described in detail; specific recommendations are made, at every step, for managing the process.

---

[6] Food and Drug Administration, Providing Regulatory Submissions to CBER in Electronic Format — Investigational New Drug Applications (INDs), February 2002.
[7] M2 EWG Electronic Common Technical Document Specification, Conference On Harmonisation Of Technical Requirements For Registration Of Pharmaceuticals For Human Use, ICH, eCTD Specification V 3.0, October 8, 2002, http://www.ich.org/pdfICH/eCTDSpecificationv3.pdf

The information presented and the procedures recommended here are based on several years of hands-on experience gained by the authors, and should be viewed as a guide and a roadmap for the regulatory electronic submissions process from a practical perspective. The reader should refer to the references cited for more specific, detailed, and up-to-date information on this subject.

It should also be noted that to conform to the scope and the objective of this publication, the current chapter focuses primarily on the marketing applications submitted to the FDA, and specifically to CDER and CBER. The process of electronic submission, however, in the other two major divisions of the FDA, namely Center for Devices and Radiological Health (CDRH) and Center for Veterinary Medicine (CVM) is emerging. Currently, there are considerable efforts to prepare these two divisions to accept full electronic submissions.

11.2 Overview of Regulations

Before the 1900s, prescribing and taking drugs was risky business for doctors and patients alike. Little was known about drugs, no scientific standards existed, and sometimes medicines caused illnesses along with severe side effects rather than curing or preventing them. The Food and Drug Act of 1906 established the first steps, in a series of many to follow, for the implementation and publishing of controls of prescription drugs. It prohibited interstate commerce in misbranded and adulterated foods, drinks, and drugs. Subsequently, several acts were passed which helped shape the current FDA drug review process. This new review process assured that drugs were safe and effective. It was lauded for years for the scientific and manufacturing quality it ensured in U.S. drugs. However, for decades, the review process drew criticism for taking too long. Getting beneficial drugs on the market quickly was just as much a part of FDA's public health mandate as keeping unproven and dangerous drugs off of the market. Early in the 1990s, the FDA started reforming the drug review process to speed the delivery of new drugs to consumers while preserving high standards of quality and safety.

To obtain added resources for reform, the FDA, Congress, and the Pharmaceutical industry negotiated the Prescription Drug User Fee Act (PDUFA)[8] of 1992. These much needed financial resources, by way of the user fees derived from the drug companies, enabled the Agency to hire additional scientists to review marketing applications for drugs. As part of the negotiations, the FDA on its part agreed to phase in ambitious performance goals such as reviewing priority new drugs in six months or less and standard new

---

[8] Food and Drug Administration Prescription Drug User Fee Act of 1992 (PDUFA), 1992, http://www.fda.gov/opacom/laws/fdcact/fdcact7c.htm

drugs in a year or less. The FDA also standardized policies, improved communications, and streamlined many burdensome rules and regulations. Influenced by the positive results, the PDUFA that was originally chartered for 5 years was extended in 1997 by the FDA for additional 5 years (PDUFA II).[9]

Subsequently in 1997 the congress passed the FDA Modernization Act (FDAMA) "To amend the Federal Food, Drug, and Cosmetic Act and the Public Health Service Act to improve the regulation of food, drugs, devices, and biological products, and for other purposes."[10]

This act embraced some of the most sweeping changes to the Food, Drug, and Cosmetic Act in 35 years. The act contained changes in how user fees were assessed and collected. For example, fees were waived for the first application for small businesses, orphan products, and pediatric supplements. The Act codified FDA's accelerated approval regulations and required the Agency to provide guidance on fast-track policies and procedures. In addition, the Agency was required to issue guidance for NDA reviewers.[1]

In 1997, the Center for Drug Evaluation and Research (CDER) and the Center for Biologics Evaluation and Research (CBER) at the Food and Drug Administration (FDA) jointly embarked upon a major undertaking to revamp the whole regulatory submissions process by mandating the acceptance of submissions in electronic format, starting in 2002.

"More Efficient Drug Development" was one of the goals set forth by the FDA's Reinvention Goals in 1997, and it was revised in 1999.[1] It stated, "By the year 2000, reinvent the drug development and review process, thereby lowering the development costs and, more importantly, reducing by an average of one year the time required to bring important new drugs to the American public. FDA will accomplish this through early and frequent consultation with product sponsors, implementation of an automated application filing process and an electronic document management system, and reauthorization of an enhanced user fee program."

On March 20, 1997, the Agency published the Electronic Records; Electronic Signatures regulation (21 CFR Part 11),[11] that "provides criteria under which FDA will consider electronic records equivalent to paper records, and electronic signatures equivalent to traditional handwritten signatures." In September 1997, CDER released the Guidance for Industry for Archiving Submissions in Electronic format. This guidance document provided details on submitting records and other documents in electronic format. According to this guidance, the electronic archival document submission should (1) display a clear, legible, easily viewed replica of the information that was

---

[9] Food and Drug Administration Prescription Drug User Fee Act of 1997 (PDUFA II), 1997, http://www.fda.gov/oc/pdufa2/5yrplan.html

[10] Food and Drug Administration Modernization Act (FDAMA), 1997, http://www.fda.gov/cder/guidance/105-115.htm

[11] Food and Drug Administration, 21 CFR Part 11 Electronic Records; Electronic Signatures; Final Rule Electronic Submissions; Establishment of Public Docket; Notice, Federal Register/Vol. 62, No. 54, March 20, 1997, p. 13430, http://www.fda.gov/ora/compliance_ref/part11/FRs/background/pt11finr.pdf

originally on paper, (2) provide the ability to print an exact replica of each page as it would have been printed in a paper submission, including retaining fonts, special orientations, table formats and page numbering, (3) include a well-structured index and the ability to easily navigate through the submission, (4) offer the ability to electronically copy text and images, and (5) serve as a substitute for paper copies.

In summary, the FDA's expedited drug approval initiative, through the adoption of electronic submissions is aimed at:

- Assisting the reviewer community in meeting PDUFA goals
- Providing reviewers with intuitive, standard presentations and tools
- Establishing electronic submissions standards and guidance
- Providing the ability to manage all submission types
- Enabling FDA to meet their PDUFA, FDAMA, and MDUFMA (Medical Device User Fee and Modernization Act) mandates and timelines
- Decreasing administrative processing time
- Decreasing processing time in order to facilitate reviewer access to regulatory submissions through the use of electronic routing and the secure transmission of regulatory documents

Realizing the new trend and encouraged by the potential benefits of electronic submissions, many sponsor companies and contract research organizations (CROs) have opted to implement this process from the very beginning and FDA started to receive more and more submissions in electronic format. As a result, the reduction in paper volumes decreased by 20% from 1997 to 1998, 30% from 1998 to 1999, and 50% from 1999 to 2000.[12]

According to the CDER 2002 Report to the Nation,[13] "The number of new drug applications submitted electronically continues to grow. Last year's electronic submissions were double the number submitted in the previous year. Overall, we had more electronic submissions last year than in the previous four years combined." This trend was presented by Levin (2002)[14] in Figure 11.1.

The report added that "The number of participating companies and the number of applications with electronic components continues to grow. About 70% of newly filed new drug applications have an electronic component and two thirds are completely electronic. About 17% of new or

---

[12] Levin, R., Industry Experience with Electronic Submissions — CDER Perspectives CDER, 2000, http://www.fda.gov/cder/regulatory/ersr/ersr4.pdf

[13] Food and Drug Administration, CDER 2002 Report to the Nation: Improving Public Health Through Human Drugs, 2002, http://www.fda.gov/cder/reports/rtn/2002/rtn2002.htm

[14] Levin, R., Electronic Submissions to the FDA 5th Annual Electronic Document Management Conference, Barcelona, Spain, September 23, 2002, http://www.fda.gov/cder/regulatory/ersr/2002_09_23_tutorial_talk/tsld001.htm

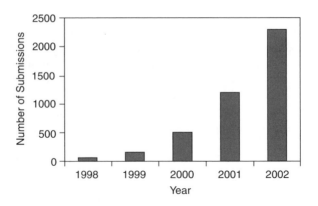

FIGURE 11.1
Number of electronic NDA submissions to CDER.

expanded use applications have an electronic component with 85% being completely electronic."[13]

11.2.1 Milestones in the Implantation of Electronic Submissions

- **September 1992**; Prescription Drug User Fee Act (PDUFA)
- **March 1997**; Electronic Records; Electronic Signatures Act (21 CFR Part 11)
- **September 1997**; FDA extended the PDUFA (PDUFA II)
- **November 1997**; FDA Modernization Act (FDAMA)
- **January 1999**; Guidance for Industry: Providing Regulatory Submissions in Electronic Format — General Considerations
- **January 1999**; Guidance for Industry: Providing Regulatory Submissions for New Drug Applications (NDA)
- **November 1999**; Guidance for Industry: Providing Regulatory Submission to the Center for Biologics Evaluation (CBER) in Electronic Format — Biologics Marketing Applications (BLA)
- **January 2001**; Guidance for Industry: Providing Regulatory Submissions in Electronic Format — Prescription Drug Advertising and Promotional Labeling
- **May 2001**; Guidance for Industry: Providing Regulatory Submissions in Electronic Format — Post-Marketing Expedited Safety Reports
- **March 2002**; Guidance for Industry: Providing Regulatory Submissions in Electronic Format — Investigational Drug Applications (IND)
- **June 2002**; FDA extended the PDUFA II (PDUFA III)

- **October 2002**; ICH M2 EWG — published the final specifications for the Electronic Common Technical Document eCTD
- **October 2002**; Medical Devices User Fee and Modernization Act (MDUFMA)[15] — amended the 1938 Federal Food, Drug, and Cosmetic Act.

The next section presents a history and background of the electronic submissions activities within the different divisions of the FDA.

11.3 History and Background

The overall effort of implementing a process for regulatory submissions — expressly, the computer assisted new drug applications (CANDA) or product license applications (CAPLA) — has been the focus of both CDER's and CBER's activities since the 1980s. Initially, each division embarked on the effort separately, until the 1997 consensus unified the effort and standardized these processes to include all types of submissions. Currently, some efforts have begun at CDRH and CVM to allow electronic submission of specific applications. A brief history of each division's undertakings is presented in this section.

In a parallel development, a process of standardization and harmonization of global dossier submissions, under the auspices of the International Conference on Harmonization (ICH), is gaining momentum. A brief background on the formation of the ICH and the harmonization process, manifested through the development of the Common Technical Document (CTD) and the electronic CTD (eCTD), is presented at the end of this section.

11.3.1 CDER

The advent of desktop computers along with the multitude of software applications that followed have mobilized the life sciences industry in general, and the drug development process in particular. Starting in early 1980s a new philosophy evolved around a concept called CANDA that was described by the FDA as basically "… any method using computer technology to improve the transmission, storage, retrieval, and analysis of data submitted to the FDA as part of the drug approval process."[16]

---

[15] Food and Drug Administration, Medical Devices and User Fee Modernization Act (MDUFMA) 2002, http://www.fda.gov/cdrh/mdufma/mdufma2002.html
[16] Dobbs J.H., The CANDA: An Overview. In: Mathieu M., ed. *CANDA: A Regulatory, Technology and Strategy Report.* Waltham, MA: Parexel International Corporation; 1992, pp.1–12.

The CANDA process, initially embraced by CDER, went through several iterations and testing during the period between 1984 and 1988. The first prototype of a CANDA system was developed in 1984 by Research Data Corporation for Abbott Laboratories to assist them in the clinical review of two NDAs[17] submitted to the Cardio–Renal Division. In September 1988, convinced by the benefits of the new process from their 4-year survey results, the FDA officially established the CANDA process by providing the basic guidelines,[18] thus allowing pharmaceutical companies and interested parties to submit sections of their NDA electronically.

The success and dynamics of CANDA brought a new wave of changes and excitement both to the FDA and the life sciences industry. As with any major change, it also created its own challenges and pitfalls. CANDAs were originally envisioned to include only submission of documents and data related to a new drug. However, often the process involved loading all custom software applications, along with the documents and data associated with a new drug, into computer systems and shipping them to the FDA for review. The main reason for such a practice was the incompatibility of the systems that were used to produce a submission (on the sponsor side) and those used at FDA for review purposes. Typically, the industry had access to more advanced systems than the FDA, thus calling for the sponsor to supply the entire system.

Although the new process was a better alternative to paper submission, soon after the implementation of CANDA, the FDA was faced with a major dilemma. Due to the fact that standard formatting was not defined for the submission of CANDAs, the agency was flooded with submissions of varying formats that were created using the different technologies and software applications which accompanied each new drug dossier. This required that the FDA reviewers receive training on variety of different hardware and software systems, which further complicated the review process and ultimately created new bottlenecks that, to some extent, impeded the perceived automation gains.

The status of the CANDA initiative and its level of industry acceptance was described in detail in two reports[19,20] published by PAREXEL/Barnett in 1992 and 1995. These reports detailed the projected future technical issues related to this process in terms of establishing a standardization scheme. The publication of CDER CANDA guidance documents in 1992 (first edition)[21]

---

[17] Ross R., Galle S., and Collom W., Regulatory Submissions: From CANDA/CAPLA to 2002 an Beyond *Drug Information Journal*, Vol. 34, 2000, pp. 761–774.

[18] U.S. Department of Health and Human Services, Food and Drug Administration: CANDA Guidance Manual. Second Edition. Rockville, MD, 1994.

[19] Mathieu M., Ed., CANDA: A Regulatory, Technology and Strategy Report. Parexel International Corporation, Waltham, MA, 1992.

[20] Collins M, Ed., CANDA 1995: An International Regulatory and Strategy Report. Parexel International Corporation, Waltham, MA, 1995.

[21] CANDA Guidance Manual. First Edition. Rockville, MD: U.S. Department of Health and Human Services, Food and Drug Administration: 1992.

and 1994 (second edition) (see footnote 18) further clarified the Agency–Industry communications related to CANDA submissions.

The CDER's Submission Management and Review Tracking (SMART) initiative in 1995, targeted the verification and enhancement of the review technologies and strategies that the Agency had been evaluating over the previous decade.[22] An important objective of SMART was to minimize, or eliminate altogether, the hardware and software system(s) provided by the sponsors for the review process, thus limiting the items provided to the Agency exclusively to electronic documents and information. Another objective of the initiative was to advocate the implementation of CANDA as an ongoing process during the life cycle of drug development and not necessarily toward the end of the spectrum.

In March 1997, the FDA laid the foundations for electronic submissions to replace the entire paper-based submissions (see footnote 11). Specifically, the final rules for accepting electronic records and electronic signatures (21 CFR Part 11) were published in the Federal Register, which set the standards for electronic records for the FDA and its regulated industries. This proved to be a major improvement to the existing process, which had previously accepted electronic submissions only as a supplement to the earlier paper submissions. In addition, for the first time, the Sponsor companies were allowed to use the portable document format (PDF) for their submission documents,[23] an option that in 1999 became the *de facto* standard.

In a parallel effort, in early 1997, the FDA and industry asked the Congress, during the Prescription Drug User Fee Act (PDUFA) reauthorization process, to mandate the Agency to develop a paperless, electronic submissions system for all types of applications.[24]

In September 1997, CDER published the Archiving Submissions in Electronic Format – NDAs guideline that specifically focused on providing directions and requirements to accommodate the archival copy for submission of the CRT and CRF sections of the application. In April 1998, CDER issued a new guidance that provided information for submitting a complete electronic format NDA for the archival copy (see footnote 17).

In 1997, CDER and CBER joined efforts to streamline the whole regulatory submissions process by mandating the acceptance of regulatory submissions in electronic format, starting in 2002. As a result, during 1999, the FDA released several guidance and specification documents (see footnotes 2, 3, and 4) on full electronic submissions related to the NDA and BLA that are still in effect today. In November 2001, CDER released the draft guidelines for the electronic ANDA (see footnote 5) for marketing generics, which became final in June 2002.[25]

---

[22] Flieger, K., Getting SMART: Drug Review in the Computer Age, Food and Drug Administration, 1994, http://www.fda.gov/fdac/features/895_smart.html

[23] Adobe Acrobat., PDF as a Standard for Pharmaceutical Electronic Submissions, White Paper, 2003, http://www.adobe.fr/products/acrobat/pdfs/pharmaceutical.pdf

[24] Mathieu M., New Drug Development: A Regulatory Overview, PAREXEL International Corp, 4th ed., Waltham, MA, 1997.

11.3.2 CBER

In the late 1980s, observing and learning from the CDER's experience, CBER initiated its own Computer Assisted Product Licensing Application (CAPLA) process. One important observation and conclusion made by CBER was the need to provide some standards for CAPLA submissions, which was lacking in CANDAs. In July 1990, CBER issued a brief guidance document for the sponsors and manufacturers of new biological products, outlining the information to be provided to the Agency when a CAPLA was planned. In this document titled Points to Consider: Computer Assisted Submissions for License Applications,[26] the FDA provided the first standards for the formatting and content of any such submission. It also described the CAPLA review process (CAPLAR) at CBER. The first official CAPLA, however, was submitted before the document was released. In 1989, Genentech submitted the first CAPLA to the Division of Cytokine Biology, which included the summary reports, line listings, SAS datasets, and clinical data tables and summaries as the electronic components.[27]

In 1991, CBER adopted a new approach for the review of CAPLAs by developing a single reviewing system, thus eliminating the need for training reviewers on several different systems. Before the end of 1991, CBER had developed the first set of concrete objectives for a complete electronic submission process. McCurdy (1993) presents a very detailed description of the CBER's 1991 system-based initiatives and what followed in a book published by PAREXEL.[27]

In June 1998, CBER published draft guidelines for CRTs, CRFs, and for Biologic License Applications/Product License Applications/Establishment License Applications (BLA/PLA/ELA) (see footnote 17). Subsequently, as mentioned earlier, in 1999, CBER joined efforts with CDER to finalize the general guidelines for electronic submissions. The final guidelines (see footnote 4) for an electronic BLA were released in November 1999.

In February 2002, CBER released a new guideline (see footnote 6) for the electronic applications for investigational new drugs (IND), where sponsors were encouraged to submit pilot applications to assist the FDA with troubleshooting and enhancing the review process.

In recent years, with the passing of the PDUFA II and the Food and Drug Administration Modernization Act (FDAMA) in 1997, CBER's goals for the review of the above submissions changed.[28] The Acts mandated expedited

---

[25] Food and Drug Administration., Guidance for Industry Providing Regulatory Submissions in Electronic Format — ANDAs (issued 6/2002, posted 6/27/2002).

[26] FDA Center for Biologics Evaluation and Research, Points to Consider: Computer Assisted Submissions for License Applications, CBER Guidance, July 1990.

[27] McCurdy L., CBER and Computer-Assisted Product License Applications, Chapter 15 in *Biologics Development: A Regulatory Overview, Mathieu M. Ed.*, PAREXEL International Corp, Waltham, MA, 1993.

[28] Food and Drug Administration, Electronic Secure Messaging v2.0, Working Instructions for Industry — Draft, Center for Biologics Evaluation and Research, Electronic Regulatory Submission and Review, May 6, 2002.

review of license applications and INDs. To fulfill these mandates, the agency created the Electronic Regulatory Submission and Review (ERSR) Program. Within CBER, the ERSR's Electronic Document Room (EDR) and Electronic Secure Messaging (ESM) systems help to address some of the requirements for these mandates.

ESM assists in fulfilling the ERSR goals of enabling secure electronic correspondence between CBER and its industry partners. A secure communications channel between CBER and industry enables the submission of electronically signed and encrypted regulatory amendments in a fully automated fashion. ESM was made available in October 2002 to the industry by CBER as a pilot project accepting only amendments to BLA with the goal to expand this service to other divisions within FDA.[29] Features of ESM included:

- **Scope** — Delivery/Receipt of Regulatory Documents and Correspondence
- **Limitation** — Limited to sponsors with Electronic Submissions
- **Focus** — Receipt of regulatory submissions to preexisting electronic application
- **Performance Enhancement** — Regulatory documents sent from sponsors on the West Coast via secure email to CBER are received by the application Regulatory Project Managers (RPM) in less than 12 min.

In addition to electronic delivery, ESM provides the following:

- Electronic signature
  - Digital signatures fully compliant with 21 CFR Part 11.
  - Utilizes Adobe and VeriSign certificates, with future plans for additional vendor support.
- e-Routing
  - Provides fully electronic workflow for the routing of IND and BLA submissions.
  - Simple electronic forms (paper based forms presented as electronic formwork) presented to RPMs. These forms allow RPMs to perform direct data entry of regulatory information into corporate databases.
  - Notifies reviewers of new submissions.

---

[29] Fauntleroy, M.B., "E-Sub Update" BIO Annual Conference, Washington, D.C., June 25, 2003, www.fda.gov/cber/summaries/bio062303mf_pt1.pdf

11.3.3   CDRH

In March 1996, the Center for Devices and Radiological Health (CDRH) published its first electronic submission related guidance document.[30] This guide presented an outline for a manufacturer to follow in preparing an abbreviated report, or abbreviated supplemental report, for Cephalometric devices intended for use with diagnostic x-ray equipment.

A recent initiative at CDRH is the proposed reengineering of the FDA medical device Registration and Listing (L&R) system,[31] where the goal is to develop a simplified, more efficient system meeting the needs of the FDA, industry, and the public. The first Grassroots Meeting of the FDA and industry representatives was held in May 1999, where the goals and the objectives of this initiative were reiterated and a course of action was proposed.

Currently, CDRH is accepting medical device applications in electronic format.[32] The Office of Device Evaluation (ODE) is currently developing formal guidelines regarding electronic submissions. Until they are finalized, CDRH is requesting the industry to give prior notification of their desire to submit an application in electronic form. This lead-time is required in order to discuss any special considerations with the sponsor prior to development of the documents.

11.3.4   CVM

The Center for Veterinary Medicine (CVM) has developed and implemented methods to accept electronic files as legal, original submissions for review.[33] Specifically, after the publication of FDA's Final Rule on Electronic Records; Electronic Signatures (21 CFR Part 11) in March 1997, a pilot project was developed for this purpose.

This project was intended to increase the efficiency of the review process of the investigational new animal drug file (INAD), the new animal drug application (NADA), the investigational food additive petition (IFAP), and the food additive petition (FAP) by providing for the electronic submission of Notices of Claimed Investigational Exemption (NCIE). The purpose of the pilot project was to determine the practicality and feasibility of electronic submission and review as an alternative to the current paper-based processes.

---

[30] Food and Drug Administration, *A guide for the submission of an abbreviated radiation safety report on cephalometric devices intended for diagnostic use* Center for Devices and Radiological Health (CDRH), March 1996.

[31] Benesch B.H. and Norman J.G., *Proposed Reengineering of The FDA Medical Device Registration And Listing (L&R) System* Center for Devices and Radiological Health (CDRH), March 2003.

[32] Food and Drug Administration, *Electronic Submissions — General Information*, The Center for Devices and Radiological Health (CDRH), 2003, http://www.fda.gov/cdrh/elecsub.html

[33] Food and Drug Administration, Electronic Submissions Project, Center for Veterinary Medicine, 2003, http://www.fda.gov/cvm/index/esubs/esubstoc.html

The pilot began September 8, 1997, with 12 companies participating, and an interim review[34] was concluded after three months. In March 1998, the CVM extended the pilot to increase participation to additional industries while the final notice was prepared for the electronic submission docket.

The CVM then drafted guidance and planned to expand the electronic submission capability into other reporting-type submissions. After meeting Government Paperwork Reduction Act requirements, guidance documents were posted on the CVM's Web page and their availability was published on the Agency Electronic Submissions Dockets in February of 2001. These actions increased the scope of the project to include Requests for a Meeting or Teleconference and Agendas, Notices of Final Disposition of Slaughter for Human Food Purposes, and Notices for Final Disposition of Animals Not Intended for Immediate Slaughter. Several guidelines on electronic submissions are planned for publication by CVM in the near future.

11.3.5 ICH and Global Submissions

Around the time when NDA and BLA specifications were being developed, a new concept was being cultivated by the Global Regulatory Agencies to standardize and expedite the process of submitting marketing applications to different regions. The efforts that ensued culminated in the formation of the International Conference on Harmonization for Registration of Pharmaceuticals for Human Use (ICH) in 1990 to oversee and implement such an initiative.

The ICH is a unique project that brings together the regulatory authorities of Europe, Japan, and the United States and experts from the pharmaceutical industry in the three regions to discuss scientific and technical aspects of product registration in order to reduce the requirements and eliminate the duplications involved during the research and development of new medicines. The next few paragraphs, adapted from the ICH Website,[35] summarize the process by which the ICH and its expert working groups (EWG) were formed. In addition, they describe the implementation steps and the current status of the CTD and eCTD.

The European community pioneered harmonization of regulatory requirements in the 1980s, as the European Union (EU) moved towards the development of a single market for pharmaceuticals. The success achieved in Europe demonstrated that harmonization was feasible. At the same time there were multilateral discussions between Europe, Japan, and the U.S. on possibilities for harmonization. It was, however, at the World Health Organization (WHO) Conference of Drug Regulatory Authorities (ICDRA), in Paris, in 1989, that specific plans for action began to materialize. Soon after, the authorities convened to discuss a *Joint Regulatory–Industry* initiative on

---

[34] Food and Drug Administration, Office of New Animal Drug Evaluation Center for Veterinary Medicine. Electronic Submission Pilot Project Report Three Month Report, December 8, 1997.
[35] International Conference on Harmonization, The ICH Harmonisation Process 2003, http://www.ich.org/ich4.html

international harmonization, and ICH was conceived. It was eventually established in April 1990 in Brussels.

11.3.5.1   Common Technical Document (CTD)

At the first Steering Committee meeting of the ICH, the *terms of reference* were agreed upon. It was decided that the *topics* selected for harmonization would be divided into three categories namely: safety, quality, and efficacy to reflect the three criteria which are the basis for approving and authorizing new medicinal products. It was also agreed that six-party *expert working groups* (EWGs) should be established to discuss scientific and technical aspects of each *harmonization topic*. Eleven such topics were identified for discussion at the First International Conference on Harmonization. One of the topics considered in the agenda was the creation of a common technical document (CTD) for preparing the marketing dossier in different regions. The ICH adopted a *harmonization process*, for each topic, which included the following five steps:

Step 1: *Consensus Building*

Step 2: *Start of Regulatory Action*

Step 3: *Regulatory Consultation*

Step 4: *Adoption of a Tripartite Harmonized Text*

Step 5: *Implementation*

The compiled text of the draft CTD reached Step 2 of the ICH process at the steering committee meeting in July 2000. A final CTD was completed in November 2000 (Step 4). A schematic illustration of a CTD and its modules are shown in Figure 11.2. The E.U. and Japan regulatory authorities required submission in CTD format starting July 2003. Although not required in the U.S., the FDA is favorably recommending that the sponsors of marketing applications submit them in the CTD format.

11.3.5.2   Electronic Common Technical Document (eCTD)

The electronic Common Technical Document (eCTD) reached Step 2 in June 2001 and after reaching Step 4 in February 2002, the final eCTD specification document was published. The ICH defines the eCTD as "… an Interface for Industry to Agency" and the desired method for the "transfer of regulatory information while at the same time taking into consideration the facilitation of the creation, review, life cycle management, and archival of the electronic submission. The eCTD specification lists the criteria that will make an electronic submission technically valid. The focus of the specification is to provide the ability to transfer the registration application electronically from Industry to a Regulatory Authority" (see footnote 7).

One of the major differences of the eCTD, compared to the paper CTD, was the incorporation of the XML (extensible markup language) technology and introduction of an XML backbone file to serve as an overall table of

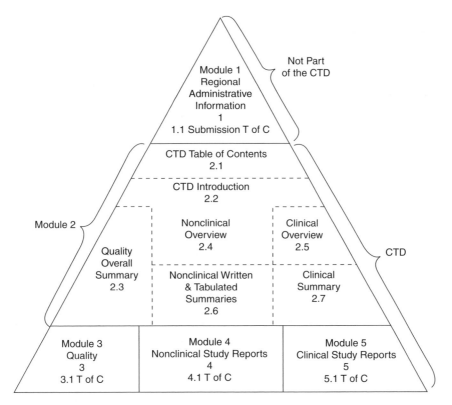

FIGURE 11.2
Schematic illustration of the CTD format.

contents (TOC). Another difference was the inclusion of all the regional specific requirements into a separate module (Module 1). Table 11.1 shows a high level comparison of paper and electronic CTDs. The common modules of the eCTD (Modules 2 through 5) were finalized in September 2002 during the Washington, D.C., meeting. An illustration of the eCTD modules is also presented in Figure 11.2. The final E.U. regional module (Module 1 — E.U.) reached Step 5 in March 2003. The draft U.S. regional module (Module 1 — U.S.) was released in July 2003; and the Japan regional module (Module 1 — Japan), originally scheduled to be released before July 2003, was not available at the time of publishing of this book.

11.4 FDA Submission Types

Based on the recent guidelines and specifications pertaining to reviewing and archiving, currently FDA divisions accept, or plan to accept, submissions listed in Table 11.2 in a fully electronic format.

TABLE 11.1

Comparison of CTD and eCTD Submission Formats

Item Submission Format	CTD Paper	eCTD Electronic
Specifications/guidance	Regional modules are not addressed It describes only Modules 2 to 5	ICH M2 EWG has produced a specification for the eCTD that is applicable to all modules Module 1 specifications addressed by regional authorities (E.U., U.S., Japan)
Submission life cycle	It does not cover details related to amendments or variations to the initial application	Covers the entire lifecycle of a product: initial applications, subsequent amendments, supplements and variations
File Formats	N/A	PDF, XML, and some regional specific files (e.g., SAS datasets, Word, WP, Excel, etc.)
Overall table of contents	In paper format	In XML backbone format

TABLE 11.2

Electronic Submission Types and Their Formats

Application Type	Submission	
	Format	Electronic
NDA	NDA & CTD	eNDA & eCTD
SNDA	SNDA	eNDA
BLA	NDA & CTD	eBLA & eCTD
ANDA	NDA	eNDA & eCTD
IND	IND	eIND

The detailed contents and directory structures of these submissions are presented in Section 7.

11.5 Planning a Regulatory Submission

Traditionally, the sponsor companies started thinking about a plan for electronic submission only as they approached the end of the drug development spectrum. This often created tremendous amount of distress, panic, and complications for the people (normally regulatory affairs groups) that were responsible for preparing the electronic version of the dossier. Learning from their own experience, or observing their peers, many sponsors realized the benefits of developing an early plan and a strategy for the marketing approval of their product. It is highly recommended that the sponsor start the planning activities as early as Phase I to facilitate better control of the overall submission process. Several requirements should be addressed when planning a regulatory submission.

Table 11.3 provides a checklist of the most common requirements for the planning stage. The checklist will aid in planning the electronic submission tasks and identify the needs of the sponsor to decide on a future course of action for proceeding with the submission process. The following section describes some of the general requirements in more detail.

11.5.1 Regulatory Requirements

There are several documents that the sponsor should acquire and maintain for reference purposes during the course of any submission. They include the FDA guidance documents, minutes of FDA meetings, and other specific and relevant documents/guidelines.

Currently, the majority of the FDA guidance documents are intended to assist the applicant/sponsor during the preparation of regulatory submissions in electronic format to CDER and CBER.

The guidance documents on electronic submissions discuss both the general issues and the topics specific to each submission type. For the common parts, they discuss issues such as acceptable file formats, media, and submission procedures that are applicable to all submission types. In some cases, the guidance for one center differs from that of the other due in part to differences in procedures and computer infrastructures. The FDA diligently works to minimize these differences wherever possible. For the specific parts, the guidance documents delineate the directory structure, file and folder naming convention for the submission items, and specific formats that need to be followed for creating item level table of contents (TOCs) or elements. In later sections of this chapter, we will discuss the details associated with each item in different submissions and will make specific recommendations on the formatting of the involved documents.

The Agency guidance documents on electronic regulatory submissions are be updated regularly to reflect the evolving nature of the technology involved and the experience of those using this technology. Thus, it is strongly recommended that the people involved in the eSubmissions visit the FDA Website for up-to-date information. For a list of guidance documents on electronic submissions that have been developed or are under development, see the Reference section of this book.

Other very important documents that should be available and referred to are the minutes of any FDA meetings (e.g., pre-NDA, pre-IND, etc.). This is extremely important as it outlines and specifies the agreements reached with the review division in terms of providing the quantity and substance of the information and its format, especially when it deviates from the standard guidelines.

11.5.1.1 Recommended General Considerations for PDF Files

This section describes key components from general recommendations for publishing PDF files (extracted from Providing Regulatory Submissions in Electronic Format — General Considerations, January 1999)[2] which will

TABLE 11.3

Checklist of Items for Planning a Regulatory Submission

Item	Sub Item(s)	Status
Regulatory requirements	Type and scope of the submission FDA guidance documents Minutes of FDA meeting(s) Other specific documents/guidelines	
Personnel resources	eSubmission team • Project Leader/Project Manager • Team Leaders • Process Area Specialists Roles and responsibilities Work flow	
Tools and technologies	Software • Adobe® Acrobat® • Office productivity tools (e.g., word processor, spreadsheet, etc.) • Scanning Software • SAS® and SAS® Viewer • XML Editor • Other necessary software applications specific to company Hardware • Industry standard desktop PCs • Scanner(s) • Large screen monitors • CD RW drives • High speed printer(s) • Copier(s) 21 CFR Part 11 Compliance and System Validation EDMS or file server with defined storage, version control, backup and security Publishing system or acrobat plug-ins tools	
eSubmission process	Process checklist Submission Process • Authoring • Publishing (*see* Publishing process) • Final compilation • Overall quality assurance • Submission Publishing process • Scanning • PDF conversion • Bookmarking and hypertext linking0 • Document information fields • Pagination • Document level quality control • Compilation • Quality assurance • Full-Text indexing • Optimization	

assure creating PDF files with formats that are compliant with the Agency requirements for review and archival purposes. It will be beneficial here to provide a brief overview on PDF. The following two paragraphs are extracted from the Acrobat white paper on PDF (2003)[23] and are intended to provide some background information to the reader.

11.5.1.1.1 What is PDF?

The term Portable Document Format, or PDF, was coined to illustrate that a file conforming to this specification can be viewed and printed on any platform — UNIX®, Mac OS, Microsoft® Windows®, and several mobile devices as well — with the same fidelity. A PDF document is the same for any of these platforms. It consists of a sequence of pages, with each page including the text, font specifications, margins, layout, graphical elements, and background and text colors. With all of this information present, the PDF file can be imaged accurately for the screen and the printing device. It can also include other items such as metadata, hyperlinks, and form fields.

PDF is a publicly available specification, regardless of the fact that Adobe created it and advances the specification through subsequent releases. Many people confuse PDF, the data format, with Adobe Acrobat, the software suite that Adobe sells to create, view, and enhance PDF documents. In 1993, the first PDF specification was published at the same time the first Adobe Acrobat products were introduced. Since then, updated versions of the PDF specification continue to be available from Adobe via the Web. The current version of PDF specification at the date of this publication is version 1.4 and is available at http://partners.adobe.com/asn/developer/acrosdk/docs.html. All of the revisions for which specifications have been published are backward compatible, that is, if your computer can read version 1.4, it can also read version 1.3 and so on. Since Adobe chose to publish the PDF specification, there is an ever-growing list of creation, viewing, and manipulation tools available from other vendors. [*Note:* Currently Adobe is shipping PDF version 1.5.]

11.5.1.1.2 Version

The PDF files must be capable of being read by Acrobat Reader version 3.0 with a search plug-in without the necessity for additional software.

11.5.1.1.3 Fonts

All the fonts used should be embedded in the PDF files to ensure that those fonts will always be available to the reviewer. Three techniques that help limit the storage space taken by embedding fonts include:

- Limiting the number of fonts used in each document
- Using only True Type or Adobe Type 1 fonts
- Avoiding customized fonts

The agency believes that the Times New Roman 12-point font is adequate in size for reading narrative text. Although sometimes tempting for use in tables and charts, fonts smaller than 12 points should be avoided whenever possible. FDA recommends the use of a black font color. Blue font may be used for hypertext links.

11.5.1.1.4 Page Orientation

Pages should be properly oriented prior to saving the PDF document in final form to ensure correct page presentation.

11.5.1.1.5 Page Size and Margins

The print area for pages should fit on a sheet of paper that is 8.5 inches by 11 inches. A margin of at least 1 inch on all sides should be allowed to avoid obscuring information if the pages are subsequently printed and bound.

11.5.1.1.6 Source of Electronic Document

PDF documents produced by scanning paper documents are usually inferior to those produced from an electronic source document. Scanned documents are more difficult to read and do not allow search or copy and paste text for editing. They should be avoided if at all possible. When using optical character recognition (OCR) software, it should be verified that all imaged text converted by the software is accurate.

11.5.1.1.7 Methods for Creating PDF Documents and Images

For creating PDF documents a method should be selected that produces the best replication of a paper document. Documents that are available only in paper should be scanned at resolutions that will ensure the pages are legible both on the computer screen and when printed, while limiting the size of the PDF file. It is recommended scanning at a resolution of 300 dots per inch (dpi) to balance legibility and file size.

11.5.1.1.8 Hypertext Linking and Bookmarks

Hypertext links and bookmarks are techniques used to improve navigation through PDF documents. Hypertext links can be designated by rectangles using thin lines, by blue text, or by using invisible rectangles for hypertext links in a table of contents to avoid obscuring text.

In general, for documents with a table of contents, bookmarks and hypertext links should be provide for each item listed in the table of contents including all tables, figures, publications, other references, and appendices. In general, including a bookmark to the main table of contents for a submission or item is helpful. Make the bookmark hierarchy identical to the table of contents.

Hyperlinking throughout the body of the document to supporting annotations, related sections, references, appendices, tables, or figures that are not located on the same page is helpful and improves navigation efficiency.

Use relative paths when creating hypertext linking to minimize the loss of hyperlink functionality when folders are moved between disk drives. Absolute links that reference specific drives and root directories will no longer work once the submission is loaded onto agency network servers. When creating bookmarks and hyperlinks, choose the magnification setting Inherit Zoom so that the destination page displays at the same magnification level that the reviewer is using for the rest of the document.

11.5.1.1.9 Page Numbering

Only individual documents should be paginated. If a submission includes more than one document, it is not needed to provide pagination for the entire submission.

It is easier to navigate though an electronic document if the page numbers for the document and the PDF file are the same. To accomplish this, the initial page of the paper document should be numbered page 1. (See in this chapter Section on Pagination.)

11.5.1.1.10 Document Information Fields

Document information fields are used to search for individual documents and to identify the document when found. (See in this chapter Section on Document Information Fields.)

11.5.1.1.11 Open Dialog Box

The Open dialog box sets the document view when the file is opened. The initial view of the PDF files should be set as Bookmarks and Page. If there are no bookmarks, the initial view should be set as Page only. Set the Magnification and Page Layout to default.

11.5.1.1.12 Security

No security settings or password protection should be included for PDF files. Printing, changes to the document, selecting text and graphics, and adding or changing notes and form fields all should be allowed.

11.5.1.1.13 Indexing PDF Documents

Full text indexes should be used to help find specific documents and/or search for text within documents. Adobe Acrobat or Acrobat Catalog (in the earlier versions) is one example of a tool that can be used to index PDF documents. When a document or group of documents is indexed, all words and numbers in the file and all information stored in the Document Information fields are stored in special index files that are functionally accessible using the search tools available in Acrobat. Portions of a document that are imaged are not indexed. Even if the document only contains images, the text in the Document Information fields of the file will be indexed.

The table of contents file for a section should be associated with the corresponding full text index file. This means that when the table of contents file is opened, the index file is automatically added to the available index list and is ready to be used.

11.5.1.1.14   *Plug-Ins*

It is acceptable to use plug-ins to assist in the creation of a submission. However, the review of the submission should not require the use of any plug-ins in addition to those provided with Acrobat Reader.

11.5.1.1.15   *Electronic Signatures*

Currently, FDA is developing new procedures for archiving documents with electronic signatures. Until those procedures are in place, a paper copy that includes the handwritten signature must accompany documents such as certifications for which regulations require an original signature.

11.5.2   Personnel

For any project, a submission team should be assembled and the roles and responsibilities of the members clearly identified at the initiation phase. These items are discussed subsequently.

11.5.2.1   *Submission Team*

The submission team is typically a composite representation of the following individuals and skill sets:

- Project Leader

  Generally the Regulatory Director, Project Manager, or Submission Manager
- Team Leaders

  Typically one person from each of the following disciplines:
  - Regulatory Affairs and Dossier Publishing
  - Nonclinical
  - Clinical/Medical
  - Chemistry and Manufacturing
  - BioStatistics and Data Management
  - Information Technology (IT)
  - Quality Assurance
  - Marketing and Risk Management
- Process Area Specialists

  Authors, reviewers, QA specialists, publishing specialists, scanning specialists, etc.

11.5.2.2 Roles and Responsibilities

The team members' roles and responsibilities should be clearly defined at both the Item and Document levels. The sample template shown in Table 11.4 (for a BLA) can be used to define team-level responsibilities along with appropriate timelines.

11.5.2.3 Work Flow

The preparation of any electronic submission involves a team-based process encompassing multiple tasks and steps. This process requires collaboration between individuals from different departments within an organization and other client representatives (e.g., CROs, contractors, consultants, etc.) that contribute to different parts of a project. For instance, a document from its inception goes through several stages before it is finalized and fully ready to be included in a submission. A typical scenario may include authoring, quality control (QC), scanning, publishing, compiling, and final quality assurance (QA), and preparing media stages. Extrapolating this process to many documents that are handled by several people simultaneously makes management of the dynamics of this process quite challenging. In order for these functionalities to work smoothly and in a timely fashion, a work flow for guiding the team members is a must.

11.5.3 Tools and Technologies

Any electronic submission project requires a set of specific hardware and software tools and technologies. Depending on the long-term goals of a company and the scope and size of each project, these requirements may vary significantly from one project to another. Thus, for a given project, these requirements should be identified and efforts extended to meet those requirements. Hence, a minimum level of compliance with these requirements should be established to ensure the eSubmission capabilities for a mid-size project. Table 11.3 shows a list of tools and technology items essential for the eSubmission process. A description of each item follows.

11.5.3.1 Software

The following is a recommended list of software:

- Adobe® Acrobat® 4.05 or later
- Acrobat® Plug-Ins (provided by third party vendors)
- Office Productivity Tools (e.g., word processor, spreadsheet, etc.)
- Scanning software
- SAS® and SAS® Viewer 8.2 or later (for data management and statistical programming groups)

TABLE 11.4

A Sample of eSubmission Items/Tasks Checklist

Item/Task	Deliverable Components	Responsible Group	Target Date
Item 1	BLA TOC, Roadmap, Cover letter, etc.	Regulatory/publishing	
Item 2	Labeling	Clinical/regulatory	
—	—	—	
—	—	—	
Item 20	—	—	
Security and Network Backup		IT	
Media preparation	CD-ROM or tape	IT/regulatory	
Overall QC of the submission media	Quality assurance report	Regulatory, QA, publishing	
Other			

- XML editor (or an application capable of creating XML backbone for eCTD)
- Other necessary software applications specific to company

11.5.3.2   Hardware

The following is a recommended list of hardware:

- Network system with security, backup and virus-protection capabilities
- Pentium IV — 1 GHz or higher processor PCs with a CD burner, a large (40 GB) hard drive, and at least 256 MB of RAM for the scan station
- 18- to 20-inch monitors for scan station and publishing PCs
- High-speed scanner(s) with automatic feeder (duplex option recommended)
- Color scanner/printer (optional)
- High-volume and high-speed printer(s) with PostScript option
- Photocopier(s)

11.5.3.3   21 CFR Part 11 Compliance and System Validation

In March 1997, the FDA issued final regulations (Part 11) that provided criteria for acceptance by the FDA, under certain circumstances, of electronic records, electronic signatures, and handwritten signatures executed to electronic records as equivalent to paper records and handwritten signatures executed on paper (see footnote 11). These regulations, which apply to all FDA program areas, were intended to permit the widest possible use of electronic technology, consistent with the FDA's responsibility to protect the public health.

21 CFR Part 11 regulations address any electronic document or record that is part of a regulated system. These regulations therefore apply to regulatory submissions, as well as all GMP, GCP, GLP, and QA/QC data. They cover issues such as validation, audit trail, legacy systems, copies of records, record retention, security and electronic signatures. This meant that all systems would be required to maintain prior revisions of data and documents.[36] Furthermore, it will also be necessary to keep a record of the changes as to who made a change and when, and describe what the old and new data are. These rules will force companies to rethink their business process as well as to examine their current systems.

Since Part 11 became effective in August 1997, significant discussions have ensued between industry, contractors, and the agency concerning the interpretation and implementation of the rule.[37] Several concerns have been raised, particularly in the areas of Part 11 requirements for validation, audit trails, record retention, record copying, and legacy systems. As a result, in February 2003, the FDA issued a new draft guidance, announcing that it intends to exercise enforcement discretion with respect to the validation, audit trail, record retention, and record copying requirements of Part 11. However, records must still be maintained or submitted in accordance with the underlying predicate rules. It was also mentioned that the FDA intends to exercise enforcement discretion and will not normally take regulatory action to enforce Part 11 with regard to systems that were operational before August 20, 1997, the effective date of Part 11 (commonly known as existing or legacy systems) while Part 11 is undergoing reexamination.

A new guidance document was released in August 2003 which reflects the current thinking of the FDA on this subject.

11.5.3.4 Electronic Document Management System

The efficient management and publishing of submission content is a requirement — not an option — for the life sciences enterprise. Life sciences organizations need to securely and efficiently control the flow of submission content, authorize and verify recipients, and track changes in compliance with regulatory agencies.

Electronic document management provides a secure and organized structure for storing and retrieving documents. The system can be designed to match the specific needs of any group or the entire company.

The benefits of an electronic document management system (EDMS) are many, and the features may include:[38]

---

[36] Prelude Computer Solutions, Inc., Electronic Submissions — Whitepaper, Prelude Computer Solutions, Parsippany, NJ, 2002.

[37] Food and Drug Administration, Draft Guidance for Industry on Part 11, Electronic Records, Electronic Signatures — Scope and Application; Department of Health and Human Services, February 2003, http://www.fda.gov/cder/gmp/cd0314.pdf

[38] Bartsch, G.U., Introduction to Electronic Document Management — Whitepaper, *Prelude Computer Solutions*, Parsippany, NJ, 2003.

- Access Control — Controls access to documents
- Accessibility — Provides control over all versions of a document and allows quick access to the final version
- Overwriting Protection — Eliminates overwriting of prior versions
- Edit Control — Allows locking documents while being modified so that only one person is able to make changes at any time
- Audit Trail — Allows viewing the name of the person who has modified a document and the time of the modification(s)
- Version Control — Allows maintaining prior versions of documents (life-cycle)
- Retrieval — Allows searching for documents based on key attributes
- Workflow: Create, Review, and Approve — Provides routing documents for review and approval

The purpose of an EDMS is to provide a repository for the documents, as well as the security and tools to review and approve them.

It is important to note that many of the small- to medium-sized companies presently lack EDMS due to the high costs associated with implementing and maintaining such an elaborate system. These companies, therefore, operate based on file servers, and have to address the requirements regarding the work flow, storage, security, version control, and backup within that framework. These items are described in proceeding sections. Although this chapter addresses issues related to both the EDMS and file servers, the emphasis is on the latter case where EDMS is not present.

11.5.3.5 Publishing Systems

Depending on the level of sophistication and comprehensiveness, there are different publishing tools and systems for regulatory submissions. Brown et al. (2002)[39] have described the following levels of sophistication for regulatory publishing systems:

- Level 1: Pen typewriters
- Level 2: Word processing software (SW)
- Level 3: Combination of word processing SW with ability to convert to PDF/XML
- Level 4: Combination of word processing SW, PDF/XML conversion capability, and tools for publishing (e.g., Acrobat plug-ins)
- Level 5: Off-the-shelf publishing software with word processing and PDF/XML conversion capabilities, and tools for publishing

---

[39] Brown, M., Inose C., and Ramos C., Regulatory Publishing, *Regulatory Affairs Journal*, Vol. 13, No. 10, October, 2002.

TABLE 11.5

Comparison of Main Features of Level 4 and 5 Publishing Systems

		Publishing System	
Item No.	Attribute Description	Level 4	Level 5
1.	Integrated within an EDMS (i.e., Requires EDMS)	No	Yes
2.	Provides audit trail (Identifying users, document status, version control, and change control)	No	Yes
3.	Provides report and other document templates for authoring	No	Yes
4.	Allows authentication of digital or electronic records	No	Yes
5.	Allows security on files, databases and repositories	No	Yes
6.	Automatic indexing (bookmark creation)	Yes	Yes
7.	Automatic hyperlinks to tables, figures, references, and other sections or documents, etc.	Yes	Yes
8.	Automatic table of contents (TOC) creation	Yes	Yes
9.	Automatic thumbnails creation	Yes	Yes
10.	Automatic pagination	Yes	Yes
11.	Batch PDF processing	Yes	Yes
12.	Document information fields creation	Yes	Yes
13.	Provides ability to modify hyperlinks attributes (color, style, rectangle visible, etc.)	Yes	Yes
14.	Provides ability to modify bookmark fonts attributes	Yes	Yes
15.	Validates the bookmarks and hyperlinks status and provides their number in a document (or in a submission)	Yes	Yes
16.	Provides both paper and electronic submissions	Yes	Yes

Source: From Brown, M., Inose C., and Ramos C., Regulatory Publishing, *Regulatory Affairs Journal*, Vol. 13, No. 10, October, 2002.

The first three levels are considered either outdated or impractical, thus are not used as often as the last two levels, and are not covered here.

Typically, a Level 5 solution is considered a complete start-to-end publishing system that has many built-in attributes that are essential for any publishing process, while a Level 4 solution provides the basic features required for a publishing process within a very cost-effective framework. The main features of these systems are contrasted in Table 11.5.

Acquiring, implementing and maintaining a complete publishing system (Level 5), along with training a knowledgeable worker who will use it, requires a considerable amount of financial and human resources. Many small- to medium-sized companies cannot afford such costs and consequently resort to Level 4 solutions. The following sections are geared towards a Level 4 publishing solution.

11.5.3.6   *Selecting a New System*

The process of selecting and implementing a new system can be extremely challenging for a company that intends to acquire and/or integrate a new technology into their existing infrastructure. It also requires careful planning along with prudent and calculated projections. Once the feasible solutions are identified, the ramification of such changes and the impact of each alternative solution should be carefully considered. The following are suggested general steps that should be taken during the selection and implementation of any new system (see footnote 36).

- Evaluate the current business process and workflow.
- Identify a set of needs/requirements.
- Identify and compare alternatives.
- Develop a plan for purchasing, support, and maintenance.
- Formulate a partial implementation (pilot project) plan.
- Develop a plan and strategy for full implementation and training.
- Validate the system.

Depending on the circumstances of the project, each step may require additional (more detailed) examination during the selection and implementation process.

It is important to note that PDF, featured with navigational review aids such as bookmarks and hyperlinks, is the foundation, and the common denominator in all of the electronic submissions. As a result, the selection of the PDF publishing system is an extremely important mission. Based on their experience with different submissions, the authors recommend a PDF publishing solution which is modular and is based on open architecture. Such a flexible system that also produces quality PDF files can easily accommodate the needs of eIND, eBLA, eNDA, and eCTD.

11.5.3.7   *Storage*

For companies with EDMS, the source documents will be stored in a repository and accessed by authorized personnel, while constantly maintaining the audit trails and version controls. If a company does not have such a system, the source and the final published documents can be stored and maintained in a file server using an appropriate directory structure under a designated network share. An example of such a directory structure, consisting of three subfolders — Working, Final, and Knowledge Base — is shown in Figure 11.3, and described below.

11.5.3.7.1   *Working (Folder)*

The purpose of this directory is to provide the users with a working area where they can create, modify, and update documents. It also allows them, when necessary, to create additional temporary directories and to maintain version control by creating documents with different naming convention in the Working folder.

11.5.3.7.2   *Final (Folder)*

This area holds the final submission documents and maintains the directory structure for the submission type. When the PDF documents are finalized

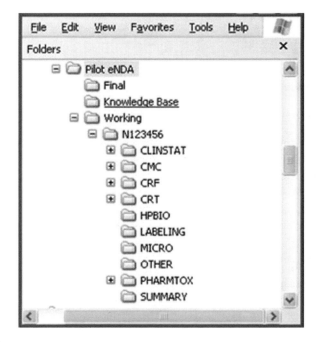

FIGURE 11.3
A recommended directory structure configuration when working with file servers.

in the Working area, they will be copied to their designated folder under the Final folder structure.

11.5.3.7.3 *Knowledge Base (Folder)*

This folder is typically used to share information related to the submission project. In addition, it may hold a Checklist, meeting agendas and minutes, and other relevant documents. A Guidance subfolder will contain necessary guidance documents from the Agency to provide the relevant and up-to-date reference information to the team members.

11.5.3.8 Security

Security is based on the roles and responsibilities defined by the project team. The IT representative is responsible for assigning appropriate privileges to team members in coordination with the Team Leader and Systems Administrator. Also, the IT representative is responsible for managing the backup of the project area on a regular basis, based on the Standard of Operations (SOP) for Network Security and Backup.

11.5.3.9 Version Control

This is an automatic process for the EDMS; however, for file servers it becomes the responsibility of the team members to maintain the versions throughout the process, following the SOP for version control (defined during the project initiation).

11.6 The Electronic Submission (eSubmission) Process

In order for the publishing process to proceed effectively and smoothly, it is of the utmost importance for the eSubmission team members to possess the knowledge of the basic steps involved in any project. As outlined in Table 11.3, the eSubmission process, in general, involves the following steps:

- Inventory of Submission Items (Checklist)
- Authoring
- Publishing
- Quality Assurance
- Final Compilation
- Submission

Figure 11.4 illustrates a workflow for a typical eSubmission publishing process.

The following scenario outlines the steps for a typical regulatory publishing process:

(Note: this assumes that there is no EDMS or publishing system in place.)

1. Create an eSubmission team.
2. Define roles and responsibilities of the team members.
3. Identify all the tools and technologies to be used in the project and provide appropriate training and technical support for team members.
4. Identify a work flow for the project.
5. Identify a storage location for the project related files.
6. Compile an inventory of all the documents to be submitted and record them in the Checklist.
7. Finalize authoring of each source document and update the Checklist accordingly.
8. Perform quality control and quality assurance (QA/QC) in every step to check and verify the status of documents; update the Checklist.
9. Convert all the documents into regulatory compliant format (e.g., PDF document with appropriate navigational items).
10. Compile individual sections of the submission after all the documents for that section are finalized.

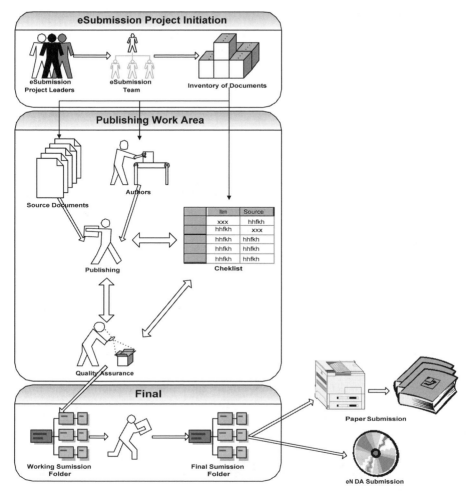

FIGURE 11.4
Illustration of steps involved in a typical eSubmission publishing process.

11. Perform QA/QC to verify the status of documents; update the Checklist.

12. Copy each completed PDF file from the Working folder into the appropriate location in the Final folder.

13. Apply the external hyperlinks and bookmarks and combine all of the completed sections to form the entire submission.

14. Perform QA/QC to verify the status of documents and the associated navigational items; update the Checklist.

15. Apply the finishing touch-ups (e.g., common bookmarks, DIFs, pagination, etc.) to finalize the submission items; update the Checklist.

16. Create indexes for required sections (if any).

17. Create the submission media (e.g., CDs, tape, etc.).

18. Perform the final QA/QC on the submission media to verify the status of submission items and their navigational items.

19. Print from finalized documents for paper submission and perform a QC (if paper submission is required).

20. Ship the submission media to the appropriate regulatory division.

11.6.1 Process Checklist

One of the most critical tools for managing an eSubmission project is a checklist in which all the steps in the process have been clearly delineated. This checklist will provide an opportunity to compile an inventory of submission Items and their corresponding documents that are planned for submission to the Agency. Besides listing each Item, the Checklist will identify its owner and status at any point along the submission process, as shown in Figure 11.5.

The Checklist plays an especially important role in managing the publishing stage. The success of a project will depend on careful and timely maintenance and usage of its Checklist. A typical Checklist can be a spreadsheet created using appropriate components for a specific submission type, based on the granularity defined by the guidance and specifications documents for that submission type.

During the initial meetings the team members should identify and build a list of all the source documents. The list is categorized based on the appropriate FDA form for that submission (e.g., 356h for NDA/BLA/

	A	B	C	D	E	F
1	Item #	Item	Team Leader	Target Date	Submission Date	Comments
2						
3		Submission to FDA		Overall status of the submission by Item		
4	1	Table of contents (Index)				
5	2	Labeling				
6	3	Summary				
7	4	CMC				
8	5	PharmTOX				
9	6	HP/BIO				
10	7	Microbiology				
11	8	Clinical				
12	9	Safety Update				
13	10	Statistical				
14	11	CRT				
15	12	CRF				
16	13	Patent information				
17	14	Patent certification				
18	15	Establishment description				
19	16	Debarment certification				
20	17	Field copy certification				
21	18	User fee cover sheet				
22	19	Financial disclosure				
23	20	Others				

FIGURE 11.5
Item level eSubmission process checklist.

	A	B	C	D	E	F	G	H	I	J
1	Item	Index	eSUB Location	Author	Responsibility	Notes / Status	Source Name	Location of Information J:\eSUB\Working\97-01	Source Format (elec/paper)	Source QA
2		RoadMap	roadmap.pdf				roadmap.doc		electronic	
3		Form 356H	B000000.001\356h.pdf				356h.pdf		Paper	
4		Cover Letter	B000000.001\cover.pdf				cover.doc		Paper/electronic	
5	1	NDA/BLA Table of Contents	B000000.001\blatoc.pdf				NDA/BLATOC.doc		electronic	
6	1	Table of contents (Index)	main folder							
7	2	Labeling	labeling							
8		I. Labeling history	Labeling/history.pdf							
9		II. Labeling text								
10		a. Proposed labeling text	Labeling/proposed.pdf							
11		b. Currently used labeling text	Labeling/current.pdf							
12		c. Last approved labeling text	Labeling/approved							
13		III. Final printed package insert	Labeling/pi.pdf							
14		IV. Carton label	Labeling/carton.pdf							
15		V. Container label	Labeling/contain.pdf							
16	3	Summary	summary							
17	4	Chemistry	cmc							
18		I. Drug Substance	Cmc/substan.pdf							
19		II. Drug Product	Cmc/product.pdf							
20		III. Investigational Formulations	Cmc/invest.pdf							
21		IV. Environmental Assessment	Cmc/environ.pdf							
22		V. Methods Validation	Cmc/methval.pdf							
23		VI. Batch Records	Cmc/batch							
24		rt105	Cmc/batch/rt105.pdf							
25		rt106	Cmc/batchrt106.pdf							
26		VII. Publications	n/a							
27	5	Nonclinical pharmacology and toxicology section	pharmtox							
28		I. Summary	Pharmtox/pharmsum.pdf							
29		II. Pharmacology studies	Pharmtox/pharm							

FIGURE 11.6
Document level publishing process checklist.

ANDA, 1571 for IND, etc.). Each document is logged under the appropriate section and under the designated item, and their status will be updated along the entire publishing process. Once the inventory of all source documents is completed, team members will be assigned at the document level. A sample document-level publishing process Checklist is shown in Figure 11.6. The Project Leader and the Team Leaders should constantly update the Checklist to monitor the status of the Items and individual documents, and the progress of the project.

11.6.2   Authoring

The essential components of any regulatory submission are the documents with which the submission is built. These documents are created in various departments in the sponsor company and may come from different collaborating partners, CROs and other consultants. Therefore, it is of utmost importance for an organization to acquire a set of standard tools that will guide and assist those involved in authoring of documents for the life cycle of a drug product. In addition to word processing software, which is a basic requirement, the following are essential elements for any authoring project:

- Standard style and format guides
- General and specific templates —internal (e.g., study protocols, amendments)

- Specific templates based on FDA or ICH requirements (e.g., clinical study reports)

The standard Style and Format Guides will assure that the final documents have all the attributes required for creating automatic TOC, bookmarks, links, and references based on the defined Heading and TOC styles. This will also become extremely useful when converting the documents to PDF format by transferring the above navigational aids.

Another important tool is development of templates for internal purposes or for submission purposes. Both FDA and ICH have developed a number of guidelines and specification documents regarding the specific items to be included for different sections of a submission (e.g., clinical study report template, etc.). Following these specifications during the creation of the documents will assure conformance to the Agency requirements and will eliminate any delays or confusion.

11.6.3   Publishing

The Publishing Process, a subset of eSubmission Process, can involve the following steps when working in a traditional File Server setup. These steps show the most common order of the workflow in the publishing process; however, depending on the circumstance of the project, and policies and priorities of the sponsor company, the orders can be altered, combined, deleted, or new steps added.

- Scanning
- PDF Conversion
- Bookmarking/Linking
- Document Information Fields
- Pagination
- Item Level Compilation
- Optimization
- Quality Assurance
- Full-Text Indexing

11.6.3.1   Scanning

Occasionally, the source format for a set of documents that should be provided to the Agency with a submission is paper only. This could be the case for reference publications, case report forms (CRFs), study protocols and amendments, documents related to chemistry, and manufacturing and controls (CMC), etc. Although scanning is generally discouraged by the Agency, in some cases it is inevitable. In those cases, the original paper documents should be scanned into PDF, bookmarked, and linked based on the guidelines provided by the Agency. This will ensure compliance with the readability, file size, navigational aids, and other requirements outlined in the guidance documents.

Scanning can be performed and PDF files can be created directly using Acrobat or any other custom software. Some of the more sophisticated scanning tools provide additional capabilities for bookmarking/linking via Optical Character Recognition (OCR) and for Process Automation, albeit at a cost.

11.6.3.2   PDF Conversion

The regulatory agencies accept PDF as the format for the transmission of submission files, thus all source documents, regardless of their original format (e.g., electronic, web page, paper, image, etc.) should be converted to PDF before their inclusion in the submission. Acrobat provides two different conversion methods (utilities): PDFWriter and Acrobat Distiller. In general, PDFWriter converts files more quickly and is recommended for simple text-only documents. On the other hand, Distiller allows for more control over the process and provides higher quality output and is recommended for documents containing text, figures, and color images.

PDF files can be created from virtually any application by using Acrobat, or similar software. Generally, in office productivity suites, the PDFMaker macro will be available after the installation of the Acrobat, and can be used for PDF conversion in those applications.

11.6.3.3   Bookmarking/Linking

As outlined by the general guidelines of the Agency, each PDF document should contain appropriate bookmarks and links to improve the navigation through the documents and the submission as a whole. As noted in the Authoring section, following an appropriate style and formats guide for creation of the original electronic documents will ensure that the majority of these navigational items get created automatically during the PDF conversion stage. There are multitudes of Acrobat plug-ins tools that will automate the creation of these navigational items (e.g., common bookmarks, pagination, CRFs, TOCs, etc.). It should be noted that no additional plug-in tools should be required for the reviewer at the Agency to be able to navigate the documents.

11.6.3.4   Document Information Fields

The Agency requires that the document information fields (DIFs) for every single PDF file be completed with proper information. Before creating the final indexes for different Items in the submission, the DIFs for individual files should be checked to ensure proper indexing and referencing. Reference should be made to individual Items sections in a submission for detailed description, instructions, and some examples on the information for completing DIFs.

11.6.3.5   Pagination

All the PDF documents should be appropriately paginated for proper navigation. Occasionally, the Agency may request some of Items or the entire submission in both electronic and paper format. Therefore, it is strongly recommended that the pagination of the electronic documents should be such that printing them will produce an equivalent or identical paper submission. Including Volume and Page number is a typical format used in such scenarios, with each volume containing about 300 to 400 pages. General guidelines should be consulted for more detailed pagination specifications.

11.6.3.6   Document Level Quality Control

After each PDF document is finalized in the Working folder, the following quality control items should be performed to ensure its integrity and compliance with the Agency requirements:

- Document Information Fields are complete and accurate.
- Thumbnails are created.
- The file size does not exceed the permitted limit.
- Table of contents reflects the style and format guides.
- Links and bookmarks are created for required items in the document.
- Magnification Option for all bookmarks and links is set to Inherit Zoom.
- Destination for every (internal) link and bookmark is set properly.
- Links and bookmarks associated with an action are correctly performed.
- Attributes of links are in accordance with the Agency's guidelines (e.g., CBER vs. CDER).
- No security level has been applied to the documents.

11.6.3.7   Compilation

The following steps are recommended for compiling the components of an electronic submission:

11.6.3.7.1   Item Level Compilation

As the files and their contents, including TOCs, are finalized for an individual Item in the Working folder, they should be copied into the similarly named folder(s) in the Final directory. This will allow the submission team members to perform quality control and take additional steps (e.g., full-text indexing, common bookmarking, QC, etc.) towards the final preparation. These steps are described later in this section.

11.6.3.7.2 *Finalizing Item and Overall Table of Contents Links and Bookmarks*

Once all of the files are copied into the Final submission folder, the external links and bookmarks in the Item TOC, as well as overall TOC should be created for those missing and the existing ones should be verified for accuracy.

11.6.3.7.3 *Common Bookmarks*

To facilitate the navigation and review process in a submission, the Agency encourages creating additional bookmarks in every document to direct the reviewer to the Item TOC (e.g., CMCTOC, CLINTOC, etc.), overall TOC (e.g., NDTOC, BLATOC, etc.), and to the Roadmap (for CBER submissions only).

11.6.3.8 **Creating Full-Text Indexes**

A full-text index is a searchable database of all the text in a document or set of documents. Depending on their versions, either the Acrobat or Acrobat Catalog can be used to create a full-text index of the PDF documents or document collections. Follow the general guidelines for creating indexes for each individual Item.

11.6.3.9 **Optimization**

The PDF documents go through several publishing steps before becoming final. The size of the files may increase due to the way they were saved. Optimization allows decreasing the file size to an optimum level, without compressing it. This is especially important when working with Version 4 of Adobe Acrobat. Therefore, it is a good practice to optimize the PDF files before sending them out either to the Agency or to other users. Along with optimization, the options for Creating Thumbnails, and File Open can be selected on a library of PDF files at the same time.

11.6.4 **Scanning for Viruses**

Normally, all networked computers have some sort of virus-scanning software installed in them that is periodically updated by the IT division. Regardless, after all the files in the Working directory are finalized and are copied to the Final directory, it is a good habit to perform a virus check to ensure that the files submitted to the regulatory Agency are clean.

11.6.5 **Overall Quality Assurance**

Although initial QC is required in every step of the publishing process, as instructed by the process checklist, a thorough review should be performed to ascertain the validity and correctness of the submission documents, and their various properties. Specifically, it should be verified that:

- Document Information Fields are complete and accurate.
- Thumbnails are created.
- Full-Text indexes have been created for all the required folders.
- The file sizes do not exceed the permitted limit.
- Common bookmarks are present both on the Item and the Submission levels.
- Magnification Option for all Bookmarks and Links is set to Inherit Zoom.
- Destination for every link and bookmark is set properly.
- Links and bookmarks associated with an action is correctly performed.
- Attributes of links are in accordance with the Agency's guidelines (e.g., CBER vs. CDER).
- For external links and bookmarks, the destination path is correct and there is no reference to a network drive (i.e., absolute path).
- No security level has been applied to the documents.

11.6.6   Creating Submission Media and Final QC

After checking all of the items in the above checklist, depending on the size of the submission, a CD(s) or a tape containing all the submission documents should be created. Any commercially available application can be used for creating the submission media. If more than one CD is used, they should be named properly and sequentially (e.g., CD-001, CD-002, etc.). Also the submission number (e.g., N123456 for NDA) should be used for the media (e.g., CD-ROM) title. Once the media is created, a final QC should be performed, preferably on a PC that is not connected to the network, to ensure that the media is functioning correctly, the reviewer can access all of the files, and there is no reference to the network drive for bookmarks and links.

After testing the validity and the integrity of the media it should be sent to the appropriate division in the Agency for review. It is important to include the FDA contact name with the package.

11.7   Electronic Submissions

As the drug development industry and the regulatory agencies advance towards a complete electronic submission frontier, new regulations and technologies are utilized to expedite the process of publishing, review, and approval of marketing/licensing applications.

Currently FDA divisions accept, or plan to accept, the submission types discussed in the following sections. They present only a summary of the guidelines and specification applicable to these submissions. The reader is strongly encouraged to consult the FDA guidance documents specific to each submission type.

11.7.1   eIND

CBER published the industry guidance document for eIND in February 2002 (see footnote 6). The FDA intends to update guidance on electronic submissions regularly to reflect the evolving nature of the technology and the experience of those using this technology. As Agency develops guidance on electronic IND submissions in the Common Technical Document (CTD) format, they intend to harmonize current guidance on eIND with the eCTD guidance.

The following sections describe some of the specific features of the eIND submission.

11.7.1.1   eIND Highlights

- Facilitates the submission of INDs in electronic format as well as ensure quick and easy information access for the reviewer.
- Features an IND main folder that is used throughout the life cycle of the application.
- Includes a table of contents (TOC) and bookmark-driven navigational construct that is similar to the structure employed in CBER's electronic marketing application.
- Assigns numeric prefixes to individual PDF file names. The numeric prefix should reflect the amendment number in which the file was submitted for review.
- Facilitates cross-referencing to another IND.
- Features the use of the roadmap.pdf file.

The following are some of the important items to consider while working on a submission. As eIND has specific requirements, it is recommended that the reader refer to eIND guidelines (see footnote 6) for more details.

11.7.1.2   Folder and File Names

Guidance provides specific naming convention for the folders (see Figure 11.7) and subfolders of the submission, TOC files, and the roadmap.

For file names not specifically described, it is recommended that the sponsor use the following naming conventions:

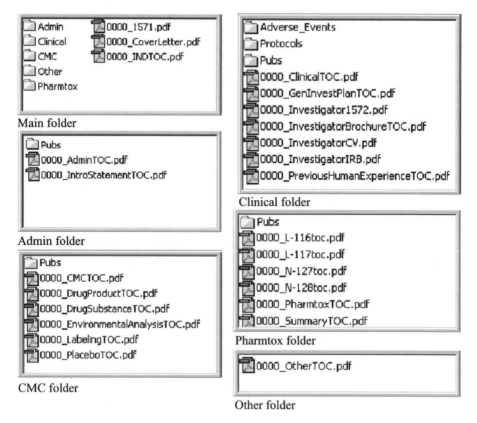

FIGURE 11.7
Naming convention and directory structure for an example eIND.

- Include the submission serial number for the file in the initial 4 numbers of the file.

- Use a descriptive name for the file up to a total of 28 characters. This is a total of 32 characters including the 4-digit serial number.

- Use the appropriate 3-character extension for the file (e.g., pdf, xpt).

- Be consistent with the file names. For example, if the protocol number is used as part of the name of the original protocol, the same name should also be used for the protocol revision. For example, protocol 1234 provided in amendment number six could be named 0006_1234.pdf. The revised protocol submitted as part of amendment 125 would be named 0125_1234.pdf.

11.7.1.3　*Bookmarks and Hypertext Links*

Refer to the common requirements section (11.5.1.1.8) for details on bookmarks and links. In addition, the reader should be aware of these specific instructions:

- For a reference list at the end of a document, provide a hypertext link from the item listed to the appropriate PDF publication file.
- Avoid linking items across submission folders.
- Include a bookmark to the roadmap, the submission's main TOC, and the folder's TOC at the highest level of the bookmark hierarchy for documents that are supplied as part of the submission.

11.7.1.4 Cross References to Other INDs

At times, IND submissions are supported by a cross-reference to another IND [21 CFR 312.23(b)]. The following points should be considered for such cases.

- The utility of the electronic IND submission will be increased if all reference materials are supplied with the IND submission.
- These files should be handled in the same manner as other electronic files submitted to the IND. For example, the files should be generated from electronic source rather than from scanned paper documents if at all possible. If the electronic source file is not available, a scanned copy will be acceptable.
- If an electronic IND or other form of documentation already exists in CBER, and the appropriate letters of authorization are supplied, the IND review team will be granted access to those documents.
- If the files chosen for referencing have been provided in electronic format, include the main folder name in which the document resides in place of the volume number required under 21 CFR 312.23(b).
- Provide copies of the appropriate letters of authorization in the "admin" folder of the submission.

11.7.1.5 Submission Management

Timely communications with the appropriate center and office staff prior to the submission of an electronic document are essential. Remember the following important points:

- Sponsor should notify the FDA in writing of their intent to submit an electronic IND at least three months prior to the target arrival date for the application. Upon receipt and review of the written notification, the Division staff will schedule a teleconference to discuss the proposed electronic dossier.
- Sponsor should submit a CD-ROM, containing mock-up text and data, conveying their interpretation of the guidance for review by Center staff 45 days before the submission target date. *(Note: The*

sponsor or drug team is required to send a demo only once, i.e., no need to provide demo for subsequent submissions.)

• Establish the secure e-mail system

Because the review of an initial IND submission must be completed in 30 days, it is essential that the electronic IND submission functions smoothly. The CD-ROM demonstration is a critical part of ensuring that smooth function. The CD-ROM demonstration should facilitate discussions of the planned regulatory submission through the presentations of mock-up text, tables, graphics, and data to CBER from the sponsor. The CD-ROM demonstration will:

• Present CBER with an opportunity to ensure that documents are presented in a standard format across all electronic IND applications

• Present an opportunity for feedback from the review team on the presentation of regulatory information (e.g., dataset structures, hypertext links, bookmarking, and document quality)

• Present an opportunity for CBER's technical staff to provide feedback on how well the proposed submission structure is consistent with the guidance

11.7.1.6 Application Structure

An IND is a compilation of many small submissions collected over an extended period of time. Frequently, during the review of an IND submission, a reviewer will need to refer to earlier submissions. To help reviewers navigate through the entire application, a directory that includes a list of not only the files for the current submission but all of the previously submitted files should be included with each new submission as well.

This list should be presented in reverse chronological order by submission as part of a PDF file called roadmap.pdf. This file is linked to the submission's main table of contents, which is, in turn, linked to the TOC provided in each subfolder. Figure 11.8 shows a sample roadmap file.

11.7.2 eANDA

This type of submission is used for marketing application approval for generics. The details of the content and format of this application are described in the FDA guidance document Guidance for Industry Providing Regulatory Submissions in Electronic Format — ANDAs in June 2002. The submission process for an eANDA closely follows that of an eNDA, except that it is shorter.

Regulations in 21 CFR 314.94 provide general requirements for submitting ANDAs to CDER. Currently, FDA Form 356h outlines the components required in the submission of an abbreviated new drug application. This

ELECTRONIC ROADMAP: I-CureAll

IND Serial Submission Number	IND Submission Date	Submission Content	CD-ROM Serial Number	Link to TOC
I12345, 0002	05-may-2003	Cover Letter 1571 Table of Contents Protocols (Protocol 1234, amendment 1)	CD-2.01	0002_AmendTOC.pdf
I12345, 0001	05-mar-2003	Cover Letter 1571 Table of Contents Chemistry, Manufacturing, & Controls (amended Drug Product and Drug Substance documents)	CD-1.01	0001_AmendTOC.pdf
ABC Pharma I-CureAll, 0000	05-jan-2003	Cover Letter 1571 Table of Contents Introductory Statement General Investigative Plan Investigator Brochure Protocols Chemistry, Manufacturing, & Controls Pharmacology and Toxicology Previous Human Experience Additional Information	CD-0.01 CD-0.02 CD-0.03	0000_INDTOC.pdf

FIGURE 11.8
An example roadmap for an eIND.

form is available on the Internet at (http://aosweb.psc.dhhs.gov/forms/fdaforms.htm). The following general issues should be considered for the electronic submission of ANDAs.

- **Consistency With New Drug Application (NDA) Guidance** — The FDA has tried to make the guidance for ANDA consistent with the NDA guidance including general issues about refusal to receive or file an application, providing the field copy, electronic signatures, and review aids, if submitted electronically.

- **Archival Copy** — Currently, the Agency accepts the archival copy of an ANDA in an electronic format. If the sponsor decides to provide an ANDA in electronic format, then the entire submission, and all subsequent supplements and amendments, should also be in electronic format. This will reduce confusion and improve review efficiency.

- **Review Copy** — The sponsor is required to submit a review copy of an ANDA in addition to the archival copy. If the archival copy is in electronic format, a separate review copy is not required.

- **Supplements and Amendments** — The recommendations in the guidance apply equally to the original submission, supplements, and amendments to ANDAs.

TABLE 11.6

Items of an ANDA as Described on FDA Form 356h

Item	Description	Folder Name
	Cover letter	ANDA
	Regulatory basis of submission	ANDA
2.	Labeling	Labeling
4.	Chemistry	CMC
6.	Human pharmacokinetics (Bioequivalence)	HPBIO
11.	Case report tabulations	CRT
12.	Case report forms	CRF
14.	Patent certification	Other
16.	Debarment certification	Other
17.	Field copy certification	Other
19.	Financial information	Other
20.	Other	Other

- **Other Considerations:**

  - *Page Numbering:*
    Page numbers should be added to individual documents; pagination across all PDF documents is not necessary.

  - *Indexing PDF Documents:*
    Creating full text indexes for eANDA is not necessary.

  - *Sending in the Electronic Submission To Be Archived:*
    The eANDA archival copy, should be sent to the CDER OGD Document Room (OGDDR).

  - *The Type of Media That Should Be Used:*
    See General Considerations guidance for information on media.

  - *Preparing the Media:*
    See General Considerations guidance for information on preparing the media.

- **Questions on ANDA Electronic Submissions** — Questions regarding the preparation of eANDAs should be directed to the Electronic Submissions Technical Support ESUB@CDER.FDA.GOV.

- **Folders** — All documents and data files for the electronic archival copy should be placed in a main folder using *ANDA* as the folder name. Inside the main folder, there should be six subfolders: *labeling, cmc, hpbio, crt, crf,* and *other.* (See Table 11.6 for the items and folder organization.) Documents and data files that belong to an item should be placed in the assigned subfolder.

- **Cover Letter** — The cover letter should be included per NDA guidance.

- **Basis for the ANDA submission** — The information should be provided for the comparison of the generic drug and the reference-listed drug, conditions for use, active ingredients, and route of administration. This information should be presented in a single PDF file named *regbasis.pdf* and placed in the *ANDA* folder. This document should have a TOC listing each one of the required items listed above. As part of the comprehensive table of contents, bookmarks should be created for each item listed in the TOC.

- **FDA Form 356h** — The FDA Form 356h should be provided as described in the NDA guidance.
- **ANDA Table Of Contents (Index)** — A comprehensive table of contents for the submission, named *andatoc.pdf*, should be created and placed inside the main ANDA folder.

The submission should contain the documents and data files for the appropriate items listed on FDA Form 356h. The detailed information on how to create each item in electronic format is provided in the guidance to industry (see footnote 5). These items include:

- Item 1: Table of Contents
- Item 2: Labeling
- Item 4: Chemistry, Manufacturing, and Controls (CMC)
- Item 6: Human Pharmacokinetics and Bioavailability
- Item 11: Case Report Tabulations (CRTs)
- Item 12: Case Report Forms (CRFs)
- Other Items: Items 14, 16, 17, 19, and 20, if applicable

11.7.3   eNDA

In this section the organization and structure of the submission for an electronic new drug application is discussed. It is strongly recommended that the reader refer to guidance document for detailed information.

11.7.3.1   *Organization*

- All documents and datasets for the electronic archival copy should be placed in a main folder using the NDA number (e.g., N123456) as the folder name. (The NDA number should be obtained prior to submission.)
- Inside the main folder, all of the documents and datasets should be organized by the NDA Items as described on page 2 of FDA Form 356h.
- Each Item has an assigned subfolder where documents and datasets belonging to the Item are placed. See Table 11.7 below for the Items and Folder organization and naming convention.

TABLE 11.7

Items of an NDA as Described in Form FDA 356h

Item	Description	Folder Name
1.	Table of contents (Index)	Main folder
2.	Labeling	Labeling
3.	Summary	Summary
4.	Chemistry section	CMC
5.	Nonclinical pharmacology and toxicology section	PharmTox
6.	Human pharmacology and bioavailability/bioequivalence section	HPBIO
7.	Clinical microbiology section	Micro
8.	Clinical section	Clinstat
9.	Safety update report	Update
10.	Statistical section	Clinstat
11.	Case report tabulations	CRT
12.	Case report forms	CRF
13.	Patent information	Other
14.	Patent certification	Other
15.	Establishment description	Other
16.	Debarment certification	Other
17.	Field copy certification	Other
18.	User fee cover sheet	Other
19.	Financial disclosure information	Other
20.	Other	Other

11.7.3.2　*Folder Structure*

Figure 11.9, shows the Main folder and subfolders of an example eNDA submission, N123456, and its contents.

11.7.3.3　*Comprehensive Table of Contents*

Regulations at 314.50(b) require a "comprehensive index by volume number and page number ..." The comprehensive table of contents, hypertext links, and bookmarks in the electronic version play the same role as the comprehensive index by volume number and page number required in the paper copy. Bookmarks and hypertext links are essential for efficient navigation through an electronic submission. For electronic submissions, the comprehensive table of contents contains three levels of detail and the appropriate hypertext links and bookmarks. (Note: CDER may refuse to file a submission that does not contain a comprehensive table of contents with hypertext links and bookmarks.) The first level of detail simply lists the items in the NDA as shown on page 2 of FDA Form 356h. Figure 11.10 presents a sample table of contents for the NDA/eNDA.

11.7.3.4　*Required Files/Folders*

- This main table of contents should be a single page and should be provided as a single PDF file. The file containing the TOC for the

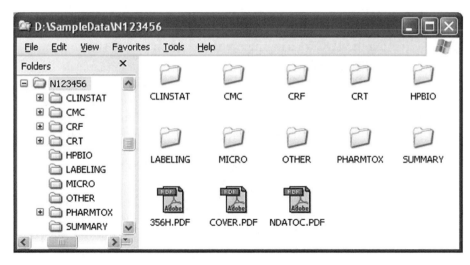

FIGURE 11.9
A sample eNDA directory structure.

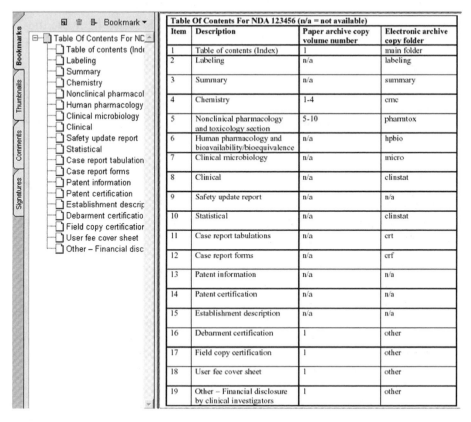

Table Of Contents For NDA 123456 (n/a = not available)			
Item	Description	Paper archive copy volume number	Electronic archive copy folder
1	Table of contents (Index)	1	main folder
2	Labeling	n/a	labeling
3	Summary	n/a	summary
4	Chemistry	1-4	cmc
5	Nonclinical pharmacology and toxicology section	5-10	pharmtox
6	Human pharmacology and bioavailability/bioequivalence	n/a	hpbio
7	Clinical microbiology	n/a	micro
8	Clinical	n/a	clinstat
9	Safety update report	n/a	n/a
10	Statistical	n/a	clinstat
11	Case report tabulations	n/a	crt
12	Case report forms	n/a	crf
13	Patent information	n/a	n/a
14	Patent certification	n/a	n/a
15	Establishment description	n/a	n/a
16	Debarment certification	1	other
17	Field copy certification	1	other
18	User fee cover sheet	1	other
19	Other – Financial disclosure by clinical investigators	1	other

FIGURE 11.10
A sample NDA/eNDA table of contents.

original NDA should be named ndatoc.pdf. The file containing the TOC for an amendment should be named amendtoc.pdf and the file containing the TOC for a supplement should be named suppltoc.pdf.

- The second level of detail contains a TOC for each Item (e.g., labeling, CMC, CRT, etc.). Provide the appropriate bookmarks and hyperlinks for each document or dataset listed to the appropriate file.

- The third level of detail is the TOC for each document or dataset. For each document, provide bookmarks for each entry in the document's table of contents to the appropriate location. For datasets, provide a data definition table (*define.pdf*) as a key to the elements being used in the datasets.

- In cases where a portion of the archival copy is in paper and a portion is in electronic format, the volume number for the paper portion should be indicated. Also, the electronic portion should be placed in the appropriate folder and listed in the table of contents.

- Generally, the paper copies for Items 13 through 20 are in volume 1, and the electronic copies are in a folder named Other. The TOC shows the entire submission including the paper and the electronic portions.

- A hypertext link should be provided from the first-level TOC to the corresponding TOC for each Item. These links are essential for establishing a comprehensive table of contents for the electronic submission.

- Some items, such as Item 3 (Summary) and Items 13 to 19, are single documents and do not have their own table of contents. In such cases, the hypertext link from the first level table of contents should go directly to the document.

11.7.4   eBLA

The Directory Structure and the Contents of the eBLA is almost identical to the eNDA, as it follows the items listed in the FDA Form 356h, except for the following:

- eBLA requires the ROADMAP.pdf, similar to that described in eIND. It includes the life-cycle of the submission, in a reverse chronological order. (See Figure 11.8 above for illustration.)

- According to the eBLA guidance[4] "For electronic submissions, Item 8 and Item 10 are identical. Documents describing statistical methods should be included in Item 8. Therefore, for this Item, you only need to link the submission TOC to the CLINTOC.pdf."

  Authors' Note: Based on experience, In this Item CBER requires more statistical information, such as Analysis Datasets, SAS programs, etc. It is highly recommended that the sponsor communicate with the division representatives prior to sending the submission.

- For the eNDA, the Item 10, Statistical, is identical to Item 8, Clinical, for the content of submission dossier. For the eBLA, the Item 10 requires different content than Item 8. For example, the statistical/ SAS programs, Data Listings, and other relevant materials are required in this Item, for eBLA submissions.
- Item 7 Microbiology does not apply to CBER submissions.
- Sponsor should submit a demo CD-ROM containing mock-up text and data, conveying their interpretation of the guidance for review by Center staff prior (six months recommended) to submission target date. *Authors' Note: The sponsor or the drug team is required to send a demo only once (i.e., no need to provide demo for subsequent submissions).*

The reader is strongly encouraged to consult the appropriate guidance documents (see footnotes 2 and 4) for details.

11.7.5   eCTD

The Electronic Common Technical Document (eCTD)[40] is the Electronic Delivery Structure of the CTD and defines the creation and transfer of eSubmissions from industry to regulatory agencies.

The specification for the eCTD is based upon content defined within the Common Technical Document (CTD) issued by the International Committee for Harmonization (ICH) M4 EWG. The CTD describes the organization of modules, sections, and documents that focus on the authoring process. The structure and level of detail specified in the CTD has been used as the basis for defining the eCTD structure and content. Additional details have been incorporated into the eCTD specification.

The contents of the eCTD are:

- Documents (mainly PDF, regional file formats)
- XML backbone (replaces CTD TOC) — viewable through Web browsers
  - CTD XML file
  - Regional XML file(s)
  - Document Type Definitions (DTD) for common and regional modules

ICH M2 EWG provides specifications regarding:

- Document-type definitions (DTD)

---

[40] International Conference On Harmonisation Of Technical Requirements For Registration Of Pharmaceuticals For Human Use ICH Harmonised Tripartite Guideline — Organisation of the Common Technical Document for the Registration of Pharmaceuticals for Human Use, M4, November 8, 2000, http://www.ich.org/ICH5C.html#organisation

- Change management
- Procedures and specifications on modules

11.7.5.1   Why eCTD?

The capability to provide regulatory submissions written in the CTD format to multiple regions simultaneously is given by eCTD, thus eliminating preparing multiple dossiers for each region. Also, eCTD both eliminates paper and allows more control on managing the workflow dynamics within multiple dossiers.

- CTD limitations:
  - The CTD does not cover the full submission. It describes only Modules 2 to 5.
  - The CTD does not describe the content of Module 1.
  - The CTD does not cover details related to amendments or variations to the initial application.
- eCTD advantages:
  - eCTD specifications produced by the M2 Expert Working Group are applicable to all modules.
  - eCTD covers the entire lifecycle of a product.
- Initial applications.
- Subsequent amendments, supplements, and variations.

11.7.5.2   Process

The process of publishing for an eCTD remains the same across submission formats. Although there are some structure and compilation tasks that vary among submission formats, on the whole the majority of the content still requires PDF with navigational features. The only major difference in eCTD compared to other formats of submission is the introduction of the XML file.

Depending upon the format of the submission selected, the following examples, shown in Table 11.8, may apply.

TABLE 11.8

Comparison of Table of Contents Requirements in Different Submissions

Submission Format	Specific Requirements	Contents	Data
eNDA	TOC in PDF	PDF	SAS® v5 transport file
eBLA	TOC in PDF & Roadmap	PDF	SAS® v5 transport file
eIND	TOC in PDF & Roadmap	PDF	SAS® v5 transport file
eCTD	TOC in XML	PDF	SAS® v5 transport file (may be XML in future)

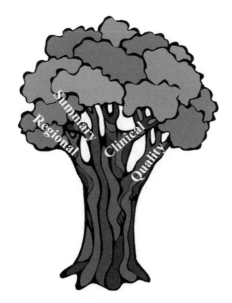

FIGURE 11.11
A tree analogy of eCTD XML backbone.

11.7.5.3 XML Backbone

The XML backbone is the TOC of an eCTD submission. It holds more information about documents than a typical Paper (e.g., NDA, CTD) or an Electronic Table of Contents (e.g., eNDA, eBLA). Often this backbone is explained using a *tree* analogy, as shown in Figure 11.11.

- The backbone is like a tree trunk
  - supported by Web browsers
- Sections or modules are branches, e.g., Module 3 (Quality)
- Documents are the leaves, e.g., List of Manufacturers

Since the eCTD is very granular in format and structure, it is anticipated that the quantity of the guidelines and specifications will continue to increase as additional refinements and innovations are made, either by the regulatory authorities, sponsors, or commercial suppliers. It is recommended that the reader frequently visit the Web sites mentioned in the References section of this chapter to obtain the latest information.

[*Note:* While this manuscript was under review, in August 2003 the FDA released a series of new regional guidance documents in which it officially announced that the FDA will accept eCTD submissions for new product applications. The reader can access these documents via the following website: http://www.fda.gov/cder/regulatory/ersr/ectd.htm.]

11.8 Summary

The FDA had long set the goal of streamlining and expediting the process for drug review and approval. Among the concepts that the FDA explored for achieving their goal was that of switching from paper to electronic media as the format for submitting marketing applications. This proved to be one of the most crucial undertakings in the FDA's strategy.

During the past couple of decades, several events including the introduction of PDUFA, FDAMA, Electronic Records; Electronic Signatures Acts, along with publishing of multiple guidance documents on electronic submissions helped shape and evolve the current process for electronic submissions. This process is a dynamic one and it is still in its evolving stages. New concepts for streamlining and expediting the drug development process, along with advancing technological tools and the establishment of new regulations and requirements are among a variety of factors that contribute to the evolution of this fast changing field.

Throughout the years, the process of regulatory submission has evolved, yet its fundamental approach, which is *collect, compile and submit*, still applies. The implementation of the electronic submission does not change the overall contents of the submissions; it only impacts the submission media (i.e., from paper to electronic). While the directory structure, file naming conventions, and *XML* backbone (for eCTD) are points of variation for different types of submissions, the core and the common denominator for all the electronic submissions is the PDF technology, and it will remain so for a foreseeable future. Hence, the process and the tools used to create the regulatory compliant PDF files are paramount.

In implementing a solution for electronic submissions, one should consider a system that not only satisfies today's needs, but is flexible enough to integrate new technologies and requirements, as they become available, for the needs of tomorrow as well.

Acknowledgments

The authors would like to acknowledge the contribution of many colleagues at Datafarm and individuals that, through their meticulous reviews, critiques, and advice, made possible the creation and publishing of this manuscript. The authors especially acknowledge Yolanda Hall, Sharyu Shah, and Frank Cerone for their many insightful suggestions and discussions during the preparation of this chapter.

Finally, the authors would like to acknowledge their families for their patience, understanding and encouragement received during this period.

12

The Practice of Regulatory Affairs

David S. Mantus

CONTENTS

12.1 Introduction

There are numerous texts (including this one), journals, Websites, conferences, and professional societies devoted to the regulation of drugs, biolog-

1-58716-007-2/04/$0.00+$1.50
© 2004 by CRC Press LLC

ics, and devices and interpretations thereof, but very few writings that speak generally to survival and success in the profession of regulatory affairs. While there are several academic centers providing graduate and certificate training in regulatory affairs, these too focus on the hardware of the matter: the laws, regulations, science, technology, and ethics of product development/marketing/regulation. What's missing? The real "fun" stuff consists of those unseen connections between all of these spheres and the balancing act of the persons who manage the connections. It's fine to know all the laws and regulations by heart (I don't, not even the regulations most applicable to my area!), but what really counts is an ability to interpret and connect, and to adapt this ability based on circumstances. This is what separates *regulation* professionals from *regulatory* professionals. This chapter is an attempt (albeit limited by scope and the author's expertise) to discuss the practice of regulatory affairs — the fundamental tools of the trade, without resorting to specific products or classes of products. The chapter is organized in a way that moves us from the most general of concepts toward the most practical. We need to start figuring out what is actually meant by regulatory affairs, then work from basics like education and attitude, through communications and documentation, and finally end with submissions.

12.2   What is "Regulatory Affairs"?

Before you can discuss the practice of regulatory affairs, you have to be sure you can define "regulatory affairs." Too often we define RA by our own limited experience — what it does at our company, in our industry, etc. To broadly define it, consider every interaction a company can have with a regulatory authority, be that authority national, state/provincial, or local. Then consider every internal department or individual that might need something from, or need to provide something to, a regulatory authority. Then consider the entire life cycle of a product, from conception to marketing (and eventual removal) and every type of product that is regulated. Consider the regulatory affairs group to be the ultimate nexus of all of these variables — the conduit between the company and the authority, over all times, for all products. Figure 12.1 is derived from several different slides I've used in lectures to encompass the field of regulatory affairs. It is an imperfect attempt, but gives some sense of scale both across a company and the life cycle of a product. It's important to remember the broad possibilities of experiences when dealing with colleagues from other companies, with unique perspectives, and sometimes narrow views of the field. There are often times when fruitful communication can only be achieved after learning each other's perspectives, and explaining one's own position in the spectrum shown in Figure 12.1.

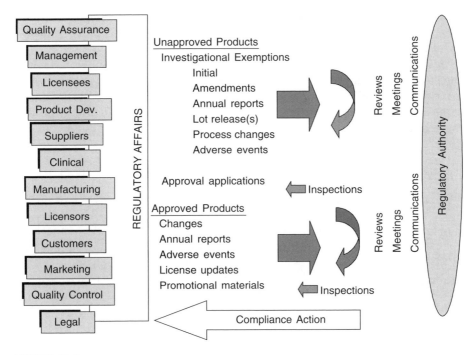

FIGURE 12.1
The spectrum of regulatory affairs.

12.3 Background and Training

12.3.1 Is There a Degree That Matters?

What is the "right" education for a regulatory affairs professional? When I first entered the field there was no "right" answer, and this was one of the reasons I entered the field. It does not require any one technical expertise, but rather the ability to distill multiple technical fields, manage human politics, and write, edit, and collate documents. I have known successful professionals with all manner of degrees (or lack thereof), and I think this diversity is one reason the profession is considered inclusive and has prospered. A trend toward specialization is a bit worrisome — a chemistry degree is not necessary to do Chemistry, Manufacture, and Controls (CMC), nor is a medical degree necessary to edit or write an Investigator's Brochure (IB). One notable trend is the growth of graduate and certificate degree programs that seek to provide "basic training" in regulatory affairs. To their credit, most of the programs provide a diverse training across multiple disciplines, in addition to some practical training across industries/product areas.

The open nature of "required training" should encourage more people to enter the RA field. I also hope the hiring managers and managers who consider existing employees' career development don't limit options due to degrees or specific training. A person whose initial training is in devices can succeed in drugs. A person without an undergraduate degree in science can develop CMC sections of submissions.[1] What matters most is an ability to question concepts and data with a critical eye and the courage to ask these questions.

12.3.2   The Importance of Self-Education

Without sounding too much like a self-help book, the importance of developing oneself can't be overstated. There are a plethora of courses and workshops across a vast spectrum of technical, legal, and regulatory matters available. Take advantage of these opportunities — what can't be applied in the short-term is liable to be useful in the long-term. Such courses also provide a great opportunity for networking. Reading about topics that are less-than-familiar or intimidating is also recommended. While this *sounds* dull as dirt, there are plenty of authors who've been able to write fairly readable nonfiction books about normally very dry topics. Seek such books out even if they are not your typical read — you'll get a good story *and* learn some things that are useful for work. Some examples include the books of John Allen Paulos.[2] These are well written tours through the world of mathematics, with few scary formulas and a lot of "back of the envelope" discussions that are useful. Another great book on statistics and decision-making is *Why Not Flip a Coin?* by H. W. Lewis. An easy read and a sometimes scary insight into how decisions are made, especially very important ones that affect millions of lives! These books on specific topics are just examples of the types of reading that one can do in one's own time that both entertain and inform. There are also books about broader topics that can help provide insights useful for regulatory work. Malcolm Gladwell's book *The Tipping Point* is a brilliant study of trends and changes in our society.[3] Mr. Gladwell has written extensively in *The New Yorker* on a wide array of topics, always using a critical analytical eye, always making it interesting, and always educating. His article "The Art of Failure" is a terrific piece on how things fall to pieces.[4] Another book from my personal reading list is *Complications* by Atul Gawande (interestingly, a friend of Gladwell's), a memoir of a surgeon's training. This last book is mentioned not because

---

[1] This is because an RA professional shouldn't be writing CMC material from scratch! They should be a conduit for this information — an editor and a reviewer. Later sections will expand on this method.

[2] Paulos has a webpage at http://www.math.temple.edu/~paulos/. One example from his book *Innumeracy* discusses diagnostics and specificity. It is a fascinatingly simple study and I've gotten a lot of mileage out of it in discussions/presentations.

[3] He has a great website at http://www.gladwell.com/ that includes all of his writings.

[4] *New Yorker*, August 21–28, 2000.

it is a technical reference, but because it provides insight into the world of physicians — the folks who study our products, prescribe them, endorse them, and critique them.

All of these books are presented as examples of the type of reading that can provide self-training that can help with regulatory work — help not only with the technical issues that arise but in the way one needs to think: broadly, critically, with an open mind, unafraid to ask questions and be questioned.

12.4 Attitude and Approach

"No." This is the most common word associated with regulatory affairs, and is even more common if you consider it the origin of "not" in the contraction "don't." As in "Don't do that," "Don't do this," and "Don't even think about that." Add "can't" into the equation and you've summed up regulatory affairs for 99% of the people who work *with* regulatory in product development. While a pervasive perception, it is fundamentally wrong, and the fact that products get approved and marketed is evidence. The perception is based on plenty of valid experiences — almost everyone can recall a regulatory person holding up a copy of the Code of Federal Regulations (CFR) and emoting that the proposed action is "in clear violation of subparagraph 345 of paragraph B of section a, subheading iii, chapter 193."[5] The author can reluctantly confess to having said such a thing (or similar) on more than one occasion. The problem is how frequently such a position is taken, and whether any other options exist in terms of opinion and contribution to a project.

12.4.1 Regulatory as Navigator

One of the most useful analogies for product development (although it can apply to any team moving toward a goal, even if that goal is abstract — such as compliance) is that of a voyage at sea.[6] Think of management (or the board of directors, or investors) as those financing the voyage — providing the ship and supplies with a specific global objective in mind, e.g., getting to Point X by Date Y. The crew of the ship consists of the various functional groups — the folks who really do the work. I'd like to say that Regulatory is the captain, but in the drug, biologic, and device industry this isn't the case. We work in the regulated health care industry, so medical issues (safety and efficacy) are paramount. So imagine Clinical (or Medical) as the captain

---

[5] Please don't look this reference up. I made it up in its entirety and any resemblance to regulations past, present or future is purely coincidental.
[6] I first wrote about this analogy when interviewed in the regulatory affairs column of *Biotechnology* magazine in the fall of 2000. I honestly can't recall the first time I heard of it.

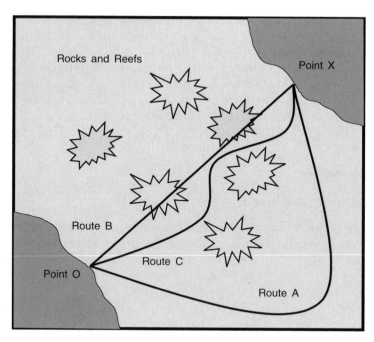

FIGURE 12.2
Getting to there from here (see text).

of the vessel, chartered with the goal stated above. The question remains: how to get from our point of origin (O) to Point X by Date Y? The navigator is usually given the job of determining the specific route to follow, and this is a very good analogy for the job of regulatory affairs. Figure 12.2 provides an overall idea of options in our imaginary scenario, and while poorly drawn, gets the message across. We're at Point O and need to get to Point X. The seas are choppy and filled with rocks and reefs. Route A is the by-the-book pathway — the "no it all" would always defer to this path. Now, in certain circumstances where time and cost are not a limiting factors Route A could be a choice. I have never yet run across such a circumstance. Route B, on the other hand, is a "full speed ahead, damn the torpedoes" sort of approach. This might be analogous to a small, inexperienced company plowing ahead despite good advice from regulatory and/or the regulators. It seems extreme, but it would appear to be more common a path than we'd like to admit. Route C is the compromise. It is a carefully planned journey with well-timed turns, more risk than Route A, but with a good chance of getting to the Point X. All three routes can be considered, and variations in between, in light of the time each takes and a comparison to the goal — Date Y. With sufficient speed (sometimes this translates into resources, but not always), Route A works. Route B covers the shortest distance, but has maximum risk of failure. Route C may require greater speed on certain legs than others to achieve the goal.

This analogy works well in considering the function of regulatory affairs in drug development — laying a strategic and tactical path to the goal. Anyone can plot the safest of courses. It takes skill and experience to plot a course that gets us there in one piece with speed and well-utilized resources. Another analogy that fits stems from a quote I once heard from a building engineer on a large bridge project. I paraphrase, but he said "Anyone can build a bridge strong enough to carry a load. It takes skill to build a bridge *just* strong enough to carry a load." The implication is that the goal is a bridge that is affordable and can be built in time, is aesthetically pleasing, and yet carries the load required. This is just like a regulatory development plan — a plan that fits budgets, timelines, and still meets the approval goals.

12.4.2   Zealotry

Far too often projects, products, and even company cultures become "religions" within an organization. A healthy positive attitude is replaced by a blind belief that success, even perfection, will be obtained. Again, while this seems like an extreme observation, many failures in drug development are rooted in an inability to see the obvious, heed prudent advice, and/or recall that we all must obey the rules. I refer to such an approach as zealotry — and it is borne from good intentions based on a strong desire for success, belief in technology/science, and the pervasive "positive at all cost" attitude of most modern businesses. In regulated product development, it can be a fatal attitude. I'm not advocating cynicism and despair, simply a healthy dose of skepticism, and a reliance on sound data and equally sound advice. Regulatory must often bear the burden of keeping proper perspective. This sometimes makes us easy targets for accusations of "negativism," but in the end a balanced approach is in the interest of the product, the company, and our careers. How do you maintain the balance? Remember that your product is one of many, your company is one of many, and all of us believe we're on *that* project, working at *that* company that just *has* to succeed! Look over our shoulders, and we see plenty of failed companies and products with very good teams in charge who believed the same things.

One of the most important times to maintain a balanced (and nonzealous) perspective is in communications with regulatory authorities, such as the FDA. Another chapter deals with the details of face-to-face meetings, so I will only touch upon the company's attitude in these interactions. The FDA has seen plenty of companies claiming to have the best technology, most dedicated clinicians, and the most brilliant management teams. One or two of them have even gotten products approved. But these approvals came based on data, not because the FDA liked the company or was in awe of their science. Stick to data, logic, and realistic approaches. The FDA will appreciate it and a more humble attitude will improve the probability of a working partnership with the Agency.

12.5   Information

Information is often considered the currency of the 21st century, and in regulatory affairs this has been the case since the earliest days of regulation. Regulatory is the interface between the company/sponsor and the outside world (in terms of regulators/regulatory authorities). As a conduit or a funnel, the regulatory department is a focal point of information, both incoming and outgoing. In order to practice regulatory and succeed, both in objective public measures (e.g., approvals) and internally (e.g., recognition and reward), recognizing the power of information and learning to manage it is critical.

12.5.1   What Information Matters?

Other chapters in this book have shown that there are considerable written resources (e.g., books, regulations) to help guide a regulatory professional. However, there are inherent limitations to this information. Published guidance, public presentations, and weekly industry newsletters cannot convey mood, body language, and subtexts. While there will be certain yes or no answers in these materials, the questions they answer do not require a regulatory person to interpret. Most questions and decisions depend on subtle judgments from regulators, and predicting these judgments, perhaps influencing these judgments, requires a mastery of information gathering and management. So the most valuable information is logically that information which is hardest to get, and is gleaned from informal conversations, emails, etc. Also included is information taken from unlikely sources or difficult-to-find sources. So how does one gather this?

12.5.2   Gathering Information

There should be no need to go over published sources of information, both commercial and governmental.[7] So what are other sources? Any opportunity to see, hear, or talk with a regulator, a more experienced drug development expert, a colleague, or a sworn enemy is an opportunity to gather information. Never be afraid to ask a question, never be afraid to approach a new person who might have information you need, and always be willing to listen. Table 12.1 provides some basic guidelines for information gathering.

So, what do I mean by novel sources or approaches? A simple anecdote relates to a project I worked on involving an older chemical entity for which no prior approval appeared to exist. The Web, the FDA, and Freedom of

---

[7] If you haven't scoured every square inch of www.fda.gov, do so. It is a treasure trove of information. If it didn't update so frequently, a book could be written about it.

TABLE 12.1

Dos and Don'ts of Information Gathering

Do	Don't
Prepare questions ahead of time	Be overly aggressive
Research who you might meet at a conference, dinner, etc. Think about what you might learn!	*As any good reporter will tell you, people prefer to talk to people who make them comfortable in an exchange that appears two-way*
Make small talk	Expect too much
There is nothing wrong with breaking the ice, finding out more about a person than what you need to know	*Regulators in particular know that the information they hold is powerful, and they're not going to tell you that you're approved in the hallway of the Minneapolis convention center*
Look again where other's have	Assume a source has been checked
Rereading or reresearching sources is OK. You may bring new perspective or a new eye for detail to the matter	*"I assumed someone already checked ... " is a very common statement. Never get caught in it*
Look where no one else would	Consider the gathering complete
Think of novel sources. This may be academic, former colleagues, old textbooks, non-FDA government agencies. You have to think of all the ways the information might be important to someone	*You should always be on the look out for new information. Just because the formal process for searching for data ended, doesn't mean you close your eyes*

Information (FOI) had no data on this entity. The assumption was that it was therefore new to the regulatory arena. Then a trip to the library and a review of a >30 year old Physician's Desk Reference (PDR) found the drug — branded and on the market prior to the modern era of regulatory approvals. Included was dosage form information, implied data on pharmacokinetics, etc. This led to a wealth of valuable information to guide the development process and to better inform research on the intellectual property of the compound.

A second anecdote relates to informal conversations with regulators. At a drug development conference recently, a box lunch was provided and served in a large ballroom. Such situations usually lead to people distributing to maximize their distance from new people and populating in clusters of familiar faces. I happened to notice the director of an FDA division that our company would probably begin working with in the next 9 to 12 months. He was in line for a poorly prepared sandwich. What followed was an informal chat over a meal on general topics related to the state of drug development (not enough truly novel chemical entities), improving communications with the industry (more frequent chats and meetings), and how quickly kids grow up nowadays. The company got face-time with the FDA, established how follow-up communications with the division work, and the potential for a collaboration started. My new friend/colleague at the Agency learned about my company, one new industry person's view of drug development, and perhaps a collaborator on a future conference session.

If it sounds simple, it is. But look around and see how few people execute it.

12.5.3 Communicating Information

What one does with information related to regulatory is as important as the information itself. Who do you tell? Who don't you tell? How do you tell it? The easiest information to share and communicate is *noncritical* information. These are findings and data from public presentations and widely available sources that simply need to be put into a logical and relevant form and shared within the organization. What about data you've found from unique sources? Something "dredged up" from an obscure FOI request based on a hunch from a former colleague you met at a conference? I would never suggest hiding these data, but there is no reason to explain openly how it was obtained. Why not keep your regulatory information gathering secrets secret?

The difficult information to communicate is critical information. This could mean anything vital to the success or failure of a project, specific and important feedback from the FDA, subtle insight that weighs heavily on the future of the company, etc. While it would be simple to just shoot an email off to the entire company, it is neither in the company's interest nor your interest to take that approach. The first thing to do is document the information carefully, so you fully understand it, and its implications. Then think of those individuals who are that combination of "need to know" and "know who else needs to know." At small start-ups, this might be the CEO or president. At larger companies, the head of clinical, a project manager, or a similar middle- to senior-level manager fits the bill. Using these first points of contacts allows the information to pass through appropriate channels.

One of the most difficult challenges is passing along negative information —bad news. There is a visceral desire to quickly get such information passed along, so oftentimes this happens carelessly, and winds up feeding rumor mills and moving outward without appropriate management. Table 12.2 provides some hints on handling such information. Don't take this as a cynical approach to regulatory, it is simple realism: just as regulatory is often the recipient of positive approval news, regulatory is the first point of contact when the FDA has to provide negative feedback.

12.6 Documentation

One of the first things one learns in regulatory and compliance is that "if it isn't documented, it wasn't done." Not following this basic principle leads to a huge number of compliance failures, and can also lead to the downfall of critical development projects. Projects in drug, device, and biologics development can take up to 10 years or more to complete and cost tremen-

TABLE 12.2

Hints for Passing Along Negative Information

1. Be accurate. Make sure your information is data-rich. If conversations were involved, quote comments verbatim. Avoid adding your own opinions to the information, supply the facts
2. Think about and research (if necessary) the implications of the "bad news" in terms of resources (costs) and time. You may or may not know the full implication of the information, but if you know a new study costing $500,000 and taking 1 year is the outcome, you might as well share it. It may also be that your first contact — the person you need to tell the information to — is not fully aware of such impacts
3. Consider an informal, first contact. This should be someone you trust implicitly. Practice your conversation, getting all of the nerves and emotions out. Make sure you're sticking to the first hint!
4. NEVER email this stuff. You may not be fully aware of the ramifications of the information, both legally and in terms of internal politics. Email puts the information in written (and therefore documented and available upon discovery) form before you've fully researched all the possible meanings and perhaps, interpretations
5. Do your best to suggest alternate paths for success. Just saying "FDA says no" doesn't help the organization. Look for ways goals can still be met. Even if all you can do is to determine what other resources might be available to help extricate the project or company from the situation, suggest it. How much better will it sound to say "FDA says no, but I'd suggest calling so-and-so at company Z, she's been in this situation before."

dous amounts of money.[8] The time involved can be up to five times longer than the average stay in a regulatory job, depending on location and industry.[9] This means projects need to outlast the people who work on them, and the only way they can do this is to have solid documentation to support them. Document progress, document decisions, document information (see above), document failures, document successes. This need to document is important at large companies where complex dynamics may move a project through the hands of multiple teams, and at small companies, where key decisions may be questioned by advisory boards, investors, potential investors, and potential partners. If you have a well thought-out defense or opinion on a key issue related to the success or failure of the company or its projects, why not write it down so others can look at it, you can share it, and it outlasts you?

12.6.1 The Memo

When I first started nonacademic work at Procter & Gamble, one of the first trainings they provided was in writing a memo. At first I thought it laughable,

---

[8] Every few years Tufts Center for the Study of Drug Development (http://csdd.tufts.edu/) does a survey that says how much and how long a typical drug takes to develop. The 2002 numbers were 7 years (on average) and $900 million. Take these numbers with a few grains of salt — they are based on a limited sample size. At a minimum they give some sense of scale for the biggest and longest projects.

[9] I've been in drug development for 11 years, and am on my fifth job. This seems excessive, but is becoming a more common trend both in biotechnology, and the economy as a whole.

but since then I believe in the power of the memo. It need not be long, it need not be in one specific format, but it should contain the following elements:

- Your name and initials and/or signature
- The recipient's name
- The date
- A subject line
- Text and references (if necessary)

What power is contained in such a document! Who said what to whom, when! It has the power to document decisions which may have taken years to come to, summarize volumes of data, and correct mistakes. This last "action" is critical to understand. We produce smoothly written standard operation procedures (SOPs), master batch production records (MBPRs), clinical protocols, and policies. It is a very common misperception that in order to comply, a company must follow the very letter of all of these standard procedures. The reality is that few, if any, actions take place perfectly in-line with written procedures. More often than not, some level of deviation occurs. The key to deviating *and* complying is to document the deviation. Use a memo! Explain what happened and why those individuals who should know, do not think it's a big deal. It sounds so simple — but read a few warning letters at the FDA web site to get a sense of how infrequently it's done.

12.6.2   Managing Documents

Volumes upon volumes have been written about document management. I seek only to remind the reader that we have to control the writing, dissemination, filing, and archiving of documents in order for them to be useful. By all means I strongly suggest doing so in the most efficient means possible. Clearly, if resources were no object, this would be a fully electronic document control and management system. I will confess that I am a poor manager of documents. Therefore I delegate and depend on others to maintain files. The concept of filing is not beyond me, I am merely poorly disciplined at starting and maintaining filing systems. Table 12.3 provides some useful hints for document management, whether the system is a fully electronic archive or an asbestos-lined fireproof cabinet.

12.6.3   Practical Example: Documenting an FDA Contact

The level of detail and the approach to documenting a contact with a regulatory authority is an ideal example of good documentation practices. It represents one of the most important functions of RA, and should reflect the professionalism and expertise of the person making the record. A generic example follows, and I've tried to add advice and ideas for each section:

RECORD OF CONTACT WITH REGULATORY AGENCY

PRODUCT IDENTIFIER: Product Code or Name			
ORIGINATOR: Your name!		**DATE OF CONTACT:** Date **TIME:** Don't laugh! Multiple calls in one day can get confusing 4 years later.	
IND Number: XX,XXX **NDA Number:** **Other File Number:**	**INITIATED BY:** **TYPE OF CONTACT:**	Company Other Email/Phone/Face-to-face	
CONTACT NAME AND TITLE: Get this right, and get every detail. If specific titles don't come up, look them up! Be sure to know where the person stands in terms of decision-making. Know the organizational chart of the division/group!		**AGENCY:** Other **CENTER:** **DIVISION:** **PHONE:** Get actual phone numbers — not general department numbers! **FAX:** **E-MAIL:**	
SUBJECT: Why did you talk?			

SUMMARY:

Describe in as impersonal a way as possible what transpired. This is not a novel or an attempt at fascinating dialogue. Stick to data. Recording verbatim comments can be incredible powerful. The specific words people choose say a lot about attitude, and this can then be relayed without editorial or subjective filtering by the reporter.

ACTION(S):

1. A clear list of actions deriving from this contact needs to be included.

DISTRIBUTION:

Regulatory File

Be sure to include all appropriate people. Some folks are extra sensitive about being left off the list!

TABLE 12.3

Document Management Ideas

---

1. Redundancy is OK. It is acceptable and even useful to maintain files in duplicate. For example, maintain an IND-specific file, where each submission to FDA is included, along with FDA feedback and supporting documents. At the same time, a chronological file of all FDA contacts can be kept, which includes FDA feedback on an IND submission. In a pinch this redundancy can save you.
2. Use any and all means to keep it simple. Color code, use multiple cabinets, label file folders elaborately. The system has to be able to outlast any one person, without an extensive training required for someone else to use the system.
3. Log files. That is to say, keep a table of contents or an index of what is in a file. This helps immensely in tracking redundancy (No. 1 above) and in keeping a system simple (No. 2 above).

What are the key concepts? Specificity and objectivity. For this type of document, your opinion should not be reflected. Accuracy and getting specific information is most important. This might take work either before or after the call but it allows a reader (and a reader who looks at this either 2,000 miles away or 2 years later) the ability to put the contact in perspective.

12.7 Submissions

Submissions to regulatory authorities are the ultimate "product" created by a regulatory department, and they also, in terms of content, format, and quality, represent the company and product. Often voluminous and spanning multiple technical areas, regulatory submissions are complex documents in every sense — from an editorial, scientific, and paper-management perspective. At the same time, these documents represent the ideal opportunity for a regulatory professional to shine — not just in the quality of the final product but in the way the document is brought together.

12.7.1 Who Writes These Documents, Anyway?

The two extremes to answer this question are both, in my opinion, wrong. At one end of the spectrum are those folks who believe the regulatory department is completely responsible for writing all submissions to regulatory authorities. At the other end are those who believe all that Regulatory does is place a postage stamp on a document written completely by the technical departments. The answer is, of course, somewhere in the middle. I will always believe that the best discussion and presentation of the data comes from those closest to the data. This means the scientists, engineers, and technicians who produce the data, do the experiments, etc. At times, it can be difficult convincing these folks why regulatory submissions need to be a priority. The key to success is recognizing:

1. Submission writing is an iterative process.
2. Submission writing is a back-and-forth process.
3. You need to lower your expectations.

Figure 12.3 illustrates the first two points. Scientists have usually gained expertise at writing scientific documents such as papers, abstracts, even technical reports. They want (and require) guidance as to what specific data need to be in a submission. Regulatory needs to point to specific regulations and guidelines that provide justification for the work, and guidance as to specific content and format. Expectations as to the quality of the work (e.g., print-ready manuscript vs. hand-written notes) and the timing of drafts are

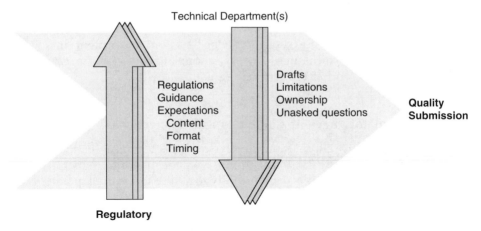

Technical Department(s)

Regulations
Guidance
Expectations
Content
Format
Timing

Drafts
Limitations
Ownership
Unasked questions

**Quality
Submission**

Regulatory

FIGURE 12.3
The process of writing submissions.

very important to resolve and to resolve early. At the same time, the technical counterparts to regulatory have their own responsibilities. They need to hit deadlines, be engaged in the process, and deliver quality work. The easiest way to achieve this is to assure *ownership* of the submission, or parts of the submission. Ownership implies an individual with responsibility and accountability for the section. This person may not do any writing, but is the one who must be sure things are delivered.

As with expectations from regulatory, gaining concurrence on owners of sections and concurrence on their responsibilities is important to establish early, and to communicate upwards through management.

The technical owners of submission writing are also responsible (or should be) for making sure that unasked questions get asked. That is to say, if key data are not requested by regulatory, or an important issue seems to go unaddressed in the document, the technical group has to mention it. The goal of every regulatory person is for this to never happen, but no one is perfect, and the submission needs to be a true collaboration.

The multiple arrows going up and down represent the multiple drafts that need to be exchanged as the process continues. These cycles of review, comment, feedback, and rewrite need to be on strict timetables, and regulatory needs to avoid being on the critical path.

The last concept on the list regarding writing was partially facetious: lowering expectations. What this refers to is reality, the odds are that you are not going to train a technical group to produce "submission-ready" output during the writing process for one submission. The amount of effort this would take leads to diminishing returns when the "polish" on a document can be done within the regulatory affairs group. I've worked with brilliant scientists who write wonderfully, if they were writing for *Nature* or *Science*. Initially I attempted to alter some of their styles when it came to summary paragraphs that sought to raise more questions instead of simply presenting data. I learned that this was just the way they wrote. It was how they knew to write for journals and editorials and one lowly regulatory submission wasn't going to alter that. Instead of focusing on style, I focused on content and data, knowing that the stylistic issues were easy enough to correct in the regulatory edits and reviews, and in the writing regulatory "owned."

12.7.2   Regulatory Review: Continuity and Connections

Most large regulatory submissions involve multiple technical sections which are written by separate technical groups. As the overall "owner" of the submission, it is regulatory's responsibility to assure the overall quality. This can usually be broken down into the concepts of continuity and connectivity.

Earlier it was implied that regulatory should avoid writing a submission — when it comes to continuity, regulatory must take the lead in writing. Sections of the document need to flow into each other, so the document appears at some level to have one voice. This is particularly important when concepts and data from multiple sections are brought together, as in introductory sections, synopses, and summary conclusions. Cut and paste doesn't cut it. The language needs to be fluid, the order of data logical.

Connectivity is a concept that is seldom recognized overtly by the regulatory community, but is in fact one of our most important responsibilities when it comes to submissions. As the owner of a submission, regulatory is really the only "person" who sees the entire document. And the document is not a linearly attached series of sections; it has multiple internal cross references and connections. For example, data on preclinical safety connects to clinical protocols in terms of dose ranges and duration of dosing. This same connection is dependent on CMC data showing that the material used for preclinical safety data is truly supportive of the material intended for use clinically. The connections within even a relatively simple document such as an investigational new drug exemption (IND) are multifold, and may be different from product to product. Who else is going to check and maintain these connections? Regulatory should have this responsibility, and is ideally positioned to manage them.

12.7.3   Presenting Data in Submissions

With the advent of electronic submission production (e.g., Word, Excel, multiple graphics packages) we far too often resort to a quick "cut and paste job" when it comes to presenting data. I would suggest that rather than blindly including graphs and tables of data, it is regulatory's job to look at these data presentations and make sure that the message behind them is clear, and that the presentation is suited to the message. If an upward trend in the data is what you want a reviewer to see, a graph is better than a table, for example. Having a y-axis that has a maximum value of 100, when all your data skirts between 0 and 10 may not make sense (of course, if your message is that the data is all well below some threshold, let's say 30, it might make sense!). Edward Tufte has written several books on the inherent value in how data is presented, and I strongly encourage you to read his books and see his lectures.[10] One of the most important concepts is to make sure the data speaks as loudly as possible, and that it speaks the right message, without being lost in the noise of the presentation. Bold colors and three or four dimensional artwork mean little if a reader cannot grasp the data, or the experiments behind the data. A classic example is when multiple experimental points (e.g., subjects in a clinical trial) are compressed into a small number of data points. The goal was clarity, but the power is lost — a reader may assume only a few experiments (or a small number of subjects) produced the data. The power of the data is thus diminished.

12.7.4   The Art of Handling Large Documents

Never underestimate the difficulty of handling large volumes of paper or even electronic files. The electronic publishing era is maturing (see the separate chapter on this topic) but the concept still holds. One of the key lessons here is to keep sections of large documents separate, until they really need to be together. This "patience with paper" avoids the need to recollate or edit multiple volumes when only a few pages are in need of work. This concept is at odds with another notion — give yourself enough time to go through the mechanics of printing and copying. When you must move ahead and some small sections (I prefer to restrict them to individual pages) are not ready, use place-holders (colored paper works well) so the pages that need last-minute replacement or fixing can be identified.

Never underestimate the value of individuals who support the handling of large documents (be they electronic or paper). All the content in the world is useless if you cannot get 10 copies on a reviewer's desk by Tuesday. Expertise in this area comes from experience. Forget to paginate a document before copying it once, and you'll remember it forever.[11]

12.8   Conclusions

This was a disjointed roller coaster ride through regulatory affairs. While not purposeful, this ride is a perfect microcosm of regulatory affairs: many topics of varying technical detail, connecting the seemingly unrelated, moments of

---

[10] Tufte's website at http://www.edwardtufte.com is almost as good as his books, which are not only educational, but works of art. Get them and read them.
[11] Imagine 3 copies of a document that has to be paginated. Imagine someone (certainly not me!) paginating all 3 copies and the last page of copy one is 340, while copy two ends at 337 and copy three finishes at 341. A lesson never forgotten.

panic, moments of boredom, but never a moment exactly like another. It is this complexity that makes the profession interesting, and it is the position of regulatory at the juncture of so many technical, managerial, and legal disciplines that makes it so vital to the industry. As a profession we need to go beyond documenting regulations and guidelines, and document how we think, why we do things one way or another, and what has worked. This chapter and this book are intended to be a small start in that direction.

13

A Primer of Drug/Device Law, or What's the Law and How Do I Find It?

Josephine C. Babiarz, Esq.

CONTENTS

Working in a "regulated" environment has many connotations, but to those of us in medical products, the "regulators" always include the Food and Drug Administration (FDA) and the Food, Drug and Cosmetic Act. (FDCA). You cannot be "in compliance" with regulations you have never read or laws you cannot find. Hence, this chapter.

1-58716-007-2/04/$0.00+$1.50
© 2004 by CRC Press LLC

In case you're unconvinced, let me give you an example. When a regulation, say the one on Informed Consent at 21 CFR Part 50,[1] requires that a participant sign and date an informed consent form, the FDA really means that the participant sign and date the form. Unless you read the regulation, you may, like a lot of nonregulatory people do, think having the participant sign the form was all you needed — that making the participant date the form was irrelevant or clearly less important. So, some folks — woe to them — might use a date stamp to memorialize when a participant signs. These folks are surprised when an FDA inspector writes up a site report, leading to a 483. After all, didn't the participant sign the form? Yes, but the regulation requires that the participant date the form. This requirement is very clear *if you read the regulation*. However, if you are looking for informed consent at 21 USC, or cannot get the current version of Informed Consent from the CFR, you do not have a chance of finding the regulation, much less reading it. (The pamphlets you pick up at the conferences for free are usually out of date; that's why they are free). Point made.

This chapter will help you know the difference between a law and a regulation and find them. Wherever possible, you will be given Internet addresses. Since these can be out of date quickly, there is also information on search engines to find what you need. You can also find the laws at most public libraries in the U.S. and certain large libraries have copies of the current regulations as well. This chapter will tell you how to do that, too. Once you understand the basics, you will be able to skim this chapter for the specific information you need to succeed.

This chapter is organized under topics, with some preliminary discussion and then a list of frequently asked questions. Intrepid regulator — forge on! You *can* find it!

1. What is a law?
2. Who makes laws?
3. What is the difference between a federal law and a state law? Which one is more important?
4. Where do I find laws?
5. How do I find current laws?
6. What is the difference between the U.S. Code and the Public Laws? How are laws published?
7. What is the difference between the Food, Drug, and Cosmetic Act and the U.S. Code?
8. Why can't I find section 510(k) in the U.S. Code?
9. Are there any state laws that apply to medical products?

---

[1] It is worth noting that the regulation is officially titled "Protection of Human Subjects," but that has not stopped regulatory professionals from identifying it as the "Informal Consent" regulation.

10. Who enforces laws?
11. What is a regulation?
12. What is the difference between a law and a regulation?
13. Which is more important — a law or a regulation?
14. What is the difference between the USC and the CFR?
15. How do I find a current regulation?
16. What is a guidance?
17. What is a "search engine" and how do I use it?

13.1 What Is a Law?

A law is a rule you have to follow. The laws can also be called *statutes*, *public laws*, *acts*, or *codes*. New laws are "enacted" (meaning they are suddenly there and you have to do something about it). Old laws are "repealed" (meaning that they really go away and you do not have to worry about them any more, like prohibition) or "amended" (meaning that they say something a little different now, and you probably need to know what changed).

13.2 Who Makes Laws?

In the U.S., a law is a rule that has been voted by an elected group of people and signed by a president, on the federal level, or a governor, on a state level.

13.3 What is the Difference Between A Federal Law and A State Law? Which One is More Important?

There are two levels of government in the U.S. — federal and state. The U.S. Constitution establishes the three branches of the federal government: the Congress, which passes the laws, the Executive, which enforces the laws and the Judiciary, which interprets the laws and decides conflicts between the branches.

The Constitution recognizes that the states of the union have their own, independent government. The states also have three branches of government, the Legislative, Executive, and Judiciary, which function in the same way as their federal counterparts.

You must comply with all the laws on each level. The Constitution and the courts prevent conflicts between the two levels of government, and each level has its own "turf" so to speak.

In the U.S., because of the Constitution and some early decisions by the U.S. Supreme Court, the federal government is supreme — a state must enforce federal laws and a state may not pass laws that interfere with any federal law. The state law is "preempted" by federal law. A perfect example of preemption is in the enforcement of the FDCA. The federal government, acting through the Congress, established criteria that a new medical device must meet before it can be cleared for marketing and sale. The FDA has developed and issued certain regulations and applications, notably the Pre-Market Approval Application and the regulations at 21 CFR Part 814 Pre-Market Approval of Medical Devices and other related regulations. These federal laws and regulations preempt the ability of the Commonwealth of Massachusetts, to develop its own state-level requirements to market and sell medical devices. So, Massachusetts could not require a medical device manufacturer to prove to the satisfaction of the Massachusetts Secretary of Health that a product under the jurisdiction of the FDCA, say a stent, is safe to use and have a separate Massachusetts license to sell the stent.

The federal law does not do away with all state law requirements, however. Federal law does *not* preempt the ability of Massachusetts to require any company or person doing business in the Commonwealth to register with the Commonwealth, pay a corporate excise tax to the Commonwealth, a property tax to the locality where the business operates, or from collecting sales tax on the sales of any devices in the Commonwealth.

There are times when the federal government actually welcomes state initiatives and works with them. A query on FDA's Website revealed an entire regulation which lists various state laws that the federal FDCA does *not* preempt: 21 CFR Part 808: Exemptions from Federal preemption of State and local medical device requirements. So, if you were going to market a medical device from a particular state, or into a particular state, you may want to know about any state laws that you must still meet before you build and ship.

As an example, let us review those Massachusetts statutes which are exempt from preemption. Quoting from 21 CFR 808.71, the regulation specifies:

> (a) The following Massachusetts medical device requirements are enforceable notwithstanding section 521 of the act because the Food and Drug Administration has exempted them from preemption under section 521(b) of the act: (1) Massachusetts General Laws, Chapter 93, Section 72, to the extent that it requires a hearing test evaluation for a child under the age of 18. (2) Massachusetts General Laws, Chapter 93, Section 74, except as provided in paragraph (6) of the Section, on the condition that, in enforcing this requirement, Massachusetts apply the definition of "used hearing aid" in Sec. 801.420(a)(6) of this chapter. (b) The following Massachusetts medical device requirements are preempted by section 521(a) of the act, and the Food and Drug Administration has denied them exemptions from preemption under section 521(b) of the act. (1) Massa-

chusetts General Laws, Chapter 93, Section 72, except as provided in paragraph (a) of this section. (2) Massachusetts General Laws, Chapter 93, Section 74, to the extent that it requires that the sales receipt contain a statement that State law requires a medical examination and a hearing test evaluation before the sale of a hearing aid.

Well, doesn't that little regulation just explain everything! Don't be too frustrated. Yes, it is not written in plain English, and besides that, the regulation does not tell you what to do. The regulation itself refers to something else, namely a clause in the Massachusetts General Laws, and even then, the regulation does not give you the whole picture, even if you knew what "notwithstanding" meant. But, since you are reading this chapter, you know how to interpret the regulation and where to find those laws, thus making sense of the regulation. Since we are talking about whether additional state requirements must be met before selling a product, your ability to find the right answer will save the company money — because you found out what had to be done on a state *and* federal level.

First, let us translate that pesky regulatory language into the way we speak. When a clause says,[2] "(a) The following Massachusetts medical device requirements are enforceable notwithstanding section 521 of the act because the Food and Drug Administration has exempted them from preemption under section 521(b) of the act," substitute the words "in spite of" for the word "notwithstanding." So, to translate that regulation: (a) The following *state* level, Massachusetts medical device requirements are still good laws that you have to follow, in spite of Section 521 of the *federal* level law called the FDCA.

Ok, so let us see what Section 521 of the FDCA says. It says,[3]

State and Local Requirements Respecting Devices
GENERAL RULE

SEC. 521. [360k][4] (a) Except as provided in subsection (b), no State or political subdivision of a State may establish or continue in effect with respect to a device intended for human use any requirement —

1. which is different from, or in addition to, any requirement applicable under this Act to the device, and

2. which relates to the safety or effectiveness of the device or to any other matter included in a requirement applicable to the device under this Act.

---

[2] 21 CRF 808.71 Ibid.

[3] Food, Drug and Cosmetic Act, Sec. 521 ff, as found via the FDA's Website, at http://www.fda.gov/opacom/laws/fdcact/fdctoc.htm

[4] To find out what the [360k] reference is all about, see the answer to question #7, what is the difference between the Food, Drug and Cosmetic Act, and the US Code.

EXEMPT REQUIREMENTS

(b) Upon application of a State or a political subdivision thereof, the Secretary may, by regulation promulgated after notice and opportunity for an oral hearing, exempt from subsection (a), under such conditions as may be prescribed in such regulation, a requirement of such State or political subdivision applicable to a device intended for human use if —

the requirement is more stringent than a requirement under this Act which would be applicable to the device if an exemption were not in effect under this subsection; or (2)the requirement —

is required by compelling local conditions, and

compliance with the requirement would not cause the device to be in violation of any applicable requirement under this Act.

Ok, so now we know that the Feds have carved out their turf. A state may not continue to enforce a law or pass a new law that is either different from or in addition to, the federal laws governing devices, nor can a state have a law that relates to the safety or the effectiveness of the device or any other device requirement under the FDCA. There are some exceptions — the Secretary of Health and Human Services (at the federal level) can make exceptions to this federal law, if the Secretary decides the state laws are a good idea. For example, an exception can be made if the Secretary decides that the state requirement is more stringent than the federal requirement. Please note that the way this exemption works — the federal secretary must decide to allow the state law to be enforced (exempted from federal pre-emption), and then, the exemption only applies to that specific state. By making this exemption, the FDA does not enforce these state-exemptions across the board.

So, without this provision in the law, there would be no exemption. We can now look at the Massachusetts law to see what that says.

Using Google®, I typed in "Massachusetts General Laws" and was rewarded with several sites. The one I ultimately chose is sponsored by the Massachusetts legislature, but there were a number of free sources I could use. Each of the free sources emphasized that they were not the "official" copy of the laws. If I had a few million dollars riding on the outcome of this law, I would pay up and get an official copy, to be sure there were no pesky little typos in the document. But for most purposes, the online access gets me the answer I need.

In order to understand the FDA's regulation, we must first read the Massachusetts laws that are effected. Those laws are in Chapter 93, Section 72 and Section 74.

By scrolling through the Table of Contents, down to Chapter 93, I learn that it deals with "Regulation of Trade and Certain Enterprises." Section 72 in particular provides:

CHAPTER 93. REGULATION OF TRADE AND CERTAIN ENTERPRISES

Chapter 93: Section 72. Purchases and sales of hearing aids, prerequisites.

Section 72. No person shall enter into a contract for the sale of or sell a hearing aid unless within the preceding six months the prospective purchaser has obtained a medical clearance.

No person shall enter into a contract for the sale of or sell a hearing aid to a person under eighteen years of age unless within the preceding six months the prospective purchaser has obtained an audiological evaluation.

No person except a person eighteen years of age or older whose religious or personal beliefs preclude consultation with a physician may waive the requirement of a medical clearance.

So, in other words, Massachusetts has passed a law that is an additional requirement on the sale of hearing aids, a medical device that is regulated by federal law. This Massachusetts law would be preempted by the federal law, because it is an additional requirement on a medical device that is being sold.
Section 74 of the Mass. General Laws says,

Chapter 93: Section 74. Sales and delivery receipts; copies of medical clearance and hearing evaluation; customer records.

Section 74. Every person who sells a hearing aid shall accompany such sale with a receipt that shall include: the name, address and signature of the purchaser; the date of consummation of the sale; the name and address of the regular place of business and the signature of the seller; the make, model, serial number and purchase price of the hearing aid; a statement whether the hearing aid is new, used or reconditioned; the terms of the sale, including an itemization of the total purchase price, including but not limited to the cost of the hearing aid, the earmold, any batteries or other accessories, and any service costs; a clear and precise statement of any guarantee or trial period; and shall also include the following printed statement in ten point type or larger: "This hearing aid will not restore normal hearing nor will it prevent further hearing loss. The sale of a hearing aid is restricted to those individuals who have obtained a medical evaluation from a licensed physician or otolaryngologist. A fully informed adult whose religious or personal beliefs preclude consultation with a physician may waive the requirement of a medical evaluation. The exercise of such a waiver is not in your best health interest and its use is strongly discouraged. It is also required that a person under the age of eighteen years obtain an evaluation by an audiologist in addition to the medical evaluation before a hearing aid can be sold to such person."

A copy of the medical clearance statement and audiological evaluation, where required, for the hearing aid shall be attached to the receipt.

Upon the date that the purchaser receives the hearing aid, the seller shall provide a delivery receipt signed by the seller and the purchaser which states the date of delivery to the purchaser of the hearing aid.

The seller shall keep records for every customer to whom he renders services or sells a hearing aid including a copy of such receipt, a copy of the medical clearance and the audiological evaluation, a copy of the delivery receipt, a record of services provided, and any correspondence to or from the customer. Such records shall be preserved for at least four years after the date of the last transaction.

So, by applying the language of the regulation to the Massachusetts General Laws, I understand that if I work for a manufacturer of hearing aids, Section 72 of the Mass General Laws is *not* preempted, that it is still valid *to the extent* there has to be a hearing test evaluation for a child under the age of 18 before the sale. In addition, Section 74 is valid *except* for the requirement that the Commonwealth required that the sales receipt for the hearing aid requires a medical examination and a hearing test evaluation prior to the sale of a hearing aid. You need to know both state and federal law, as well as how to read the regulations, if you want to manufacture and sell medical products.

There are other areas where the states regulate activities which impact your ability to comply with federal law. Federal law does not address certain really important things, like how old you need to be before you can sign a contract (or give informed consent), what medical data privacy rights you have apart from HIPAA, or what is the legal test for a defective medical product, say a pill for depression. Legal requirements for disclosures in informed consent are also found on a state level, and FDA's regulations clearly indicate that federal *and* state laws govern the document and process.

In these cases, the federal government adopts the state's definition in enforcing the federal regulation. So, let us say your state says a person can legally sign a contract at 18 years old. Another state says you have to be 21. Even if your company is located in the 18 years state, and you submit your FDA application from your state, and the FDA has reviewed and approved your informed consent form (contract), when you go to a state that says you have to be 21 to sign a contract, you need to have a parent or guardian sign for the 18-year-olds. The FDA does not preempt the local requirement of 21 years. You can have 18-year-olds sign only in a state that allows 18-year-olds to be bound to contracts. You cannot argue that the federal government preempted the age of consent where a state says you have to be 21 years old to be bound to a contract.

In conclusion, there is an interplay between federal and state laws. The correct answer to the question is that you must comply with all laws that apply to your product. Just complying on a federal level, or on a state level, is not enough.

13.4 Where Do I Find Laws?

You can find them in a lot of places, which is why saying the dog chewed your Internet connection or your library is permanently closed due to local budget cuts will not work.

First, if you are going to make a career in medical products, it is worth your while to buy a copy of the relevant FDA-enforced laws. You can buy just the FDA volume, Title 21, from a number of publishers. One is available by credit card from the U.S. Code Service, Lawyer's Edition, Lexus Law Publishing, at 701 East Water Street, Charlottesville, Virginia. This edition contains not only the laws, but also key court cases and the amendment history. You can buy updates each year, which I also recommend.

Why do I think it important to buy the book? Because I find that it saves time and keeps you organized. The Internet gives you access to information in little pieces; it can be very frustrating to use. When you have a text, you can flip easily back and forth between sections, look ahead and behind, and not have to scroll through sections or have pages reload. Additionally, you can write in a book you own, and cover it with little tabs that make you look very prepared when you go to a meeting. Folks think you read it if you have a tab on the page, and that you know what is important. You cannot bring a hard copy of your browser bookmarks to a meeting.

You can also find the laws for free. Most public libraries have copies of the U.S. Code, as well as copies of the laws of the state in which the library is located.

Public libraries keep copies of federal and appropriate state laws in the reference section (the federal laws are usually maroon volumes, organized by numbers; the states can be any color. Massachusetts laws come in either green or black, depending upon the subscription service the library chose). Knowing that libraries keep copies of the state laws (for the state the library is in) can also be very helpful, because not all states have Websites which provide their laws for free. An Internet subscription for a lawyer's service would have these state and local laws, but you might find the services very expensive, and frankly unnecessary, when you can find most things you need on the Web for free, or obtain for a minimal public record copying fee.

You can also find the U.S. laws on the Internet, using Thomas, the U.S. Congressional source for information. Thomas' web address is http://thomas.loc.gov/. A number of law schools have Web sites with useful information, and you can access most of them without paying tuition. One that I like is the Legal Information Institute of Cornell Law School; the Website is www.law.cornell.edu/

There are also Web sites, like Findlaw.com®, that can help you locate the specific law you want. Findlaw® will show you but not allow you access to laws provided by a subscription service.

There is an important trick to finding the laws, and that is to understand the two systems under which the laws are generally organized: the United States code and the Public Laws. The difference between these two is discussed under Section 13.6.

13.5 How Do I Find Current Laws?

It is actually very simple to find the current laws. You must check the publication date, and understand the source's policy for obtaining current laws. Basically, you want to be sure that any source you check is updated, so you are not reading something that is old and may have been amended, or is missing the most recent enactments.

For a book, check the title page, with the date of the copyright. If it is this year's date, it is almost current, except for any laws that have passed since the book was published. For an earlier copyright date, check if there is a back "pocket part." If the book is more than a year old, there should be an update, known as the "pocket part" inserted in the back flap or "pocket" of the book. Because there is an additional cost for the pocket part, and there are recent library budgets cuts, some libraries have cancelled their pocket part subscriptions. But it is always worth a check. You can check for updates using the Public Laws, discussed in Section 13.6.

For Internet resources, you still have to check the publication date. This is not the date of your search, at the bottom of the page you print, but is the real date that tells you when this compilation of laws was last updated. The compilation date tells you that the compilation does *not* include any laws passed after that date. For example, let us look at the U.S. Government Printing Office's Code, available on the web www. access.gpo.gov/congress/cong013.html That Website itself lets you know that certain editions of the Code are current only up to a point — the latest edition available is the 2000 Code, which contains the permanent laws as of January 2, 2001. So, while this edition would contain all of FDAMA (the Food and Drug Administration Modernization Act of 1997), this Code would not contain laws passed since January 2, 2001. Since Congress has been busy all that time passing laws, you need more than this site has to offer.

So, the site also links you to the recent permanent Public Laws, and you can get the latest information there, or through Thomas. In order to get the update to this version of the Code, you need to use the Public Laws. Before you can do that, you must understand the difference between the Public Laws and the Code, which is explained in the answer to Section 13.6.

13.6 What is the Difference between the U.S. Code and the Public Laws? How are Laws Published?

Really and truly, the U.S. Code and the Public Laws are BOTH laws passed by Congress. They are just organized in a different way. The permanent Public Laws are those laws that Congress works on and passes on a daily basis. The Public Laws are referenced by the identity number of the Congress working on them. The Congress in session on July 1, 2003 is the 108th Congress, so all of its laws begin with the numbers 108. For example, it is Public Law 108-020 that provides benefits and other compensation for certain individuals with injuries resulting from administration of smallpox counter-measures, and for other purposes,[5] which was passed in April, 2003. As one of my students phrased it, the Public Laws is like a diary, where each law is recorded on the day it is passed.[6] Congress can pass different laws on the same subject in the same year and in different years, so the only way to find out all the laws passed on a subject using the Public Laws is to read and search all of the laws. This is not particularly efficient, which is why the Library of Congress developed the U.S. Code.

The U.S. Code puts all of the Public Laws passed on any one subject into one big chapter, or Title. The Code not only puts all the Public Laws on one subject together, but also edits them to make sense. Just like you revise a term paper that your professor has corrected. If you are asked to add a footnote, or an explanatory section, you add the footnote where indicated, and the explanation in the area that it belongs. You would not do well to reprint your error-ridden term paper "as is," and then add a chapter entitled, "The Professor thinks I should add this stuff." Same thing with the Code. The librarians made the changes called for in the Public Laws before they published the Code. So, the Code paragraph numbers and section designations (like a, b, and so on) will be different than those in the Public Laws, even though the words are the same.

If that explanation was hard to follow, read on to see how the federal government explains it.

The best answer to this question is found on Thomas, the Website of the U.S. Congress.[7] Here is the inside information:

---

[5] For those of you with an insatiable need to know these things, the number of the Congress changes with each election, not calendar year. So, the 109th will coincide with the next Presidential election in 2004.

[6] Conversation with Afshin Shamooni, graduate student at the Massachusetts College of Pharmacy and Applied Health Sciences.

[7] Thomas, Legislative Information on the Internet; http:thomas.loc.gov/home/lawsmadebysec/publication.html#sliplaws.

How Our Laws Are Made

XIX. PUBLICATION

Slip Laws — Statutes-at-Large — U.S. Code

One of the important steps in the enactment of a valid law is the requirement that it shall be made known to the people who are to be bound by
it. There would be no justice if the state were to hold its people responsible for their conduct before it made known to them the unlawfulness
of such behavior. In practice, our laws are published immediately upon
their enactment so that the public will be aware of them.

If the President approves a bill, or allows it to become law without
signing it, the original enrolled bill is sent from the White House to the
Archivist of the U.S. for publication. If a bill is passed by both Houses
over the objections of the President, the body that last overrides the veto
transmits it. It is then assigned a public law number, and paginated for
the Statutes at Large volume covering that session of Congress. The
public and private law numbers run in sequence starting anew at the
beginning of each Congress and are prefixed for ready identification by
the number of the Congress. For example, the first public law of the 106th
Congress is designated Public Law 106-1 and the first private law of the
106th Congress is designated Private Law 106-1. Subsequent laws of this
Congress also will contain the same prefix designator.

Slip Laws

The first official publication of the statute is in the form generally known
as the "slip law." In this form, each law is published separately as an
unbound pamphlet. The heading indicates the public or private law
number, the date of approval, and the bill number. The heading of a slip
law for a public law also indicates the U.S. Statutes at Large citation. If
the statute has been passed over the veto of the President, or has become
law without the President's signature because he did not return it with
objections, an appropriate statement is inserted instead of the usual no-
tation of approval.

The Office of the Federal Register, National Archives and Records Administration, prepares the slip laws and provides marginal editorial notes
giving the citations to laws mentioned in the text and other explanatory
details. The marginal notes also give the U.S. Code classifications, enabling the reader immediately to determine where the statute will appear
in the Code. Each slip law also includes an informative guide to the
legislative history of the law consisting of the committee report number,
the name of the committee in each House, as well as the date of consid-

eration and passage in each House, with a reference to the Congressional Record by volume, year, and date. A reference to presidential statements relating to the approval of a bill or the veto of a bill when the veto was overridden and the bill becomes law is included in the legislative history as a citation to the Weekly Compilation of Presidential Documents.

Copies of the slip laws are delivered to the document rooms of both Houses where they are available to officials and the public. They may also be obtained by annual subscription or individual purchase from the Government Printing Office and are available in electronic form for computer access. Section 113 of Title 1 of the U.S. Code provides that slip laws are competent evidence in all the federal and state courts, tribunals, and public offices.

Statutes at Large

The U.S. Statutes at Large, prepared by the Office of the Federal Register, National Archives and Records Administration, provide a permanent collection of the laws of each session of Congress in bound volumes. The latest volume containing the laws of the first session of the 105th Congress is number 111 in the series. Each volume contains a complete index and a table of contents. A legislative history appears at the end of each law. There are extensive marginal notes referring to laws in earlier volumes and to earlier and later matters in the same volume.

Under the provisions of a statute originally enacted in 1895, these volumes are legal evidence of the laws contained in them and will be accepted as proof of those laws in any court in the U.S.

The Statutes at Large are a chronological arrangement of the laws exactly as they have been enacted. There is no attempt to arrange the laws according to their subject matter or to show the present status of an earlier law that has been amended on one or more occasions. The code of laws serves that purpose.

U.S. Code

The U.S. Code contains a consolidation and codification of the general and permanent laws of the U.S. arranged according to subject matter under 50 title headings, in alphabetical order to a large degree. It sets out the current status of the laws, as amended, without repeating all the language of the amendatory acts except where necessary. The Code is declared to be prima facie evidence of those laws. Its purpose is to present the laws in a concise and usable form without requiring recourse to the many volumes of the Statutes at Large containing the individual amendments.

The Code is prepared by the Law Revision Counsel of the House of Representatives. New editions are published every 6 years and cumulative supplements are published after the conclusion of each regular session of the Congress. The Code is also available in electronic form.

Now that you have read the theory, let us look at an example of how a Public Law is actually written, so that it can be integrated into the U.S. Code.

An easily accessible example is the FDAMA, which is specifically known as Public Law 105–115. It was passed in November 1997.

Using Thomas and the Public Law reference, I was able to obtain a copy of the FDAMA, as it was passed. The first section of the FDAMA gives instructions as to how to incorporate the FDAMA into the U.S. Code. The first Section of the FDAMA reads as follows:

Section 1. Short Title; References; Table of Contents

(a) SHORT TITLE- This Act may be cited as the `Food and Drug Administration Modernization Act of 1997'.

(b) REFERENCES- Except as otherwise specified, whenever in this Act an amendment or repeal is expressed in terms of an amendment to or a repeal of a section or other provision, the reference shall be considered to be made to that section or other provision of the Federal Food, Drug, and Cosmetic Act (21 U.S.C. 301 et seq.).

(c) TABLE OF CONTENTS- The table of contents for this Act is as follows"…

In (b), we see that the FDAMA makes express reference to the FDCA as it reads in the US Code, in Title 21. A lot of the provisions that follow are simply instructions to the editors of the U.S. Code, telling the editors what words and punctuation marks to change. One can only understand the intent and operation of the new law by making these changes and reading the now edited text. Notice that each Public Law has its own table of contents and section numbers, and that these section numbers are not the same as those in the Code. Each Public Law follows its own outline numbering system and the Code because it incorporates all changes from all Public Laws, and has a much larger outline form.

For example, the FDAMA added the fast track for drug products. The relevant Section in the FDAMA is Section 112, but the part of the Code that is effected is different. The FDAMA actually reads, at Section 112:

Sec. 112. Expediting Study and Approval of Fast Track Drugs

(a) IN GENERAL- Chapter V (21 U.S.C. 351 et seq.), as amended by section 125, is amended by inserting before section 508 the following:

Sec. 506. Fast Track Products

(a) DESIGNATION OF DRUG AS A FAST TRACK PRODUCT-

   (1) IN GENERAL- The Secretary shall, at the request of the sponsor of a new drug, facilitate the development and expedite the review of such drug if it is intended for the treatment of a serious or life-threatening condition and it demonstrates the potential to address unmet medical needs for such a condition. (In this section, such a drug is referred to as a 'fast track product.')

The FDAMA actually makes a reference to the FDCA, and changes that first. This is how the FDAMA section on Fast Track Products is added to the FDCA[8]:

Sec. 506. [356] Fast Track Products

(a) DESIGNATION OF DRUG AS A FAST TRACK PRODUCT —

   (1) IN GENERAL — The Secretary shall, at the request of the sponsor of a new drug, facilitate the development and expedite the review of such drug if it is intended for the treatment of a serious or life-threatening condition and it demonstrates the potential to address unmet medical needs for such a condition. (In this section, such a drug is referred to as a "fast track product.")

The language, as you see, is the same in both versions. The real test becomes where does one find this language in the Code? The FDA has mapped this out for you, but noting the Code section in brackets which are bolded here – Sec. 506 **[356]** –

Looking at Section 356 in 21 USC produces the following language:

SUBCHAPTER V — DRUGS AND DEVICES Part A — Drugs and Devices Sec. 356. Fast track products (a) Designation of drug as fast track product (1) In general The Secretary shall, at the request of the sponsor of a new drug, facilitate the development and expedite the review of such drug if it is intended for the treatment of a serious or life- threatening condition and it demonstrates the potential to address unmet medical needs for such a condition. (In this section, such a drug is referred to as a "fast track product.")

The words are the same; it is the classification and numbering system that changes with the source you are using. Only the Public Laws contain the instructions for actually editing the main body of law, in our case, the FDCA and by making those changes, impact the U.S. Code itself.

---

[8] Taken from the FDA's web-site, http://www.fda.gov/opacom/laws/fdcact/fdcact5a.htm, which shows the sections for both the Food, Drug and Cosmetic Act and the US Code.

13.7 What is the Difference between the Food, Drug and Cosmetic Act and the U.S. Code?

The main difference is the section numbering; the actual substance of the text is the same. The Food, Drug and Cosmetic Act is the name of a Public Law, originally passed decades ago and updated. The United States Code is the name of the compiled law, and Title 21 contains the Food, Drug and Cosmetic Act sections that regulators normally use.

13.8 Why Can't I Find Section 510(k) in the U.S. Code?

Don't panic. They have not eliminated that wonderful loop-hole, known as the "same as" or "me, too" exemption for devices. The Section number by which the provision is known refers to the FDCA. In the FDCA, the numbering system places that section at 510. When the amendments were incorporated into the U.S. Code, the appropriate numbering system was Section 360. Again, the FDA Website assists with the conversion, and indicates both section numbers for reference.

The actual provision reads as follows[9]:

510(k) Registration of Producers of Drugs and Devices

SEC. 510. [360]

(a) As used in this section....

(k) Each person who is required to register under this section and who proposes to begin the introduction or delivery for introduction into interstate commerce for commercial distribution of a device intended for human use shall, at least ninety days before making such introduction or delivery, report to the Secretary (in such form and manner as the Secretary shall by regulation prescribe) —

    (1) the class in which the device is classified under section 513 or if such person determines that the device is not classified under such section, a statement of that determination and the basis for such person's determination that the device is or is not so classified, and

    (2) action taken by such person to comply with requirements under section 514 or 515 which are applicable to the device.

---

[9] See the FDA's web-site, as noted above.

13.9 Are There Any State Laws That Apply to Medical Products?

Yes. Pharmacy laws are one of the biggest examples of how each state can and does exert control over medical products. The FDCA provides that certain medical products are available only by prescription from a physician. The FDCA goes on to say that it does not regulate physicians. The states regulate physicians and pharmacists, as well as how certain products are stored, dispensed and used. As discussed earlier, there are many instances where the federal government is pleased to let the states "work out the details," so to speak.

You should also be on the lookout for certain state laws governing biologics, which can sometimes be cloaked as privacy statutes. These have significant impact on genetic testing, data collection, and product development which relies upon such data.

13.10 Who Enforces Laws?

At times it seems like everybody does. The fact is that the executive branch of government is charged with enforcing laws. This list includes the Department of Justice, DEA agents, the FBI and State Police for criminal matters, and for our purposes, FDA inspectors for civil matters. However, an FDA inspector may stumble upon something troublesome, and refer a matter out for criminal investigation, so treat all folks carefully.

13.11 What Is a Regulation?

A regulation is a binding instruction issued by an agency (in our case, the FDA) that tells you how to interpret and comply with a law. Regulations are *must follows* — i.e., if you fail to follow a regulation, and you have an inspection, the FDA inspector must write up your failure on a 483; failures to follow regulations may end up in the "issued warning letter" section of the FDA Website, not a good place to be.

Another group of folks who are really interested in regulations and whether or not you comply with them, are the lawyers. Any injury to any person caused by any medical product is made far more lucrative if the manufacturer, sponsor, CRO, or other responsible party failed to do what the regulations required them to do. The economics are really simple —

injury plus failure to follow regulation equals money from the irresponsible (and hopefully insured) party for the injured, including the legal fees expended by the lawyer to get to the money.

13.12 What Is the Difference between a Law and a Regulation?

They come from different branches of government and have different functions. However, they each must be obeyed.

Laws come from legislative bodies, like the Congress and set policy in broad terms. Regulations come from the executive branch, and provide details on how laws are to be implemented, or obeyed. The FDA is part of the executive branch of government, and is under Health and Human Services (HHS). The HHS is a cabinet position, whose Secretary reports to the President.

Congress sometimes directs the executive branches to issue regulations. That was the case with FDAMA, where Congress decreed that regulations concerning dissemination of information on unapproved products be issued. The FDA did promulgate an initial set of regulations, which restricted the amounts and types of information manufacturers could publish concerning unapproved products. Litigation ensued over the breadth of the regulation, and the courts ultimately decided the regulation was overly broad, in that it infringed on the constitutional rights of commercial free speech, and so struck down the existing regulation.

While the courts have the power to nullify regulations that are not consistent with the statutes, or have been improperly issued (usually meaning that there has been inadequate public hearings), or exceed the agency's authority, these cases are really far and few between. Most of the time, the FDA's regulations are given great deference by a court, and are upheld.

My general advice is "Don't sue the FDA." The reason is pure economics. A lawsuit will delay your product from clearance/approval. Courts are backlogged, and delays can be substantial. Say you have a product whose potential revenues are $12 million a year — not an unrealistic estimate for many drugs worth pursuing. If you lost even 6 months (an unrealistically short time) in a court proceeding, you have lost $6 million. Even a day's delay would cost you more than $32,876. If you can work out something that the FDA will allow, some resubmission that you can do in 6 weeks, and the 6-week delay would have cost only $1.3 million, compared with the $6 million loss for the court delay, you have saved money. And that $6 million assumes you win in court and the FDA does not appeal. If the case drags on for 3 years, you have lost $36 million and more than likely, 3 valuable years of patent exclusivity. So, unless you are manufacturing cigarettes, most of the time there is not much to gain by suing.

13.13 Which Is More Important — a Law or a Regulation?

The problem for regulators is that both are equally important. Violation of laws can result in criminal penalties, but hopefully no one is reading this chapter with an eye to "cutting it close on the out-of-jail" end of things. Violation of regulations results in warning letters, which is why a lot of "old-timers" in the industry insist that "a regulation is a law you follow."

13.14 What Is the Difference Between the USC and the CFR?

The USC stands for the U.S. Code and contains *Laws*. The CFR stands for the Code of Federal Regulations and contains *Regulations*. The CFR does *not* have laws, and the USC does *not* have regulations. The USC is enacted by Congress and the CFR is the domain of the Executive branch, in our case, Health and Human Services.

A CRF has nothing to do with either one of them. CRF stands for "Case Report Form," the name for the medical and clinical trial record of a participant.

13.15 How Do I Find a Current Regulation?

You can find current regulations using the same basic skill set that you developed finding the laws.

You can go to a federal depository and get a copy of the regulations. You then check the print date and see how current it is. All new regulations must be printed in the Federal Register. You can usually find hard copies of the Register in the same public libraries that are federal depositories, and the Register will print any new final regulations that have been published since the date of the last printing of the regulations.

The U.S. government has done a remarkable job in putting its regulations on the Internet. The Federal Register is also on the Internet.

The question is, how do you find a current regulation? Starting with the CFR, check the last date that the version you are looking at, was published. For 21 CFR, it is April 1. That tells you that the version you are looking at contains regulations published, and in effect, up to March 31. To determine whether or not there are any changes to a particular regulation, search the Federal Register for any published changes to the regulation, from April 1 through the date that is important to you.

For example, say you want to know what regulation was in effect on June 30, 2003. The current edition of 21 CFR goes up to April 1, 2003. That leaves the period between April and June 30 open. You can go to the Federal Register and refine your search to the dates between April 1, 2003 and June 30, 2003 to determine if there were any changes. I like to overlap my date searches, so that I catch any changes that are in progress on the edition date. It is more than likely that the April 1 edition will contain regulations that become effective on April 1, but by starting my Federal Register search on March 31, I overlap a day and remove all doubt.

13.16   What Is a Guidance?

The FDA issues "guidance" on a number of subjects. As the lead paragraph says, the guidance represents the agency's thinking, but is not binding. That means you should read it to determine what the agency's view on a subject is or was at a particular time. The disclaimer also means that following a guidance does not guarantee that your application will be filed. Some guidances are, by the agency's own admission, hopelessly out of date, but they just have not gotten around to revising them yet. An example is the guidance on statistical databases.

You should discuss what guidances to follow at the preliminary meetings you hold with your FDA reviewers. This removes all doubt about what you are expected to do, and hopefully makes the job easier. You should always read and understand a relevant guidance before your preliminary meeting, so you can ask intelligent questions about how the guidance impacts your application. There is a central listing of guidances available from the FDA's Website. You can check your results by searching your center for applicable guidances.

13.17   What is a Search Engine and How Do I Use it?

A search engine is a computer program that looks for information on the Internet, also known as the World Wide Web. Most search engines use "text searches," which means that you type in a topic, or a few words that you want to find (called a "search string" — a "string" of words) and the search engine then takes that text and looks in various Websites for the same text. When the search engine finds your text on a Website, you have a "hit."

Search engines are sometimes called "spiders" by their programmer inventors, playing off the World-Wide-Web image. (Spiders spin webs and then crawl over them, looking for prey).

Most engines use "text," that is words, to find things. You list a word, and then the engine generally goes to the title line of a Web page to see if your word is in the title, or somewhere on that page. If your search word is there, the spider will usually bring the page back to you and display it.

Lucky for us, the spider does not bring back *every* page that matches your word. First, there are simply too many pages on the Web, and more are added every day. It may take a search engine a month to check all of the web pages that exist, so unless you are willing to wait 30 days or more, you will not get all of the most recent Web pages in your search. Next, not all Web pages are accessible to spiders. The University of California Berkley Website notes that between one-half to two-thirds of the Web is actually "invisible" to spiders and search engines. The invisible Web includes specialized searchable databases inaccessible to spiders because: (1) spiders cannot type their passwords in and 2) spiders cannot regenerate specialized database searches.[10] Additionally, most spiders have filters that remove links to hard-core pornographic content. This is obviously helpful when you are looking at products that treat breast cancer or sexual dysfunction. However, some Web designers are not very scrupulous, and often will put words in their Web page headers (lines of code generally seen by spiders more than people), so you can still end up with somebody's home page replete with family pictures and story of when they moved into their new house, or links that would be embarrassing at best, in a professional work environment. Look at your search engine hits in the privacy of your own cubicle before incorporating the results into your PowerPoint presentation and heading for the main office.

Some search engines use "computer intelligence" to find text. This means that the search engines actually look at what other people wanted to find, and if a lot of people found that site and liked it, an "intelligent" search engine will "think" that it is the one you want and let you find it as well. This process is "ranking," and used by Google® and similarly powered search engines.[11] So, if you are looking for scientific evidence that copper-lined bracelets really ease arthritis pain, any popular common search engine is going to list all the places you can buy these things, well before you hit upon that obscure article in JAMA or other serious publication about the efficacy of these bracelets.

So, user beware. A big thing to remember about search engine results — just because you did not find the information you were looking for does not mean that the information does not exist. It only means you did not find it.

There are a couple of reasons why you did not find what you were looking for. One, the information simply may not be posted on a Website that you can access for free. This is unfortunately true with many court decisions

---

[10] "Finding Information on the Internet: A Tutorial; Types of Search Tools; U.C. Berkeley Library; http://www.lib.berkeley.edu/Teaching.Lit/Guides/Internet?ToolsTable.html

[11] Some folks consider this search engine editing or "ranking" of information a serious influence on intellectual thinking and free speech, and search-engine watch-dog Websites are springing up. For example, please see www.google-watch.org

and regulations. As state funding is cut back, fewer and fewer states go to the expense of putting all their laws and court decisions online. Two, you may not have plugged in the right text for your search or chosen the right search engine.

A couple of things can go wrong with any search. You can get way too many hits, you can get the wrong hits, and you can get nothing. So, let us deal with the easy things first. Like getting too many hits. Say I want to know how much a parking fine is in the town of Arlington, Massachusetts. I type in "fine" and "Arlington." I end up with "fine arts," "fine art framing," "Arlington Heights, Virginia," "Arlington, Texas," "fine homes," "fine dining," "fine weather" — you get the picture. A search engine cannot distinguish between different meanings for words in a text search. So, the spider on my Google® search is replete with success, having found about 347,000 hits for me to peruse. I, however, have not got the information I wanted. I can only have gotten the information I wanted if the Town of Arlington, Massachusetts had a Website and that Website has the information about parking fines, and if I limited my search to "parking fines" AND "Arlington, Massachusetts." This time, the search was successful. Google® produced 763 hits, and the first one was "Traffic Rules, Article 10, Arlington, Massachusetts." When I hit on the link, I was thwarted. The message was that the Web page was temporarily out of order, had moved, etc., etc. However, Google® has a feature that bailed me out. I moved the cursor to the "Cached" line, and lo and behold, a list of parking fines appeared (it is $10 for all night parking; same as that for an expired meter). Google® has this neat feature of putting into memory — its "cache" — copies of the Web pages. So, as long as I know the Arlington Selectmen did not vote to increase parking fines last night, looking at the old Google®-saved Cache worked just fine.

A search engine will not substitute synonyms or concepts for your text. If you want to find out the gross sales of Tylenol® and its generic equivalents, you must know that "acetaminophen" is the active ingredient in Tylenol®. More to the point, you must be aware of specific terms or names used to identify concepts, laws, and regulations. Many industry folks refer to the 21 CFR Part 50 as the "Informed Consent Regulation." In fact, the true title of Part 50 is "Protection of Human Subjects." Your brain can make the connection between the two titles, but a search engine using text cannot. So, sometimes you have to peruse a table of contents to find what you are really looking for. Lastly, a text search engine will not correct spelling. So, even if you know the correct title for Part 50, and type in "protection for humane subjects," the search will not succeed.

A number of colleges and universities have wonderful tutorials on their Websites, describing search engines and how to use them. For a list of useful resources, please see the endnotes. Go try one out — it saves lots of time in the long run!

Index

A

Abbreviated New Drug Application
(ANDA), 5, 14–16
  amendments/supplements to, 293
  electronic submissions, 251, 259, 292–295
Absorption, distribution, metabolism,
excretion (ADME) studies, NDA,
92, 100, 101–102
Acceptance criteria, investigational drugs,
57
"A" codes, 15
Acrobat Distiller, 285
Acrobat Reader, 269
Action letters, FDA, 12
Active ingredients, review of, 17–18
Acts, 323
Adobe Acrobat, 269, 273
Adverse Device Effects, 169
Adverse drug reactions, suspected, (SADR),
70
Adverse events/reactions
  definition of, 67–68, 226
  and dose response, 109
  medical devices, 169, 179, 191
  reporting, 16, 48, 67–71, 226–227
  summary for NDA, 108–109
  unexpected, 68
Advertising
  medical devices, 178, 193
  regulation of, 7, 18–19
Advisory committee meetings, 117, 126
Advisory panels, PMA, 183
Alert report, 16
Ames test, 137
Analytical controls
  drug products, 98–99
  drug substances, 94–97
Analytical methods
  summarizing, 102–103
  testing, 31
Animal models, toxicology testing, 142, 143
Animal studies
  NDA, 100–101

pharmacology/toxicology information,
59–61
preclinical, biologics, 134
Annual reports
  IND, 48, 73–74
  PMA, 190
Antibodies, monoclonal
  animal models, 143
  immunogenicity of, 143
  in vivo use, 149
  pharmacokinetic effects, 140
  proof-of-concept studies, 138
  regulation of, 131
  safety concerns, 143–144
Antimicrobials, microbiological testing, 93,
106
Antitoxins, safety issues, 130, 131
Application fees
  PDUFA, 201
  waivers, 24
Application summary, NDA, 91–94
Approvable Letter, FDA, 12
Approval Letter, FDA, 12
Approval process
  accelerated, 6, 13, 204–205, 254–255,
334–335
  biologics, 133
*Approved Drug Products with Therapeutic
Equivalence Evaluations,* 14–16
Archival copy
  eANDA, 293, 294
  electronic submission of, 259
  NDA, 83, 85
  eNDA, 259, 295, 298
Audits
  clinical quality assurance, 187, 223–227
  Phase II trials, 33
Authoring, electronic documents, 283–284

B

Background reports, regulatory, 25–26, 27